Statistics for Veterinary and Animal Science

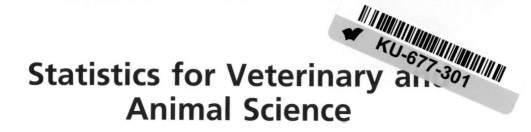
Aviva Petrie, BSc, MSc, CStat

Senior Lecturer in Statistics at the Eastman Dental Institute,
Senior Lecturer in Statistics at the Royal Veterinary College,
Honorary Lecturer in Medical Statistics at the London School of
Hygiene and Tropical Medicine,
University of London

Paul Watson, BSc, PhD, DSc, BVetMed, MRCVS

Professor of Reproductive Cryobiology,
The Royal Veterinary College,
University of London

Illustrations prepared by Alexander Hunte, CNA

Blackwell
Science

© 1999 by Blackwell Science Ltd,
a Blackwell Publishing Company
Editorial Offices:
Osney Mead, Oxford OX2 0EL, UK
  Tel: +44 (0)1865 206206
Blackwell Science, Inc., 350 Main Street,
Malden, MA02148-5018, USA
  Tel: +1 781 388 8250
Iowa State Press, a Blackwell Publishing
Company, 2121 State Avenue, Ames, Iowa
50014-8300, USA
  Tel: +1 515 292 0140
Blackwell Science Asia Pty, 54 University
Street, Carlton, Victoria 3053, Australia
  Tel: +61 (0)3 9347 0300
Blackwell Wissenschafts Verlag,
Kurfürstendamm 57, 10707 Berlin, Germany
  Tel: +49 (0)30 32 79 060

First published 1999 by Blackwell Science Ltd
Reprinted 2000, 2001, 2002

Library of Congress
Cataloging-in-Publication Data
Petrie, Aviva.
    Statistics for veterinary and animal science / Aviva
Petrie, Paul Watson; illustrations prepared by Alexander
Hunte.
      p. cm.
    Includes bibliographical references (p.) and index.
    ISBN 0-632-05025-X
    1. Veterinary medicine—Statistical methods.
  I. Watson, Paul, B. Sc. II. Title.
  SF760.S73P48 1999
  636.089′07′27—dc21   99-13540
                                                                            CIP

ISBN 0-632-03742-3
A catalogue record for this title is available
from the British Library

Set in 10/12pt Times
by SNP Best-set Typesetter Ltd., Hong Kong
Printed and bound in Great Britain by
the Alden Group, Oxford

For further information on
Blackwell Science, visit our website:
www.blackwell-science.co.uk

Contents

Preface

Although statistics is anathema to many, it is, unquestionably, an essential tool for those involved in animal health and veterinary science. It is imperative that practitioners and research workers alike keep abreast with reports on animal production, new and emerging diseases, risk factors for disease and the efficacy of the ever-increasing number of innovations in veterinary care and of developments in training methods and performance. The most cogent information is usually contained in the appropriate journals; however, the usefulness of these journals relies on the reader having a proper understanding of the statistical methodology underlying study design and data analysis.

The modern animal scientist and veterinary surgeon therefore needs to be able to handle numerical data confidently and properly. Often, for us, as teachers, there is little time in busy curricula to introduce the subject slowly and systematically; students find they are left bewildered and dejected because the concepts seem too difficult to grasp. While there are many excellent introductory books on medical statistics and on statistics in other disciplines such as economics, business studies and engineering, these books are unrelated to the world of animal science and health, and students soon lose heart. It is our intention to provide a guide to statistics relevant to the study of animal health and disease. In order to illustrate the principles and methods, the reader will find that the text is well-endowed with real examples drawn from companion and agricultural animals. Although veterinary epidemiology is closely allied to statistics, we have concentrated only on statistical issues as we feel that this is an area which, until now, has been neglected in veterinary and animal health sciences.

Our book is an introductory text on statistics. We start from very simple concepts, assuming no previous knowledge of statistics, and endeavour to build up an understanding in such a way that progression on to advanced texts is possible. We intend the book to be useful for those without mathematical expertise but with the ability to utilize simple formulae. We recognize the influence of the computer and so we avoid the description of complex hand calculations. Instead, emphasis is placed on understanding of concepts and interpretation of results, often in the context of computer output. In addition to acquiring an ability to perform simple statistical techniques on original data, the reader will be able critically to evaluate the efforts of others in respect of the design of studies, and of the presentation, analysis and interpretation of results.

The book can be used either as a self-instructional text or as a basis for courses in statistics. In addition, those who are further on in their studies will be able to use the text as a reference guide to the analysis of their data, whether they be postgraduate students, veterinary practitioners or animal scientists in various other settings. Every section contains sufficient cross-referencing for the reader to find the relevant background to the topic.

We would like to acknowledge the generosity of Penny Barber, Mark Corbett, Dr J.E. Edwards, Dr Jonathan Elliott, Dr Gary England, Dr Oliver Garden, Dr Anne Pearson, Dr P.D. Warriss, Professor Avril Waterman-Pearson, and Susannah Williams, who shared their original data with us. In places, we have taken published summary data and constructed a primary data set to suit our own purposes; if we have misrepresented our colleagues' data, we accept full responsibility. We are particularly grateful to Alex Hunte who lent us his skills in preparing the illustrations, and to Dr David Moles who assisted with the preparation of the statistical tables. We especially thank Dr Ben Armstrong, Dr Caroline Sabin and Dr Ian Martin who kindly gave us their critical advice as the text was developed. Professor John Smith was instrumental in getting us to consider writing the text in the first place, and we thank him for his continual encouragement. In addition, we acknowledge our debt to a host of other colleagues who have helped with discussions over the telephone, with their expertise in areas we are lacking, and in general encouragement to complete what we hope will be a useful contribution to the field of veterinary and animal science.

Lastly, we acknowledge with gratitude the patience and encouragement of our families. Our marriage partners, Gerald and Rosie, have endured with fortitude our neglect of them while this work was in preparation. In particular, our children, Nina, Andrew and Karen, and Oliver and Anna, have had to cope with our absorption with the project and lack of involvement in their activities. We trust they will recognize that it was in a good cause.

Aviva Petrie
Paul Watson

Chapter 1

The Whys and Wherefores of Statistics

1.1 LEARNING OBJECTIVES

By the end of this chapter, you should be able to:

- Distinguish between a qualitative and a quantitative variable.
- List the types of scales on which variables are measured.
- Explain what is meant by the term 'biological variation'.
- Define the terms 'systematic error' and 'random error', and give examples of circumstances in which they may occur.
- Distinguish between precision and accuracy.
- Define the terms 'population' and 'sample', and provide examples of real (finite) and hypothetical (infinite) populations.
- Summarize the differences between descriptive and inferential statistics.

1.2 AIMS OF THE BOOK

1.2.1 What will you get from this book?

All the biological sciences have moved on from simple qualitative description to concepts founded on numerical measurements and counts. The proper handling of these values, leading to a correct understanding of the phenomena, is encompassed by statistics. This book will help you appreciate how the theory of statistics can be useful to you in veterinary and animal science.

We, the authors, aim to introduce you to the subject of statistics, giving you a sound basis for managing straightforward study design and analysis. Where necessary, we recommend that you extend your knowledge by reference to more specialized texts. Occasionally, we advocate your seeking expert statistical advice to guide you through particularly tricky aspects.

You can use this book in two ways:

1. The chapter sequence is designed to develop your understanding systematically and we therefore recommend that, initially, you work through the chapters in order. You will find certain sections marked in small type with a symbol, which indicates that you can skip these, at a first read through, without subsequent loss of continuity. These marked sections contain information you will find useful as your knowledge develops. Chapter 13 deals with particular types of analyses which, depending on your areas of interest, you may rarely need.

2. When you are more familiar with the concepts, you can use the book as a reference manual; you will find sufficient cross-referenced information in any section to answer specific queries.

1.2.2 What are learning objectives?

Each chapter has a set of **learning objectives** at the beginning. These set out in task-oriented terms what you should be able to 'do' when you have mastered the concepts in the chapter. You can therefore test your growing understanding; if you are able to perform the tasks in the learning objectives, you have understood the concepts.

1.2.3 Should you use a computer statistics package?

We encourage you to use available computer statistics packages, and therefore we do not dwell on the development of the equations on which the analyses are based. We do, however, present the equations (apart from when they are very complex) for completeness, but you will normally not need to become familiar with them since computer packages will provide an automatic solution. Throughout the book we use, as our examples, computer output from a statistical package called SPSS. Although the layout of the output is particular to each individual package, from our description you should be able to make sense of the output from any other major statistical package.

1.2.4 Will you be able to decide when and how to use a particular procedure?

Our main concern is with the *understanding* which underlies statistical analyses. This will prevent you falling into the pitfalls of misuse which surround the unwitting user of statistical packages. We present the subject in a form which we hope is accessible, using examples showing the application of the subject to veterinary and animal science. A brief set of exercises follows each chapter, based on the ideas presented within. These exercises should be used to further check your understanding of the concepts and procedures. Answers to the exercises are given at the back of the book.

1.2.5 Use of the Glossaries of Terms and Notation

Statistical nomenclature is often difficult to remember. We have gathered the most common symbols and equations used throughout this book into a Glossary of Notation in Appendix D. This gives you a readily accessible reminder of the meaning of the terminology.

You will find a Glossary of Terms in Appendix E. In this glossary, we define common statistical terms which are used in this book. They are also defined at the appropriate places in relevant chapters, but the glossary provides you with a ready reference if you forget the meaning of a term. Terms which are in the Glossary are introduced in the text in bold type. Note, however, that there are some instances where bold is purely used for extra emphasis.

1.3 WHAT IS STATISTICS?

The number of introductory or elementary texts on the subject of statistics indicates how important the subject has become for teachers of biological sciences, if not for their students! However, the fact that there are many texts might also suggest that we have yet to discover a foolproof method of presenting what is required.

The problem confronted in biological statistics is as follows. When you make a set of numerical observations in biology, you will find the values are scattered. You need to know whether the differences are due to causes you are interested in or are part of a 'background' natural variation. You need to evaluate what the numbers actually mean, and to represent them in a way that readily communicates their meaning to others.

The subject of statistics embraces:

- The design of the study in order that it will reveal the most information efficiently.
- The collection of the data.
- The analysis of the data.
- The presentation of suitably summarized information, often in a graphical or tabular form.
- The interpretation of the analyses in a manner which communicates the findings accurately.

Strictly, this broad numerical approach to biology is correctly termed '**biometry**' but we shall adopt the more generally used term '**statistics**' to cover all aspects. Statistics (meaning this entire process) has become one of the essential tools in modern biology.

1.4 STATISTICS IN VETERINARY AND ANIMAL SCIENCE

One of the common initial responses of both veterinary students and animal science students is: Why do I need to study statistics? The mathematical basis of the subject causes much uncertainty, and the analytical approach is alien. However, in professional life, there are many instances of the relevance of statistics:

- The **published scientific literature** is full of studies in which statistical procedures are employed. Look in any of the relevant scientific journals and notice the number of times reference is made to mean ± SEM, to statistical significance, to P-values or to t-tests or Chi-squared analysis or analysis of variance. The information is presented in the usual brief form and, without a working knowledge of statistics, you are left to accept the conclusions of the author, unable to examine the strength of the supporting data. Indeed, with the advent of computer-assisted data handling, many practitioners can now collect their own observations and summarize them for the advantage of their colleagues; to do this, they need the benefit of statistical insights.

- In the animal health sciences, there are an increasing number of independent **diagnostic services** which will analyse samples for the benefit of health monitoring and maintenance. Those running such laboratory services must always be concerned about quality control and accuracy in measurements made for diagnostic purposes, and must be able to supply clear guidelines for the interpretation of results obtained in their laboratories.

- The **pharmaceutical and agrichemical industries** are required to demonstrate both the safety and the efficacy of their products in an indisputable manner. Such data invariably require a statistical approach to establish and illustrate the basis of the claim for both these aspects. Those involved in pharmaceutical product development need to understand the importance of study design and to ensure the adequacy of the numbers of animals used in treatment groups in order to perform meaningful experiments. The veterinary product licensing committees require a thorough understanding of statistical science so that they can appreciate the data presented to substantiate the claims for a novel therapeutic substance. Finally, practitioners and animal carers are faced with the blandishments of sales representatives with competing claims, and must evaluate the literature which is offered in support of specific agents.

- Increasingly, there is concern about the regulation of **safety and quality of food for human consumption**. Where products of animal origin are involved, the animal scientist and the veterinary profession are at the forefront. Examples are: pharmaceutical product withdrawal times before slaughter based on the pharmacokinetics and pharmacodynamics of the products, the withholding times for milk after therapeutic treatment of the animal, tissue residues of herbicides and insecticides, and the possible contamination of carcases by antibiotic-resistant bacteria. In every case, advice and appropriate regulations are established by experimental studies and statistical evaluation. The experts need to be aware of the appropriate statistical procedures in order to play their proper roles.

In all these areas, a common basic vocabulary and understanding of biometrical concepts is assumed to enable scientists to communicate accurately with one another. It is important that you gain mastery of these concepts if you are to play a full part in your chosen profession.

1.5 TYPES OF VARIABLE

A **variable** is a characteristic which can take values which *vary* from individual to individual or group to group, e.g. height, weight, litter size, blood count, enzyme activity, coat colour, percentage of the flock which are pregnant, etc. Clearly some of these are more readily quantifiable than others. For some variables, we can assign a number to a category and so create the appearance of a numerical scale, but others have a true numerical scale on which the values lie. We take **readings** of the variable which are measurements of a biological characteristic, and these become the **values** which we use for the statistical procedures. Both these terms are in general use, and both refer to the original measurements, the **raw data**.

Numerical data take various forms; a proper understanding of the nature of the data and the classification of variables is an important first step in choosing an appropriate statistical approach. The flow charts shown in Appendix C illustrate this train of thought which culminates in a suitable choice of statistical procedure to analyse a particular data set.

We distinguish the main types of variable in a systematic manner by determining whether the variable can take 'one of two distinct values', 'one of several distinct values' or 'any value' within the given range. In particular, the variable may be one of the following:

(a) **Qualitative/categorical variable** – an individual belongs to any one of two or more distinct categories for this variable. A *binary* or dichotomous variable is a particular type of nominal categorical variable defined by only *two* categories; for example, pregnant or non-pregnant, male or female. We customarily summarize the information for the categorical variable by determining the number and percentage (or proportion) of individuals in each category in the sample or population. Particular scales of a categorical variable are:

- **Nominal scale** – the distinct categories which define the variable are unordered and each can be assigned a name, e.g. coat colours (piebald, roan or grey).
- **Ordinal scale** – the categories which constitute the variable have some intrinsic order but there are no consistent and defined intervals between the various categories; for example, body condition scores, subjective intensity of fluorescence of cells in the fluorescence microscope, degree of vigour of motility of a semen sample. These 'scales' are often given numerical values 1 to *n*.

(b) **Quantitative variable** – consisting of numerical values on a well-defined scale, which may be:

- **A discrete (discontinuous) scale**, i.e. data can take only particular integer values, typically counts, e.g. litter size, clutch size, parity (number of pregnancies).
- **A continuous scale**, for which all values are theoretically possible (perhaps limited by an upper and/or lower boundary), e.g. height, weight, speed, concentration of a chemical constituent of the blood or urine. Theoretically, the number of values that the continuous variable can take is infinite since the scale is a continuum. In practice, continuous data are restricted by the degree of accuracy of the measurement process. By definition, the interval between two adjacent points on the scale is of the same magnitude as the interval between two other adjacent points, e.g. the interval on a temperature scale between 37° and 38°C is the same as the interval between 39° and 40°C.

1.6 VARIATIONS IN MEASUREMENTS

It is well-known that if we repeatedly observe and quantify a particular biological phenomenon, the measurements will rarely be identical. Part of the variability is due to an inherent variation in the biological material being measured. For example, not all cows eat the same quantity of grass per day even if differences both in body weight and water content of the feed are taken into account. We shall use the term '**biological variation**' for this phenomenon, although some people use the term 'biological error'. (Biological error is actually a misleading term since the variability is not in any sense due to a mistake.)

By the selection of individuals according to certain characteristics in advance of the collection of data we may be able to *reduce* the range of biological variation but we cannot eliminate it. Selection is often based on animal characteristics (e.g. species, strain, age, sex, degree of maturity, body weight, showjumpers, milking herds, hill sheep, etc.), the choice of which depends upon the particular factors under investigation. However, the result is then only valid for that *restricted population* and we are not justified in extrapolating beyond that population. For example, we should not assume that a study based on beef cattle applies to other types of cattle.

In addition to biological variation, there will most likely be differences in repeated measurements of the same subject; these are **technical variations** or **errors**, due to a variety of instrumental causes and to human error. We may properly consider them to be errors since they represent departures from the true value.

1.6.1 Biological variation

The causes of biological variation, which makes one individual differ from the next, may be obvious or subtle. For example, variations in any characteristic may be attributable to:

- Genetics – e.g. greater variability in the whole cow population compared with just Friesians.
- Environment – e.g. body weight varies with diet, housing, intercurrent disease, etc.
- Gender – sexual dimorphism is common.
- Age – many biological data are influenced by age and maturity, e.g. the quantity of body fat.

In the heterogeneous population, the biological variation may be considerable and may mask the variation due to particular factors under investigation. Statistical approaches must take account of this inherent variability. The problem for the scientist, having measured a range of results of a particular feature in a group of individuals, is to distinguish between the sources of variation.

Here are two examples of problems created by biological variation:

- Two groups of growing cattle have been fed different diets. The ranges of the recorded weights at six months of age show an overlap in the two groups. Is there a real difference between the groups?

- You have the results of an electrolyte blood test which shows that the serum potassium level is elevated. By how much must it be elevated before you regard it as abnormal?

1.6.2 Technical errors

A technical or measurement error is defined as the difference between an observed reading and its 'true' value. Measurement errors are due to factors which are, typically, **human** (e.g. variations within and between observers) or **instrumental**, but may also be attributed to differences in conditions (e.g. different laboratories).

Technical errors may be systematic or random. A **systematic error** is one in which the recorded value is consistently above (or below) its true value; the result is then said to be *biased*. When the recorded values are evenly distributed above and below the true value, **random errors**, due to unexplained sources, are said to be occurring. Random variation can be so great as to obscure differences between groups but this problem may be minimized by taking repeated observations.

(a) Human error

Human error can occur whenever a person is performing either an unfamiliar task or a routine or monotonous task; fatigue increases the chances of error. Errors due to these factors are usually random, and providing steps are taken to minimize them (e.g. practice to acquire a proper level of skill, avoiding long periods of monotonous labour and by checking results as measurements are made), they can generally be ignored.

Other sorts of human error can arise because of data handling. In large data sets, **rounding errors** rarely provide inaccuracies of importance but in small data sets these can be quite substantial. If you use a computer to manage your data, you need not be concerned about this, since computer algorithms generally avoid rounding errors by carrying long number strings even if these are not displayed.

Another recognized human error is called **digit preference**. Whenever there is an element of judgement involved in making readings from instruments (as in determining the last digit of a number on a scale), certain digits between 0 and 9 are more commonly chosen than others to represent the readings; such preferences differ between individuals. This may introduce either a random or a systematic error, the magnitude of which will depend on the importance of the last digit to the results.

(b) Instrumental error

Instrumental errors arise for a number of reasons (see Fig. 1.1). Providing we are aware of the potential problem, the causes are often correctable or reducible.

- With a *systematic offset* or *zero error*, a 'blank' sample consistently reads other than zero. It

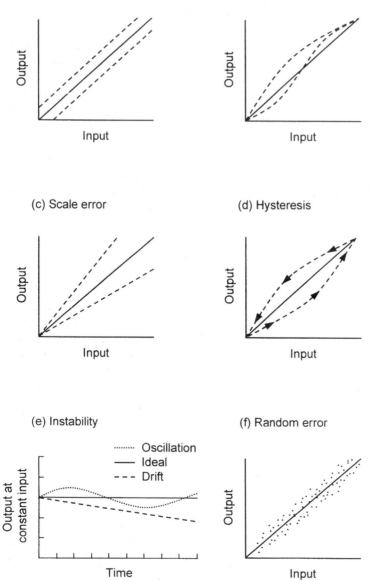

Fig. 1.1 Types of instrumental error. 'Input' refers to the true value of the measurements being recorded, 'output' refers to the recorded response, and the solid line refers to the situation when the output values equal the input values. Errors in measurement are represented by dots or dashed lines.

is common in colorimetry and radioisotope measurements (Fig. 1.1(a)).

- *Non-linearity* is a systematic error, commonly seen in performance of strain gauges, thermocouples and colorimeters (Fig. 1.1(b)).
- *Proportional* or *scale error* is usually due to electronic gain being incorrectly adjusted or altered after calibration: it results in a systematic error (Fig. 1.1(c)).
- *Hysteresis* is a systematic error commonly encountered in measurements involving galvanometers. It may require a standard measurement procedure, e.g. always adjusting input *down* to desired level (Fig. 1.1(d)).
- *Instability* or *drift*. Electronic gain calibration may drift with temperature and humidity giving rise to an intermittent but systematic error, resulting in an unstable baseline (Fig. 1.1(e)).
- *Random errors* are commonly seen in attempts to measure with a sensitivity beyond the limits of resolution of an instrument (Fig. 1.1(f)). Most instruments carry a specification of their accuracy, e.g. it is no use attempting to measure to the nearest gram with a balance accurate only to 10 grams.

Two or more of these sources of error may occur simultaneously. Technical errors of all kinds can be minimized by careful experimentation. This is the essence of **quality control** and is of paramount importance in a diagnostic laboratory. Quality control in the laboratory is about ensuring that processes and procedures are carried out in a consistently satisfactory manner so that the results are trustworthy. We introduce some additional terms in order to understand these concepts more fully.

1.7 TERMS RELATING TO MEASUREMENT QUALITY

Two terms which are of major importance in understanding the principles of biological measurement are **precision** and **accuracy**. It is essential they are understood early in a consideration of the nature of data measurement.

- **Precision** refers to how well repeated observations agree with one another.
- **Accuracy** refers to how well the observed value agrees with the true value.

To understand these terms consider the diagrams in Fig. 1.2, in which the bull's-eye represents the true value: in Fig. 1.2(a) there is poor accuracy and poor precision, in Fig. 1.2(b) there is poor accuracy and good precision, while in Fig. 1.2(c) there is both good accuracy and good precision.

It is possible to have a diagnostic method (e.g. a blood enzyme estimation) which gives good precision but poor accuracy (Fig. 1.2(b)) because of systematic error. In an enzyme activity estimation, such an error might be due to variation in temperature.

Several other terms are in use and these are defined as follows:

- **Repeatability** is concerned with gauging the similarity of replicate, often duplicate, measurements of a particular technique or instrument or observer under identical conditions, e.g. measurements made by the same observer in the same laboratory. It assesses technical errors (see Section 13.3).

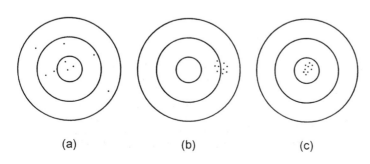

   (a)   (b)   (c)

Fig. 1.2 Diagram representing the concepts of accuracy and precision: (a) represents poor accuracy and precision, (b) represents poor accuracy but good precision, and (c) represents both good accuracy and precision.

- **Method agreement** (also called reproducibility) is concerned with determining how well two or more methods of measurement of the same quantity agree with one another, e.g. measurements made by different observers perhaps working in different laboratories and perhaps using different methods (see Section 13.3).
- **Stability** concerns the long-term repeatability of measurement. Diagnostic laboratories will usually have a reference material kept for checking stability over time.
- **Validity** is concerned with determining whether the measurement is actually measuring what it purports to be measuring. In the clinical context, the measurement is compared to a 'gold standard' (see Section 13.2).

1.8 POPULATIONS AND SAMPLES

The concept of a **population** from which our measurements are a **sample** is fundamental. A population includes all representatives of a particular group, whereas a sample is a subgroup drawn from the population. We aim to choose a sufficiently large sample in such a manner that it is representative of the population (see Sections 1.8.2, 4.2 and 12.4).

1.8.1 Types of population

In this book we usually use the word 'animal' to suggest the unit of investigation, but also we use other terms such as 'individual' or 'case'. We want you to become familiar with different terminology. A population of animals may be represented by:

- The individuals, e.g. all cattle, all beef cattle, all Herefords, all the herd.
- The measurements of a particular variable, e.g. liver weights, bone lengths, blood hormone or enzyme levels.
- Numbers of items (in a given area, volume or time), e.g. blood cell counts or faecal egg counts, counts of radioactive particle emissions.

The population may be either a **real** (or **finite**) group or a **hypothetical** (or **infinite**) group. For example, if we are interested in the growth rate of pigs in Suffolk, then the population is all pigs in Suffolk. This is a real or finite population. If, however, we want to know the effect of an experimental diet in these pigs, we will feed the test diet to a sample of pigs which now comprises the only representatives of a hypothetical population fed on the test diet. Theoretically at least, we could actually measure the entire population in finite cases, but infinite populations are represented *only* by the sample.

1.8.2 Random sampling and random allocation

We examine a sample with a view to making statements about the population. The sample must therefore be *representative* of the population from which it is taken if it is to give useful results applicable to the population at large. In order for the sample to be representative, the individuals should be selected randomly (i.e. by chance) from *all* possible members of the entire population. This concept of **random selection** is fundamental to sampling (see Section 12.4).

It is essential to use an objective method to achieve random sampling, and a method based on a random number sequence is the method of choice. The sequence may be obtained from a table of random numbers (see Table A.11) or be generated by a computer random number generator or, if only a small sequence, be generated by a mechanical method such as rolling a die.

Note that for allocating individuals into treatment groups, principles of **random allocation (randomization)** must also be employed to avoid subjective influence and ensure that the groups are comparable (see Section 5.6). Again, a random number sequence is required to provide objective allocation of individuals or treatments so that the causes of any subsequent differences in performance between the groups can be properly identified.

1.9 TYPES OF STATISTICAL PROCEDURES

Statistical procedures can be divided into **descriptive statistics** and **inferential statistics**.

- **Descriptive statistics**. We use these techniques to reduce a data set to manageable proportions, summarizing the trends and tendencies within it, in order to represent the results clearly. From these procedures we can produce diagrams, tables and numerical descriptors. Numerical descriptors include measures which convey where the centre of the data set lies, like the arithmetic mean or mode, and measures of the scatter or dispersion of the data, such as the variance or range. These are described more fully in Chapter 2.
- **Inferential statistics**. Statistical inference involves *estimation* of population parameters using sample data. A *parameter*, such as the mean or proportion, describes certain features of the distribution of a variable (see Section 4.3.2). Usually, estimation is followed by a procedure called *hypothesis testing*, which investigates a particular theory about the data. Hypothesis tests allow conclusions relating to the population to be drawn from the information in a sample. You can only use these tests properly, and so avoid the pitfalls of misinterpretation of the data, when you have a knowledge of their inherent assumptions. Some of these techniques are simple and require little expertise to master, while others are complex and are best left to the qualified statistician. Details of these procedures can be found in Chapters 6–13; the flow charts in Appendix C provide a quick guide to the choice of the correct test.

1.10 CONCLUSION

We develop the ideas presented in this chapter in subsequent chapters. As we have said, the concepts are introduced building on one another, and you will need a sound understanding of the earlier theory in order to appreciate the material presented later.

The best incentive for wrestling with statistical concepts is the need to know the meaning of a data set of your own. Remember – statistical procedures cannot enhance poor data. Providing the data have been acquired with sufficient care and in sufficient number, the statistical procedures can supply you with sound summary statements and interpretative guidelines; the interpretation is still down to you! In the chapters which follow, the emphasis is on developing your understanding of the procedures and their limitations to aid your interpretation. We hope you find the experience of getting to grips with your data rewarding, and discover that statistics can be both satisfying and fun!

EXERCISES

The statements in questions 1.1–1.3 are either TRUE or FALSE.

1.1 Biological variation:
(a) Is the main cause of differences between animals.
(b) Is the term given to differences between animals in a population.
(c) Is the reason why statistics are necessary in animal health science.
(d) Makes it impossible to be sure of any aspect of animal science.
(e) Is the term given to the variation in ability of a technician performing a monotonous task throughout the day.

1.2 A sample is *randomly* drawn from a population:
(a) To reduce the study to a manageable size.
(b) To ensure that the full range of possibilities is included.
(c) To obtain 'normal' animals.
(d) To obtain a representative group.
(e) To avoid selector preferences.

1.3 A nominal scale of measurement is used for data which:
(a) Comprise categories which cannot be ordered.

(b) Are not qualitative.

(c) Take many possible discrete quantitative values.

(d) Are evaluated as percentages.

(e) Are ranked.

1.4 Decide whether the following errors are likely to be systematic or random (S or R):

(a) The water bath which holds samples for an enzyme assay fails during incubation.

(b) A clinician reading a clinical thermometer has a digit preference for the numbers 0 and 5.

(c) The calibration on a colorimeter was not checked before use.

(d) Scales for measuring the weight of animal feed packs are activated sometimes before the sack is put on and sometimes after, depending on the operator.

(e) A chemical balance weighing to 100 mg is used to weigh quantities of 2550 mg.

1.5 Decide whether the following are either real or hypothetical populations (R or H):

(a) Milking cows in a trial for the effectiveness of a novel mastitis treatment.

(b) Horses in livery stables in the south-east of England.

(c) Fleas on dogs in urban Liverpool.

(d) Fleas on dogs treated with an oral monthly ectoparasite treatment.

(e) Blood glucose levels in diabetic dogs.

1.6 Identify the appropriate type of variable (nominal, ordinal, discrete or continuous) for the following data (N, O, D or C):

(a) The coat colour of cats: in a colony of 35 cats there were 1 white, 3 black, 7 ginger, 7 agouti, 11 tortoiseshell and 6 of other colours.

(b) The percentages of motile spermatozoa in the ejaculates of six bulls at an AI centre collected on a single day during March; they were 73, 81, 64, 76, 69 and 84%.

(c) Spectrophotometer measurements of maximum light absorbence at 280 mμ of solutions of egg yolk proteins; they were 0.724, 0.591, 0.520 arbitrary units.

(d) The motility of a series of frozen and thawed samples of spermatozoa estimated on an arbitrary scale of 0–10 (0 indicating a completely immotile sample).

(e) Plasma progesterone levels (ng/ml) measured monthly in pregnant sheep throughout gestation by means of radioimmunoassay.

(f) Kittens classified one week post-natally as either flat-chested (abnormal) or normal.

(g) The optical density of negative micrographs of fluorescent cells calculated from measurements obtained with a densitometer: the results for groups A, B, and C were 0.814, 0.986, 1.103 units, respectively.

(h) Litter sizes of rabbits during an investigation of a behavioural disturbance about the time of implantation.

(i) The body condition scores of goats.

(j) Numbers of deaths due to particular diseases per year studied in an epidemiological investigation.

(k) Radioactivity determined by scintillation counts per min in a β-counter.

(l) The gestation length (days) in cattle carrying twins and in those carrying singletons.

Chapter 2

Descriptive Statistics

2.1 LEARNING OBJECTIVES

By the end of this chapter, you should be able to:

- Explain, with diagrams, the concepts of frequency distributions.
- Interpret diagrams of the frequency distributions of both qualitative and quantitative data.
- Identify frequency distributions which are skewed to the right and skewed to the left.
- Describe and conduct strategies to compare frequency distributions which have different numbers of observations.
- List the essential attributes of good tables and good diagrams.
- Interpret a pie chart, bar chart, dot diagram and histogram and state their appropriate uses.
- Interpret a stem-and-leaf diagram and a box-and-whisker plot, and state their appropriate uses.
- Interpret a scatter diagram and explain its usage.
- List different measures of location and identify their strengths and limitations.
- List different measures of dispersion and identify their strengths and limitations.
- Summarize any given data set appropriately in tabular and/or diagrammatic form to demonstrate its features.

2.2 SUMMARIZING DATA

We collect data with the intention of gleaning information which, usually, we then convey to interested parties. This presents little problem when the data set comprises relatively few observations made on a small group of animals. However, as the quantity of information grows, it becomes increasingly difficult to obtain an overall 'picture' of what is happening.

The first stage in the process of obtaining this picture is to organize the data to establish how often different values occur (see **frequency distributions** in Section 2.3). Then it is helpful to further condense the information, reducing it to a manageable size, and so obtain a snapshot view as an aid to understanding and interpretation. There are various stratagems that we adopt; most notably, we can use:

- **Tables** to exhibit features of the data (see Section 2.4).
- **Diagrams** to illustrate patterns (see Section 2.5).
- **Numerical measures** to summarize the data (see Section 2.6).

2.3 EMPIRICAL FREQUENCY DISTRIBUTIONS

2.3.1 What is a frequency distribution?

A **frequency distribution** shows the frequencies of occurrence of the observations in a data set. Often the distribution of the observed data is called an **empirical frequency distribution**, in contrast to the **theoretical probability distribution** (see Section 3.3) determined from a mathematical model.

It is vital that you clearly understand the distinction between qualitative and quantitative variables (see Section 1.5) before you make any attempt to form a frequency distribution since the variable type will dictate the most appropriate form of display.

- When a variable is **qualitative**, then the observed frequency distribution of that variable comprises the frequency of occurrence of the observations in every class or category of the variable (see Section 2.5.1). We can display this information in a table in which each class is represented, or in a diagram such as a bar chart or a pie diagram.

  For example, if the variable represents different methods of treatments to prevent hypomagnesaemia in dairy cows, the numbers of farms observed using each method would comprise the frequency distribution. The data can be illustrated in a pie chart (Fig. 2.3).

- When the variable of interest is **quantitative** (either discrete or continuous), then the information is most easily assimilated by creating between 5 and 15 non-overlapping, preferably equal, intervals or classes which encompass the range of values of the variable. It is essential that the class intervals are *unambiguously* defined such that an observation falls into one class only; these classes are adjacent when the data are discrete, and contiguous when the data are continuous. We determine the number of observations belonging to each

class (the class frequency). The complete set of class frequencies is a frequency distribution. We present it (see Section 2.5.2) in the form of a table or a diagram such as a bar chart (discrete variable) or a histogram (continuous variable).

For example, columns 1 and 2 of Table 2.1 show the frequency distribution of the threshold response of sheep to a mechanical stimulus applied to the forelimb; Fig. 2.5 is a histogram of the data. These data reflect sensitivity to pain sensation in the extremities of sheep at pasture, and were derived as the control data in a study of the relationship of pain threshold and the incidence of foot rot; a higher threshold was associated with a greater incidence of disease (Ley *et al.*, 1995).

2.3.2 Relative frequency distributions

Although creating a frequency distribution is a useful way of describing a set of observations, it is difficult to compare two or more frequency distributions if the total number of observations in each distribution is different. A way of overcoming this difficulty is to calculate the proportion or percentage of observations in each class or category. These are called **relative frequencies** and each is obtained by dividing the frequency for that category by the total number of observations (see column 3 of Table 2.1). The sum of the relative frequencies of all the categories is unity (or 100%) apart from rounding errors.

2.3.3 Cumulative relative frequency distributions

Sometimes it is helpful to evaluate the number (the cumulative frequency) or percentage (cumulative relative frequency) of individuals which are contained in a category and in all lower categories. Generally, we find that cumulative relative frequency distributions are more useful than cumulative frequency distributions. For example, we may be interested in using the data

Table 2.1 Frequency distribution of mechanical threshold (N) of 470 sheep.

Class limits of mechanical threshold (newtons)	Frequency	Relative frequency (%)	Cumulative relative frequency (%)
1.00–1.90	9	1.9	1.9
2.00–2.90	44	9.4	11.3
3.00–3.90	88	18.7	30.0
4.00–4.90	137	29.1	59.1
5.00–5.90	69	14.7	73.8
6.00–6.90	37	7.9	81.7
7.00–7.90	21	4.5	86.2
8.00–8.90	17	3.6	89.8
9.00–9.90	19	4.0	93.8
10.00–10.90	14	3.0	96.8
11.00–11.90	4	0.9	97.7
12.00–12.90	6	1.3	98.9
13.00–13.90	2	0.4	99.4
14.00–14.90	3	0.6	100.0
Total	470	100.0	

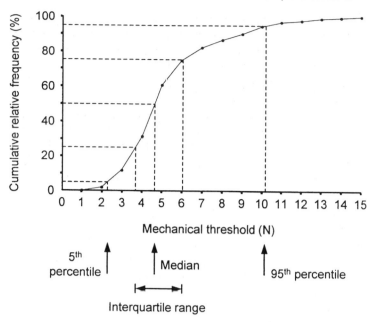

Fig. 2.1 Cumulative relative frequency polygon of mechanical threshold of sheep (data from Ley *et al.*, 1995, with permission).

of Table 2.1 to determine the percentage of sheep whose mechanical threshold is less than 7.01 newtons. We form a **cumulative relative frequency distribution** by adding the relative frequencies of individuals contained in each category and all lower categories, and repeating this process for each category. The cumulative relative frequencies are tabulated in column 4 of Table 2.1 and the distribution is drawn in the **cumulative relative frequency polygon** of Fig. 2.1.

We can evaluate the **percentiles** (often called *centiles*) of the frequency distribution from this cumulative frequency distribution. Percentiles are the values of the variable which divide the total frequency into 100 equal parts. They are used to divide the frequency distribution into useful groups when the observations are arranged in order of magnitude. In particular, the 50th percentile (called the *median* – see Section 2.6.1(b)) is the value of the variable which divides the distribution into two halves; 50% of the individuals have observations less than the median, and 50% of the individuals have observations greater than the median. Often the 25th and the 75th percentiles are quoted (these are called the *lower quartile* and *upper quartile*, re-

spectively); 25% of the observations lie below the lower quartile and 25% of the observations lie above the upper quartile, the distance between these quartiles being the *interquartile range*. The 5th and 95th percentiles enclose the central 90% of the observations. We show how to evaluate these percentiles from the cumulative frequency distribution polygon in Fig. 2.1.

2.4 TABLES

A table is an orderly arrangement, usually of numbers or words in rows and columns, which exhibits a set of facts in a distinct and comprehensive way. The layout of the table will be dictated by the data, and therefore will vary for different types of data. It is useful, however, to remember the most important principles which govern well-constructed tables; we outline them in the Box 2.1.

2.5 DIAGRAMS

A diagram is a graphic representation of data and may take several forms. It is often easier to

Box 2.1 Rules for well-constructed tables.

- Include a concise, informative, and unambiguously defined title.
- Give a brief heading for each row and column.
- Include the units of measurement.
- Give the number of items on which any summary measure (e.g. a percentage) is based.
- When providing a summary statistic (e.g. the mean) always include a measure of precision (e.g. a confidence interval – see Section 4.5).
- Give figures only to the degree of accuracy that is appropriate (as a guideline, one significant figure more than the raw data).
- Do not give too much information in a table.
- Remember that it is easier to scan information down columns rather than across rows.

Box 2.2 Rules for well-constructed diagrams.

- Keep it simple and avoid unnecessary 'frills' (e.g. making a pie chart three-dimensional).
- Include a concise, informative, and unambiguously defined title.
- Label all axes, segments, and bars, if necessary using a legend or key showing the meaning of the different symbols used.
- Present the units, the numbers on which summary measures are based, and measures of variability where appropriate.
- Avoid exaggerating the scale on an axis, perhaps by omitting the zero point, so as to distort the results.
- Include a break in the scale only if there is no other satisfactory way of demonstrating the extremes.
- Show coincident points in a scatter diagram.
- Ensure that the method of display conveys all the relevant information (e.g. pairing).

discern important *patterns* from a diagram rather than a table, even though the latter may give more precise numerical information. Diagrams are most useful when we want to convey information quickly, and they should serve as an adjunct to more formal statistical analysis. You will find the guidelines in Box 2.2 helpful when you construct a diagram.

2.5.1 Qualitative data

When data are qualitative or categorical then each observation belongs to one of a number of distinct categories or classes. We can determine the number or percentage of individuals falling into each class or category and display this information in a *bar chart* or a *pie chart*.

(a) Bar chart

A **bar chart** is a diagram in which every category of the variable is represented; the length of each bar, which should be of constant width, depicts the number or percentage of individuals belonging to that category. Figure 2.2 is an example of a bar chart. The length of the bar is proportional to the frequency or relative frequency in the relevant category, so it is essential that the scale showing the frequency or relative frequency should start at zero for each bar.

You may find in other people's work that the frequency in a category is indicated by a pictorial representation of a relevant object. Typically, this object in a veterinary study will be the animal under investigation. Such a diagram is called a **pictogram**. There is an inherent danger of misinterpretation when making crude comparisons by eye of the frequencies in different categories. Is it height or area or volume of the object which represents the frequencies? To a certain extent, this problem can be overcome by using equally sized images, so that the frequency in a category is indicated by the appropriate number of repetitions of the image. The effect is similar to a bar chart, with each 'bar' containing varying numbers of images. However, because of the potential for confusion, we do not recommend that you use pictograms to display frequencies.

(b) Pie chart

A **pie chart** is a circle divided into segments with each segment portraying a different category of the qualitative variable (see Fig. 2.3). The total area of the circle represents the total frequency, and the area of a given sector is proportional to the percentage of individuals falling into that category. A pie chart should include a statement of the percentage or actual number of individuals in

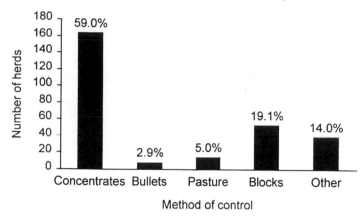

Fig. 2.2 Bar chart showing the number of herds in which specific methods of control of hypomagnesaemia were used by dairy farmers in 278 dairy herds (data from McCoy *et al.*, 1996, with permission).

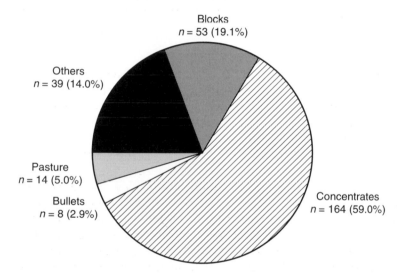

Fig. 2.3 Pie chart showing percentage of herds in which specific methods of control of hypomagnesaemia were used by dairy farmers in 278 dairy herds (redrawn from McCoy *et al.*, 1996, with permission).

each segment. Generally, we prefer the bar chart to the pie chart as the former is easier to construct and is more useful for comparative purposes, partly because it is easier to compare lengths by eye rather than angles.

2.5.2 Quantitative data

When the data are quantitative, we may show every data value, for example in a *dot diagram*, or we may display only a summary of the data, for example, in a *histogram*.

(a) Dot diagram

If the data set is of a manageable size, the best way of displaying it is to show every value in a **dot diagram/plot**. When we investigate a single quantitative variable, we can mark each observation as a dot on a line calibrated in the units of measurement of that variable, plotted horizontally or vertically.

- If the data are in a single group, the diagram will look like Fig. 2.9.
- When we are comparing the observations in two or more groups, we can draw a dot dia-

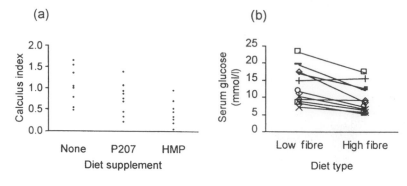

Fig. 2.4 Dot diagram showing (a) the calculus index on teeth in three groups of dogs on different diets (based on summary data from Stookey *et al.*, 1995, and (b) the change in serum glucose concentration in each of 11 diabetic dogs on high- and low-fibre diets (based on summary data from Nelson *et al.*, 1998).

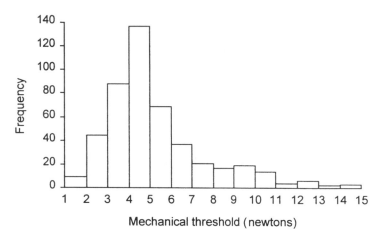

Fig. 2.5 Histogram of mechanical threshold of 470 sheep (data from Ley *et al.*, 1995, with permission).

gram with the horizontal axis designating the groups, and the vertical axis representing the scale of measurement of the variable. Then, in a single diagram, we can show the values for each group in a vertical dot plot, facilitating the comparison of groups as well as providing a visual display of the distribution of the variable in each group (see Fig. 2.4(a)).

- When an individual reading in one group bears a direct relationship to that in another group (e.g. from two litter mates, or before and after within an individual) we can join the related dots in a pair by a straight line (see Fig. 2.4(b)). The directions of the slope of the lines may indicate a difference between the groups.

(b) Histogram

The frequency distribution of a quantitative variable (see Section 2.3.1) can be displayed as a

histogram. This is a two-dimensional diagram in which the horizontal axis represents the units of measurement of the variable of interest, with each class interval being clearly delineated. We construct rectangles above each class interval so that the *area* of the rectangle is proportional to the frequency for that class. If the intervals are of equal width, then the height of the rectangle is proportional to the frequency.

The histogram gives a good picture of the frequency distribution of the variable (see Fig. 2.5). The distribution is **symmetrical** if its shape to the right of a central value is a mirror image of that to the left of the central value. The **tails** of the frequency distribution represent the frequencies at the extremes of the distribution. The frequency distribution is **skewed to the right** (positively skewed) if the right-hand tail is extended, and **skewed to the left** (negatively skewed) if the left-hand tail is extended. It is not

Frequency	Stem and leaf	
6	1 *	04&
3	1 .	&
20	2 *	111123344&
24	2 .	5566778889
40	3 *	0011111222222334111
48	3 .	5555555566666777788888899
65	4 *	000111111111222222233333334444
72	4 .	555555556666666777777788888888899999
39	5 *	000011112222334444
30	5 .	55666777889999
18	6 *	00123344
19	6 .	557778889&
9	7 *	014&
12	7 .	5689&
8	8 *	024&
9	8 .	59&
8	9 *	34&
6	9 .	56
Extremes	(9.7), (9.8), (9.9), (10.0), (10.2), (10.3), (10.4)	
Extremes	(10.5), (10.7), (10.8), (10.9), (11.0), (11.3), (11.5)	
Extremes	(11.8), (12.0), (12.3), (12.4), (12.6), (12.8), (12.9)	

Stem width: 1.00
Each leaf: 2 case(s)
& denotes a fractional leaf (i.e. one case)
* indicates that there are 2 branches for that stem unit

Fig. 2.6 Stem-and-leaf diagram of mechanical threshold of sheep (data from Ley *et al.*, 1995, with permission).

uncommon to find biological data which are skewed to the right; the distribution of the data in Fig. 2.5 is skewed to the right.

You should note that although the histogram is similar to the bar chart, the rectangles in a histogram are contiguous because the quantitative variable is continuous, whereas there are spaces between the bars in a bar chart.

(c) Stem-and-leaf diagram

We often see a mutation of the histogram, called a **stem-and-leaf diagram**, in computer output. Each vertical rectangle of the histogram is replaced by a row of numbers which represent the relevant observations. The stem is the core value of the observation (e.g. the unit value before the decimal place) and the leaf is a sequence of ordered single digits, one for each observation, which follow the core value (e.g. the first decimal place). Plotting the data in this way provides an easily assimilated description of the distribution of the data whilst, at the same time, showing the raw data. Figure 2.6 is a stem-and-leaf diagram for the mechanical threshold data for sheep.

(d) Box-and-whisker plot

Another diagram which we often see in computer output, the **box-and-whisker plot**, provides a summary of the distribution of a data set. The scale of measurement of the variable is usually drawn vertically, and the diagram comprises a box with horizontal limits defining the upper and lower quartiles (see Section 2.3.3), enclosing the central 50% of the observations, with the median (see Section 2.6.1(b)) marked by a horizontal line within the box. The whiskers are vertical lines extending from the box as low as the 2.5th percentile and as high as the 97.5th percentile (sometimes the percentiles are replaced by the minimum and maximum values of the set of observations). Figure 2.7 is a box-and-whisker plot of the mechanical threshold data for sheep. The

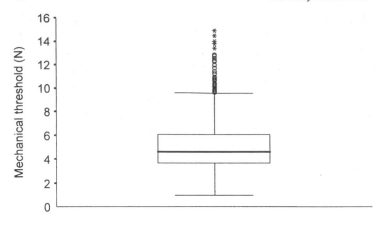

Fig. 2.7 Box-and-whisker plot of mechanical threshold of sheep (data from Ley *et al.*, 1995, with permission). Note that extreme values are indicated in the diagram.

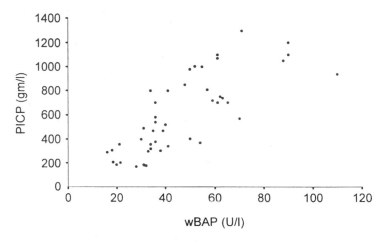

Fig. 2.8 Scatter diagram showing the relationship between two measures of bone formation: bone alkaline phosphatase activity (wBAP) and Type I collagen concentration (PICP) (redrawn from Jackson *et al.*, 1996, with permission of the publisher WB Saunders Company).

box-and-whiskcr plot is particularly useful when a number of data sets are to be compared in a single diagram (see Fig. 7.2).

(e) Scatter diagram

The **scatter diagram** is an effective way of presenting data when we are interested in examining the relationship between two quantitative variables. The diagram is a two-dimensional plot in which each axis represents the scale of measurement of one of the two variables. Using this rectangular co-ordinate system, we relate the value for an individual on the horizontal scale (the *abscissa*) to the corresponding value for that individual on the vertical scale (the *ordinate*) by marking the relevant point with an appropriate

symbol, such as a cross or circle (see Fig. 2.8). Coincident points should be identifiable. We can discern possible relationships between the variables by observing the scatter of points, and then we may join the points to produce a line graph, or draw a line which best represents the relationship (see Chapter 10).

2.6 NUMERICAL MEASURES

Using a visual display as a means of describing a set of data helps us get a 'feel' for the data, but our impressions are subjective. It is usually essential that we supplement the visual display with the appropriate numerical measures which summarize the data. If we are able to determine some form of average which measures the central tendency of the data set, and if we know how widely scattered the observations are in either direction from that average, then we will have a reasonable 'picture' of the data. These two characteristics of a set of observations measured on a quantitative variable are known as **measures of location** and **measures of dispersion**.

Note that it is customary to distinguish between measures in the population (called *parameters*) and their sample estimates (called *statistics*) by using Greek letters for the former and Roman letters for the latter (see the Glossary of Notation in Appendix D).

2.6.1 Measures of location (averages)

The term **average** refers to any one of several measures of the **central tendency** of a data set.

(a) The arithmetic mean

The most commonly used measure of central tendency is the **arithmetic mean** (usually abbreviated to the **mean**). It is obtained by adding together the observations in a data set and dividing by the number of observations in the set.

If the continuous variable of interest is denoted by x and there are n observations in the sample, then the sample mean (pronounced x bar) is

$$\bar{x} = \frac{\sum x}{n}$$

Example
The following are plasma potassium values (mmol/l) of 14 dogs:

4.37, 4.87, 4.35, 3.92, 4.68, 4.54, 5.24, 4.57, 4.59, 4.66, 4.40, 4.73, 4.83, 4.21

$$\bar{x} = \frac{63.96}{14} = 4.57 \text{ mmol/l}$$

- The mean has the disadvantage that its value is influenced by outliers (see Section 5.9.2). An **outlier** is an observation whose value is highly inconsistent with the main body of the data. An outlier with an excessively large value will tend to increase the mean unduly, whilst a particularly small value will decrease it.

- The mean is an appropriate measure of central tendency if the distribution of the data is symmetrical. The mean will be 'pulled' to the right (increased in value) if the distribution is skewed to the right, and 'pulled' to the left (decreased in value) if the distribution is skewed to the left.

(b) The median

Another frequently used measure of central tendency is the **median**. The median is the central value in the set of n observations which have been arranged in **rank order**, i.e. the observations are arranged in increasing (or decreasing) order of magnitude. The median is the middle value of the ordered set with as many observations above it as below it (see Box 2.3). The median is the 50th percentile (see Section 2.3.3).

Example
The weights (grams) of 19 male Hartley guinea pigs were:

314, 991, 789, 556, 412, 499, 350, 863, 455, 297, 598, 510, 388, 642, 474, 333, 421, 685, 536

If we arrange the weights in rank order, they become:

297, 314, 333, 350, 388, 412, 421, 455, 474, **499**, 510, 536, 556, 598, 642, 685, 789, 863, 991

The median, shown in bold, is the $(19 + 1)/2 = 10$th weight in the ordered set; this is 499 g.

- The arithmetic mean and the median are close or equal in value if the distribution is symmetrical.

Box 2.3   Calculating the median.

- *If n is odd*, then the median is found by starting with the smallest observation in the ordered set and then counting until the $(n + 1)/2$th observation is reached. This observation is the median.
- *If n is even*, then the median lies midway between the central two observations.

- The advantage of the median is that it is not affected by outliers or if the distribution of the data is skewed. Thus the median will be less than the mean if the data are skewed to the right, and greater than the mean if the data are skewed to the left.
- A disadvantage of the median is that it does not incorporate all the observations in its calculations, and it is difficult to handle mathematically.

(c) The geometric mean

If we take the logarithm (either to base 10 or to base *e*) of each value of a data set which is skewed to the right, we usually find that the distribution of the log-transformed data becomes more symmetrical. In this case, the arithmetic mean of the log-transformed values is a useful measure of location. However, it has the disadvantage that it is measured on a log scale. We therefore convert it back to the original scale by taking its antilogarithm; this is the **geometric mean**. The distribution of biological data, if not symmetrical, is frequently skewed to the right; we would then calculate the geometric mean to represent an average value.

For example, Fig. 2.9 shows the distribution of the weights of the guinea pigs (the example in Section 2.6.1(b)), illustrated in a dot plot, first as the untransformed data (Fig. 2.9(a)) and then as the log-transformed data (Fig. 2.9(b)). You can see that the transformation improves symmetry, and the geometric mean is smaller than the arithmetic mean and closer to the median. It is important to realize we apply the transformation to

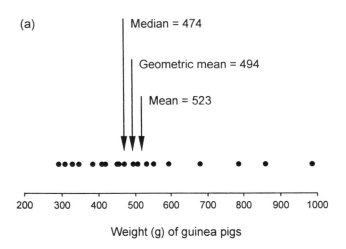

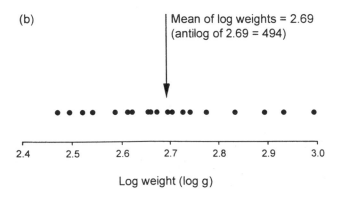

Fig. 2.9   Dot plots for (a) the weights, and (b) the $\log_{10}$ weights of 19 guinea pigs.

each value of the raw data and *not* to the class limits of grouped data, even when the data are presented as a frequency distribution. Figure 2.10(b) shows the effect of this log transformation on the distribution of the mechanical threshold data summarized in Table 2.1 and displayed in Fig. 2.10(a). The mean of the log mechanical threshold data is 0.6778 log newtons; the antilog of this mean, the geometric mean, is 4.76 newtons. Note that the arithmetic mean is 5.25 newtons and the median is 4.65 newtons. You can see that the distribution is more symmetrical, and the geometric mean represents the central tendency of the transformed data much better than the arithmetic mean of the untransformed data.

- The geometric mean is always less than the arithmetic mean if the data are skewed to the right.
- The geometric mean is usually approximately equal to the median if the data are skewed to the right. We often prefer to use the geometric mean rather than the median for right-skewed data because the properties of the distribution of the mean (from which the geometric mean is calculated using the log data) are more useful than those of the median.

(a) Histogram of raw data

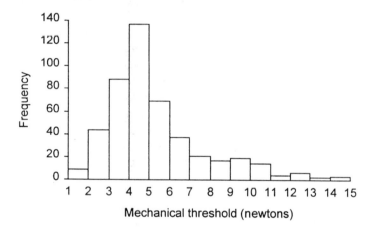

(b) Histogram of log data

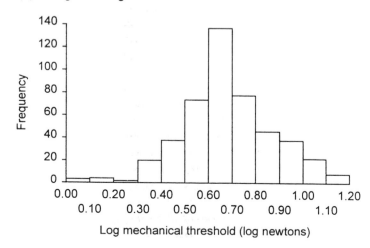

Fig. 2.10 Histograms of the mechanical threshold of sheep showing (a) the raw data, and (b) the $\log_{10}$ transformed data (data from Ley *et al.*, 1995, with permission).

(d) The mode

A well-known but infrequently used measure of central tendency is the **mode**. It is the most commonly occurring observation in a set of observations. The mode often has a different value from both the arithmetic mean and the median. The **modal group** or **modal class** is the group or class into which most observations fall in a histogram.

In the mechanical threshold data of Table 2.1 and Fig. 2.5, the modal group represents values between 4.01 and 5.00 newtons. In another context, we might use the mode to indicate the most common litter size in a breed of dogs, e.g. the most common litter size of bearded collie dogs is seven.

For the following reasons, statisticians tend not to favour the mode as a tool for summarizing data:

- The mode is determined by disregarding most of the observations.
- The mode depends on the accuracy with which the data are measured.
- Some distributions do not have a mode whilst other distributions may have more than one mode. A distribution which has a single mode or modal group is called **unimodal**; a distribution which has two humps (i.e. modes or modal groups) separated by a trough is called **bimodal** even if the frequency of occurrence of the observations in the two modes or modal classes is not equal.

2.6.2 Measures of dispersion (spread)

There are a number of measures of the spread of the data, each of which has different attributes.

(a) The range

The **range** is defined as the difference between the largest and smallest observations. In the mechanical threshold data, the range is 13.9 newtons, being the difference between the maximum value of 14.9 newtons and the minimum value of 1.00 newton.

- The range is an easily determined measure of dispersion of the observations of a quantitative variable.
- It gives undue weight to extreme values and will, therefore, overestimate the dispersion of most of the observations if outliers are present.
- The range tends to increase in value as the number of observations in the sample increases.

(b) The interquartile range

The **interquartile range** is the range of values which encloses the central 50% of the observations if the observations are arranged in order of magnitude. It is defined as the difference between the first and third quartiles (see Section 2.3.3). In the mechanical threshold data, the interquartile range lies between 3.68 and 6.10 newtons (see Fig. 2.1).

- The interquartile range is influenced neither by the presence of outliers nor by the sample size.
- It suffers from the disadvantage, in common with the range, of ignoring most of the observations, being calculated from just two of them.

(c) The variance

The **variance** is determined by calculating the *deviation* of each observation from the mean. This deviation will be large if the observation is far from the mean, and it will be small if the observation is close to the mean. Some sort of average of these deviations therefore provides a useful measure of spread. However, some of the deviations are positive and some are negative, depending on whether the observation is greater or less than the mean, and their arithmetic mean is zero. The effect of the sign of the deviation can be annulled by squaring every deviation, since the square of both positive and negative numbers is always positive. The arithmetic mean of these squared deviations is called the variance.

In fact, when we select a sample of *n* observations from our population, we divide the sum of the squared deviations in the sample by $n - 1$ instead of n. It can be shown that this produces a better estimate (i.e. *unbiased*, see Section 4.4.3) of the population variance. Thus, the sample variance, s^2, which estimates the population variance, σ^2, is given by

$$s^2 = \frac{\sum (x - \bar{x})^2}{n-1}$$

We rarely calculate the variance from first principles in this age of hand-held calculators and computers, and so we make no attempt here to show the mechanics of the calculation.

Example

The plasma potassium data of 14 dogs, for which the mean was calculated as 4.57 mmol/l (Section 2.6.1(a)), gives a sample variance of

$$s^2 = \frac{1.32297}{13} = 0.10177 \, (\text{mmol/l})^2$$

If you were reporting the variance, you would probably correct it to one decimal place more than the original data. This variance would therefore be reported as $0.102 \, (\text{mmol/l})^2$.

- The variance uses every available observation.
- Although the variance is a sensible measure of spread, it is not intuitively appealing as its dimensionality is different from that of the original measurements.

(d) The standard deviation

The **standard deviation** (often abbreviated to SD) is equal to the square root of the variance. The standard deviation may be regarded as an average of the deviations of the observations from the arithmetic mean. It is often denoted by s in the sample, estimating σ in the population, and is given by

$$s = \sqrt{\text{Variance}} = \sqrt{\frac{\sum (x - \bar{x})^2}{n-1}}$$

We can calculate the standard deviation on a calculator rather than by substituting the actual

observations into the above formula. (Note: most calculators have two SD function keys, one for the population SD and one for its estimate from the sample. These may be marked as σ (for the population) and s (for the sample). On some calculators, you may find them marked as σ_n (for the population) and s_{n-1} or σ_{n-1} (for the sample). The use of σ_{n-1} is confusing because it is contrary to the generally accepted convention of nomenclature.)

Example

In the plasma potassium data of 14 dogs used as the example of the calculations of the mean and the variance

$$s = \sqrt{0.10177} = 0.319 \, \text{mmol/l}$$

- The standard deviation (SD) uses all the observations in the data set.
- The SD is a measure of spread whose dimensionality is the same as that of the original observations, i.e. it is measured in the same units as the observations.
- The SD is of greatest use in relation to a symmetrically distributed data set which follows the Gaussian or Normal distribution (see Section 3.5.3). In this case, it can be shown that the interval defined by the (mean ± 2 SD) encompasses the central 95% (approximately) of the observations in the population. In the example above, the interval is $4.57 \pm 2(0.319)$, i.e. from 3.93 to 5.21 mmol/l.
- For data which are Normally distributed, four times the standard deviation gives us an indication of the *range* of the majority of the values in the population. In the plasma potassium example, this is $4 \times 0.319 = 1.28$ mmol/l.

Sometimes the standard deviation is expressed as a percentage of the mean; we call this measure the **coefficient of variation** (CV). It is a dimensionless quantity which can be used for comparing relative amounts of variation. However, these comparisons are entirely subjective because its theoretical properties are complex, so we do not recommend its use.

2.7 THE REFERENCE RANGE

Sometimes we are interested in describing the range of values of a variable which defines the healthy population; we call this the **reference range** or the **reference interval**. Because of the problem caused by outliers, we calculate the reference range as the interval which encompasses, say, the central 90%, 95% or 99% of the observations obtained from a large representative sample of the population. We usually calculate the values encompassing 95% of the observations; the reference values is then defined by the mean ±1.96 SD (the 1.96 is often approximated by 2) provided the data have an approximately Normal distribution (see Section 3.5.3). If the data are not Normally distributed, we can still calculate the reference range as the interval defined by the 2.5th and 97.5th percentiles of the empirical distribution of the observations.

We can use the reference range to determine whether an individual animal may be classified as belonging to the population of healthy animals. If the animal under consideration has a value for this variable which lies outside the specified range for the healthy population, we may conclude that the animal is unlikely to belong to the normal population and is a diseased animal. For example, plasma creatinine values above the reference range of 40 to 180 μmol/l were used to diagnose renal failure in cats in a study by Barber and Elliott (1998).

Note that the reference range is sometimes called the normal range. The latter term is best avoided because of the confusion between 'normal' implying healthy and 'Normal' in the statistical sense describing a particular distribution. In this book we distinguish the two by small and capital letters but they may still be misconstrued.

EXERCISES

The statements in questions 2.1–2.4 are either TRUE or FALSE.

2.1 An appropriate diagram to show the frequency distribution of a continuous variable is:

(a) A histogram.
(b) A pie chart.
(c) A stem-and-leaf plot.
(d) A bar chart.
(e) A box-and-whisker plot.

2.2 An appropriate measure of central tendency for continuous data which are skewed to the right is:
(a) The arithmetic mean.
(b) The geometric mean.
(c) The antilog of the arithmetic mean of the log-transformed data.
(d) The median.
(e) The 50th percentile.

2.3 The standard deviation:
(a) Is a measure of spread.
(b) Is the difference between the 5th and 95th percentiles.
(c) Is greater than the range of the observations.
(d) Measures the average deviation of the observations from the mean.
(e) Is the square of the variance.

2.4 The reference range (containing 95% of the observations) for a particular variable:
(a) Cannot be calculated if the data are skewed.
(b) May be used to determine whether or not an animal is likely to be diseased if its value for the variable is known.
(c) Can be evaluated from a small sample of data.
(d) Is equal to the mean ± SD if the data are Normally distributed.
(e) Is equal to the difference between the largest and smallest observations in the data set.

2.5 The following data show the resting pulmonary ventilation in 25 adult sheep (l/min):

8.3	8.0	9.9	6.1	5.5
10.3	6.5	7.6	7.6	7.6
6.9	10.3	7.8	7.3	8.9
10.1	7.6	9.1	8.3	4.8
10.2	6.5	9.1	7.0	11.9

Draw histograms of the data with:
(a) Class interval 1.0 l/min, lowest class 4.25–5.24 l/m.

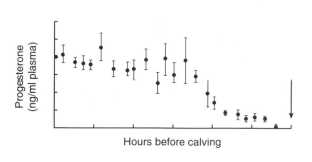

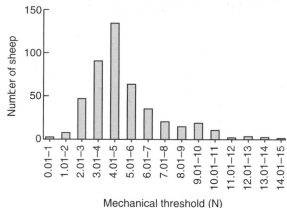

(a) Progesterone concentrations measured in plasma from cows in the period before calving (mean ± SEM)

(b) Distribution of mechanical thresholds in 470 sheep

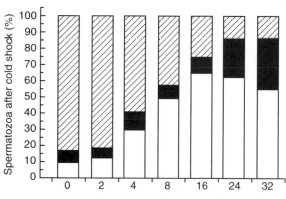

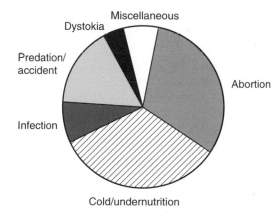

(c) Categorization of boar spermatozoa into ☐ live acrosome-intact, ■ live acrosome-damaged, and ▨ dead subgroups after cold shock at various times after ejaculation

(d) Relative importance of different causes of lamb deaths

Fig. 2.11 Illustrations taken from the literature: (a) reproduced from Parker *et al.* (1988), with permission; (b) reproduced from Ley *et al.* (1995), with permission; (c) reproduced from Tamuli and Watson (1994), with permission; and (d) redrawn from Merrell (1998) *Sheep Veterinary Society Congress Times* with permission of the publisher.

(b) Class interval 0.2 l/min, lowest class 4.80–4.99 l/m.

(c) Class interval 5.0 l/min, lowest class 4.50–9.49 l/m.

All the histograms should appear on the same sheet of graph paper and should not be superimposed. Use the same scales for all of them. Which is the most appropriate histogram for demonstrating the distribution of the data? Explain your answer.

2.6 Figures 2.11(a)–(d) have errors in their presentation. Identify the incorrect features and suggest what is required to rectify the errors.

2.7 The following data, 44.4, 67.6, 76.2, 64.7, 80.0, 75.0, 34.2, 29.2, represent the infection of goats with the viral condition *peste des petits ruminants*, expressed as the percentage morbidity in Indian villages (from Kulkarni *et al.*, 1996). Calculate the median.

2.8 Calculate the mean and the median of the following data set. What evidence is there for concluding that the data are or are not symmetrically distributed?

Body weights of 16 weanling female mice in grams:
54.1 49.8 24.0 46.0 44.1 34.0 52.6 54.4
56.1 52.0 51.9 54.0 58.0 39.0 32.7 58.5

2.9 Use a calculator with statistical functions to calculate the range, the variance and the standard deviation of the sample data below:

The vitamin E concentration (μmol/l) in 12 heifers showing clinical signs of an unusual myopathy (from Gunning & Walters, 1994):
4.2 3.3 7.0 6.9 5.1 3.4 2.5 8.6 3.5 2.9 4.9 5.4

Probability and Probability Distributions

3.1 LEARNING OBJECTIVES

By the end of this chapter, you should be able to:

- Calculate the mathematical probability of the occurrence of particular outcomes in simple events, such as dice-throwing, coin-tossing.
- Elaborate the simple rules of probability: (a) addition rule, (b) multiplication rule, and illustrate each with a simple example.
- Explain a probability density function.
- List the properties of the Normal distribution.
- Describe the Standardized Normal Deviate.
- Explain how you might verify approximate Normality in a data set.
- Define situations when a Lognormal distribution might apply.
- Define conditions under which measurements show a Binomial distribution, and give an example.
- State when a Binomial distribution is approximated by a Normal distribution.
- Define conditions under which measurements show a Poisson distribution, and give an example.
- State when a Poisson distribution is approximated by a Normal distribution.

3.2 PROBABILITY

3.2.1 The relevance of probability to statistics

So far, we have discussed the processes involved in summarizing and displaying the results obtained from a group of animals. The approaches, collectively known as **descriptive statistics**, are an important first step to any analysis. However,

usually we want to generalize the results from a representative sample to the larger population from which they came; that is, we want to make *inferences* about the population using the sample data.

For example, suppose the mean and standard deviation of serum iron concentration in a random sample of 59 Simmental cows is $27.64\,\mu mol/l$ and $6.36\,\mu mol/l$, respectively. It is unlikely that the results obtained in this sample are identical to those which would be observed in the population of Simmental cows. However, we want to use this information to infer something about this population. There is invariably some doubt associated with the inferences drawn about the population; this doubt is quantified by a **probability** which is fundamental to statistical inference as it provides the link between the sample and the population. We discuss the concepts of **inferential statistics** in Chapter 4 when the notion of sampling and sampling distributions is introduced, and develop the theory in subsequent chapters. Here we introduce the concepts of probability.

3.2.2 Definitions of probability

There are several approaches to defining a probability:

- We can take the **subjective** or personal view of probability which is to regard it as a measure of the strength of belief an individual has that a particular event will occur. For example, 'That cow has a 60% chance of calving tonight'. Whilst this approach to defining a probability has the advantage that it is possible to assign a probability to any event, this is more than offset by the fact that different people are likely to assign different probabilities to the same event, often influenced by irrelevant considerations.

- A second approach to defining a probability relies on having an understanding of the theoretical **model** defining the set of all possible outcomes of a trial; we evaluate the probability solely on the basis of this model, without recourse to performing the experiment at all. It is often called an ***a priori*** probability. So, for example, we know that there are two equally likely outcomes when an unbiased coin is tossed: either a head or a tail. This is the model from which we can deduce that the probability of a defined event, obtaining a head, say, is 1/2 = 0.5.

- The third approach to defining a probability, and the one used in statistical inference, is to regard a probability as the proportion of times a particular outcome (the event) will occur in a very large number of 'trials' or 'experiments' performed under similar conditions. The result of any one trial should be independent of the result of any other trial, so whether or not the event occurs in any one trial should not affect whether or not the event occurs in any other trial. For example, if we were interested in estimating the probability of a litter size greater than three in a colony of guinea pigs, we would have to count the number of such litters over a lengthy period, say a year, and divide it by the total number of litters. This is the **frequency** definition of probability because it relies on counting the frequency of occurrence of the event in a large number of repetitions of similar trials. The probability defined in this way is thus the *relative frequency* of the event in repeated trials under similar conditions.

It is interesting to note that the various definitions of probability are not entirely distinct. The proportion of times that an event would be observed if an experiment were to be repeated a large number of times approaches the *a priori* probability. So, if a coin were tossed five times, we would not be very surprised to observe four heads; however if the coin were tossed 1000

times, we would be more likely to observe approximately 500 heads. Thus, the values for the probability defined using both the *a priori* approach and the frequency approach coincide when the experiment is repeated many times. Similarly, the subjective view of probability cannot be divorced from the frequency view as the former is usually based on experience which in turn relies on previous occurrences of similar events. For example, the likely incidence of liver fluke infestation can be forecast on the basis of the previous year's rainfall, and is founded on a large database of rainfall/fluke incidence relationships.

3.2.3 Properties of a probability

It is clear that, since a probability is defined as a relative frequency or a proportion, its numerical value must lie between 0 and 1.

- A probability of 0 means that the event *cannot* occur.
- A probability of 1 (unity) means that the event *must* occur.

We often convert probabilities into percentages (with a range 0–100%) or express them as ratios (e.g. a 1-in-3 chance of an event occurring). Sometimes we focus our interest not on a particular event occurring but on that event *not* occurring, i.e. on the *complementary event*. It follows from the properties of a probability that the probability of the event not occurring is 1 minus the probability of the event occurring. So, if the probability of a kitten contracting feline viral rhinotracheitis after vaccination at 9 and 13 weeks of age is 0.04 (in a particular location and time), then the probability of being adequately protected is 0.96.

3.2.4 Rules of probability

Two simple rules which govern probabilities are:

- **Addition rule**: When two events are *mutually exclusive*, implying that the two events cannot occur at the same time, then the probability of *either* of the two events occurring is the *sum* of the probabilities of each event.

For example, assuming that a carton of dog biscuit shapes contains equal numbers of the five different shapes, the probability of picking either a diamond shape or a round shape from the carton is the sum of the probability of a diamond (1/5) and the probability of a round (1/5) which is 2/5 or 0.4.

- **Multiplication rule**: When two events are *independent*, so that the occurrence or non-occurrence of one event does not affect the occurrence or non-occurrence of the other event, then the probability of *both* events occurring is the *product* of the individual probabilities.

For example, if a Friesian cow is inseminated on a particular day and sustains the pregnancy, then the probability of her calving by 278 days later (the mean gestation period) is 0.5. If two Friesian cows are inseminated on the same day (and both sustain the pregnancy), then the probability of both of them calving by 278 days later is $0.5 \times 0.5 = 0.25$.

3.3 PROBABILITY DISTRIBUTIONS

3.3.1 Introduction

We introduced **empirical frequency distributions** in Section 2.3; these allow us to assimilate a large amount of *observed* data and condense them into a form, typically a table or a diagram, from which we can interpret their salient features. Another type of distribution is a **probability distribution**; this is a *theoretical* model which we use to calculate the probability of an event occurring. The probability distribution shows how the set of all possible mutually exclusive events is distributed, and can be presented as an *equation*, a *chart* or a *table*. We may regard a probability distribution as the theoretical equivalent of an empirical relative frequency distribution, with its own mean and variance.

A variable which can take different values with given probabilities is called a **random variable**. A probability distribution comprises all the values that the random variable can take, with their associated probabilities. There are numerous probability distributions which may be distinguished by whether the random variable is **discrete**, taking only a finite set of possible values, or **continuous**, taking an infinite set of possible values in a range of values (see Section 1.5). A discrete random variable with only two possible values is called a **binary** variable, e.g. pregnant or not pregnant, diseased or healthy.

3.3.2 Avoiding the theory!

We discuss some of the more common distributions in this chapter although, for simplicity, we omit the mathematical equations which define the distributions. You do not need to know the equations for the procedures we describe in this text, since the required probabilities are tabulated.

We are aware that much of the theory associated with probability distributions presents difficulties to the novice statistician. Moreover, it is possible to perform analyses on a variable without this knowledge. We have therefore chosen not to present more details of these distributions than we believe are absolutely necessary for you to proceed. Advanced statistics texts and many elementary texts cover this in more detail.

3.4 DISCRETE PROBABILITY DISTRIBUTIONS

3.4.1 Definition

Box 3.1 defines a discrete probability distribution. An example of a *discrete* random variable is seen in simple Mendelian inheritance. Consider the

Box 3.1 Definition of a discrete probability distribution.

A discrete probability distribution attaches a probability to every possible mutually exclusive event defined by a discrete random variable; the sum of these probabilities is 1 (unity).

(a)

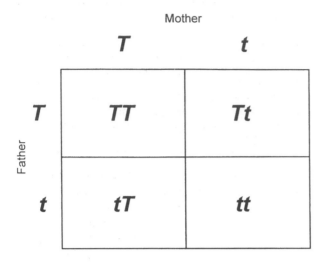

(b)

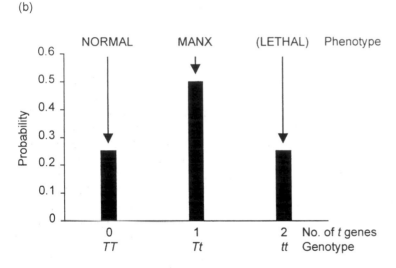

Fig. 3.1 The genetic characteristics of cats whose parents are each of Manx genotype *Tt*: (a) four possible genotypic outcomes, and (b) probability distribution of the number of *t* genes, the random variable which determines the phenotype of the cat.

situation where we have a pair of alleles represented by *T*, the dominant allele, and *t*, the recessive allele. In Manx cats the recessive mutant, *t*, is associated with the tailless condition but the homozygous recessive combination, *tt*, is lethal and these embryos do not develop. The heterozygous condition, *Tt*, results in the tailless Manx cat, and the homozygous *TT* condition is the normal cat with a tail. When two Manx cats are mated, there are four equally likely genotypic outcomes: *TT*, *Tt*, *tT* and *tt* (see Fig. 3.1(a)).

Figure 3.1(b) is a chart of the discrete probability distribution of the recessive allele, *t*. The probability distribution for this random variable is the complete statement of the three possible phenotypic outcomes with their associated probabilities. In the chart, the horizontal axis describes the set of the three possible outcomes defining the random variable, and the vertical axis measures the probability of each outcome. Each probability is represented by a bar; the sum of the three probabilities attached to the possible outcomes is unity (i.e. 0.25 + 0.5 + 0.25 = 1). As can be seen in Fig. 3.1(b), in this case there are only three viable genotypes (*TT*, *Tt*, *tT*), giving rise to a ratio of phenotypically Manx cats to normal cats of 2:1. It is easy to see that the diagrammatic representation of a probability distribution bears a strong resemblance to the empirical bar chart in which the vertical axis represents relative frequency, as in Fig. 2.2.

There are many different discrete probability distributions. The two distributions which are particularly relevant to biological science are the **Binomial** and **Poisson** distributions. As we explain in Section 3.6.1, these two discrete distributions are often approximated by a continuous distribution.

3.4.2 The Binomial distribution

The Binomial distribution is relevant in the situation in which we are investigating a *binary* response. There are only two possible outcomes to what we shall term a 'trial': either the animal is pregnant or it is not; either the animal shows clinical signs of infectious disease or it does not. It is common in statistical theory to use the terminology 'success' in a trial to represent the situation when the individual possesses the characteristic (e.g. disease) or the event occurs (e.g. pregnancy). Likewise, 'failure' is used to represent the complementary event, i.e. the situation when the individual does not possess the characteristic (e.g. is disease-free) or the event does not occur (e.g. not pregnant). We define the Binomial distribution in Box 3.2.

So for example, suppose we take blood samples from six cattle randomly selected from the population. Each animal in the population is either seropositive for *Leptospira* (success) or not (failure), i.e. we have a binary response variable. We know that the prevalence of *Leptospira* in the cattle population is approximately 30% (this is π). We can use this information and

Box 3.2 The Binomial distribution.

> The random variable in the Binomial distribution represents the number of successes in a series of n independent trials in which each trial can result in either a success (with probability, π) or a failure (with probability, $1 - \pi$). In theory, there are n possible outcomes in this situation as it is possible to observe either 1 success or 2 or 3 or . . . up to n successes in the n trials. The Binomial distribution attaches a probability to each outcome. Its mean and variance are $n\pi$ and $n\pi(1 - \pi)$, respectively.

our knowledge of the Binomial distribution to attach a probability to each of the possible outcomes – the probability that none is positive for *Leptospira*, or alternatively, that 1, 2, 3, . . . , up to 6 are positive. These probabilities are, respectively, 0.1176, 0.3025, 0.3241, 0.1852, 0.0595, 0.0102 and 0.0007, which, when added, sum to 1 (apart from rounding errors).

(a) The importance of the Binomial distribution

The Binomial distribution is particularly important in statistics because of its role in analysing *proportions*. A proportion is derived from a binary response variable, e.g. the proportion of animals with disease if each animal either has or does not have the disease. We can use our knowledge of the Binomial distribution (usually its Normal approximation, see Section 3.6.1) to make inferences about proportions (see Sections 4.7 and 9.3.1). As an example, Little *et al.* (1980) used the differences in the proportions of Leptospiral positive antisera in groups of aborting and normal animals to investigate the role of Leptospiral infection in abortion in cows. It was shown that the aborting cows had a significantly higher proportion of *Leptospira* positive antibody levels than the normal animals.

3.4.3 The Poisson distribution

Another discrete probability distribution which occurs in veterinary and animal science is the Poisson distribution. We define the Poisson distribution in Box 3.3.

Box 3.3 The Poisson distribution.

> The random variable of a Poisson distribution represents the *count* of the number of events occurring randomly and independently in time or space at a constant rate, μ, on average. The mean and variance of the distribution are equal to μ.

For example, using the Poisson distribution, we can attach probabilities to a particular count – the number (say, 5550) of scintillation events caused by a radioactive sample in a scintillation counter in unit time, or the number (say, 35) of blood cells in unit volume of a diluted sample, or the number (say, 60) of parasitic eggs per unit volume or weight of faecal sample, or the number (say, 12) of poisonous plants per quadrant across a field. Usually, for convenience, we employ the Normal approximation to the Poisson distribution for analysing these data (see Section 3.6.1). □

3.5 CONTINUOUS PROBABILITY DISTRIBUTIONS

3.5.1 Relationship between discrete and continuous probability distributions

In order to understand the relationship between discrete and continuous probability distributions:

- Refer to Fig. 3.2(a), an example of a very simple discrete probability distribution. All possible events are represented on the horizontal axis. The vertical length of each line represents the probability of the event. Since all events are represented, and the total probability must equal unity, the sum of the lengths of all the lines also equals 1.
- Refer to Fig. 3.2(b), an illustration of a discrete probability distribution in which there are a large, but still finite, number of possible discontinuous values of the random variable. Again, the sum of the lengths of all the lines equals unity.
- Now refer to Fig. 3.2(c). This figure represents the probability distribution of a continuous random variable. In contrast to a discrete probability distribution, here the variable can take an infinite number of values so it is impossible to draw separate lines. The shaded

Box 3.4 Properties of a continuous probability distribution.

> - A continuous probability distribution is defined by a probability density function.
> - The total area under the probability density function is 1 (unity).
> - The probability that the continuous random variable lies between certain limits is equal to the area under the probability density function between these limits.

area now represents the total probability of unity. The curve which defines the area is called a **probability density function** which is described by an equation. Box 3.4 summarizes the properties of a continuous probability distribution.

3.5.2 Calculating probabilities from the probability density function

If the variable of interest is continuous, then the probability that its value lies in a particular interval is given by the relevant area under the curve of the probability density function (see Fig. 3.3). We can determine the area under the curve for a range of values of the random variable by a mathematical process (called integration) applied to the equation. Rather than having to do this, there are special tables which relate areas under the curve to probabilities for the well-known continuous distributions, such as the **Normal, Student's *t*, Chi-squared** and *F*-distributions, each defined by its own equation.

3.5.3 The Normal (or Gaussian) distribution

(a) Empirical distributions and Normality

The **Normal** or **Gaussian distribution**, named after C.F. Gauss, an eighteenth century German mathematician, is the most important of the continuous distributions because of its role in sampling theory which we will consider in Chapter 4. The term 'Normal' is not meant to imply that the

(a) Discrete random variable taking only three values

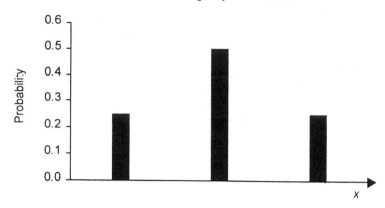

(b) Discrete random variable taking 15 values

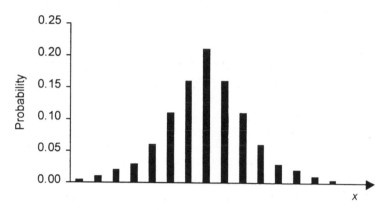

(c) Probability density function of a continuous random variable

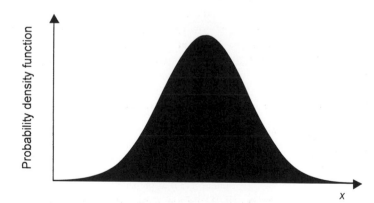

Fig. 3.2 The probability distribution of discrete and continuous random variables.

probability distribution of the random variable is typical, even though it is a good approximation to the distribution of many naturally occurring variables, or that it represents a 'non-diseased' group of individuals. To distinguish the Normal distribution from any other interpretation of normal, we use an upper case N in the former instance throughout this book.

(a)

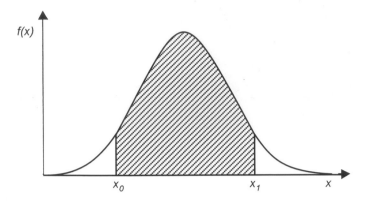

(b)

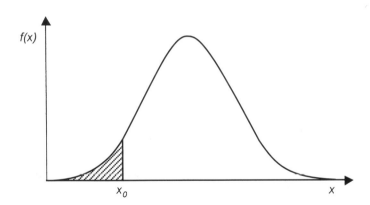

(c)

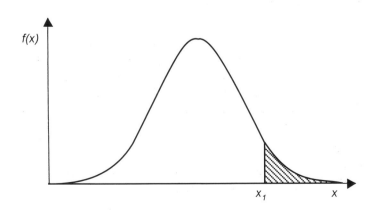

Fig. 3.3 Relationship between the area under the probability density function, $y = f(x)$, for the random variable, x, and probability. The total area under $f(x)$ is 1; the shaded area in (a) represents Prob $\{x_0 < x < x_1\}$, (b) Prob $\{x < x_0\}$ (c) Prob $\{x > x_1\}$.

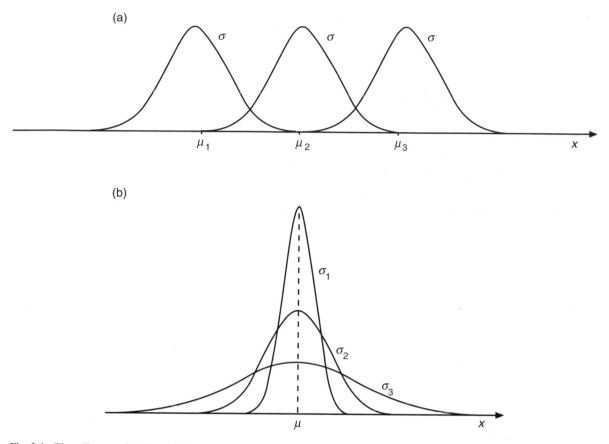

Fig. 3.4 The effect on the Normal distribution of changing the parameters μ and σ: (a) different means, $\mu_1 < \mu_2 < \mu_3$, same standard deviation, σ, and (b) different standard deviations $\sigma_1 < \sigma_2 < \sigma_3$, same mean, μ.

The Normal distribution is a theoretical distribution. We often find that observations made on a variable in a group of individuals have an empirical frequency distribution which is similar to a Normal distribution. We then make the assumption that the distribution of that variable in the population is Normal. If this is a reasonable assumption, we can use the properties of the Normal distribution to evaluate required probabilities. For example, the 6 furlong finish times for Thoroughbreds on Louisiana racetracks have an empirical distribution which is approximately Normal (Martin *et al.*, 1996). We show, in Section 3.5.3(c), how we can use the 6 furlong finish time to calculate the probability that a racehorse has a finish time greater than 77 s.

(b) Description

As well as possessing the property, in common with other continuous distributions, that the area under the curve defined by its probability density function is unity, the Normal distribution has several useful properties. These are listed in Box 3.5 and demonstrated in Figs 3.4(a) and (b).

(c) Areas under the curve and the Standard Normal distribution

In order to calculate the probability that a value of the variable, x, is greater than x_1, (see Fig. 3.3(c)), you can use Table A.1. We will take you through a four-step process:

Box 3.5 Properties of the Normal distribution.

- The Normal distribution is completely described by two parameters: the mean and the standard deviation. These are usually denoted by the Greek letters μ and σ, respectively. The mathematical formula for the probability density function is omitted for simplicity.
- It is unimodal.
- It is symmetrical about its mean. This implies that the curve to the right of the mean is a mirror image of the curve to the left of the mean. It is often described as 'bell-shaped'.
- Its mean, median and mode are all equal.
- If the standard devation remains unchanged, increasing the value of the mean shifts the curve horizontally to the right. Conversely, decreasing the value of the mean shifts the curve horizontally to the left (see Fig. 3.4(a)).
- A decrease in the standard deviation of the curve makes the curve thinner, taller and more peaked. Conversely, an increase in the standard deviation makes the curve fatter, shorter and flatter (see Fig. 3.4(b)).
- The limits $(\mu - \sigma)$ and $(\mu + \sigma)$ contain 68.3% of the distribution (see fig. 3.5(a)).
- The limits $(\mu - 1.96\sigma)$ and $(\mu + 1.96\sigma)$ contain 95% of the distribution (see Fig. 3.5(a)). This fact is often used in the calculation of a reference range (see Section 2.7).
- The limits $(\mu - 2.58\sigma)$ and $(\mu + 2.58\sigma)$ contain 99% of the distribution (see Fig. 3.5(a)).

1. Recognize that the probability that x has a value greater than x_1 is equal to the area under the Normal distribution curve to the right of x_1.
2. Define the mean and the standard deviation of your Normal distribution. In general terms, we call these μ and σ, respectively.
3. Convert this Normal distribution into a **Standard Normal distribution** (see Fig. 3.5(b)) which has a mean of 0 and a standard deviation of 1 (unity). This is the distribution of a new variable, z, which is called a **Standardized Normal Deviate (SND)**. In general terms

$$z = \frac{x - \mu}{\sigma}$$

and in this particular example, the value of the SND which corresponds to x_1 is

$$z_1 = \frac{x_1 - \mu}{\sigma}$$

4. Use Table A.1 to determine the specified area. Instructions for the procedure are given with the table which has an accompanying illustrative diagram. It is important to realize that:

(a) The Standard Normal distribution is symmetrical around its mean of zero. Thus the tail area to the right of a value z_1 is the same as the tail area to the left of $-z_1$; equivalently, the probability that $z > z_1$ is equal to the probability that $z < -z_1$. Table A.1 provides the sum of these two tail area probabilities for various values of z. The values of z are sometimes called **critical values** or **percentage points**, as each defines a percentage of the total area under the probability density function.

(b) To obtain the area to the right of z_1 from Table A.1, we have to divide the probability obtained from the table by 2. This is because the probabilities in the table relate to both tails of the Standard Normal distribution, whereas here we are interested only in the right tail.

(c) You should be aware that the Standard Normal distribution is not always tabulated in the same way as Table A.1. For example, you might find that only the right tail or the left tail area is tabulated. However, you can always determine the probability that is required for your problem by subtraction and/or multiplying or dividing by 2, as long as you remember that the Standard Normal distribution is symmetrical and that the total area under the curve is 1.

Suppose we want to apply this theory to a practical example; we know that the 6 furlong finish time for Thoroughbreds on Louisiana racetracks is approximately Normally distributed in the population with a mean of 75.2 s and a standard deviation of 2.2 s (Martin *et al.*, 1996). We want to determine the probability of a racehorse having a finish time of greater than, say, 77.0 s. The value of z corresponding to $x_1 = 77.0$ is

(a)

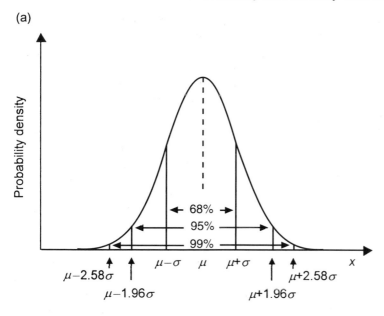

(b)

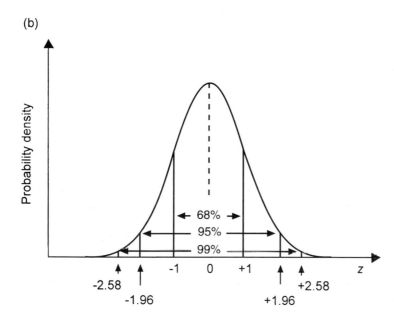

Fig. 3.5 Areas under (a) the Normal curve; the random variable, x, has mean = μ and standard deviation = σ, and (b) the Standard Normal curve; the random variable, $z = (x - \mu)/\sigma$, has mean = 0 and standard deviation = 1.

$z_1 = (77.0 - 75.2)/(2.2) = 0.82$. Since we are only interested in the probability in the upper tail of the distribution, the required probability is half the tabulated two-tailed probability. Thus, the probability is $0.5 \times 0.4122 = 0.2061$; we would expect about 21% of the racehorses to have finish times greater than 77.0 s.

(d) Determining the Standardized Normal Deviate from a defined probability

It may be that we are interested not in evaluating a probability (area under the curve) from a particular value of the SND, z, but in the reverse procedure, i.e. in determining the value of z from a specified probability. Naturally, it is possible to do this from Table A.1 but, for simplicity and convenience, we give the z values for some common probabilities in Table A.2. We show z values both for the situation in which the probability of interest corresponds to the sum of the right- and left-hand tail areas (a **two-tailed probability**), and for the situation in which all the probability of interest corresponds only to the right-hand tail area (a **one-tailed probability**). Two-tailed probabilities are more often relevant than one-tailed probabilities; we discuss this in Section 6.3 in relation to one- and two-sided tests of hypotheses. Note that we may also require a z value in order to calculate a confidence interval (see Sections 4.5.2 and 4.7).

Suppose we want to know the two values of z which encompass the central 95% of the distribution; this leaves 2.5% of the distribution in each tail, i.e. 5% of the entire distribution is in the two tails. Thus we enter Table A.2 and note that the value of z which corresponds to a two-tailed probability of 0.05 is 1.96. You can now see how the value given in the penultimate bullet point of Box 3.5 is derived.

(e) Establishing Normality

The assumption of Normality is important if we wish to use the properties of the Normal distribution to calculate relevant probabilities. We stress, however, that although the assumption of Normality is inherent in many statistical procedures, the procedures are often valid providing the data are *approximately* Normally distributed.

- The easiest approach to establishing approximate Normality is to produce a histogram of the empirical frequency distribution and determine, by eye, whether the distribution appears unimodal, bell-shaped and symmetrical. This subjective approach is often adequate but it does not work well when the number of observations is small, say, less than 20.
- We can use more formal ways of establishing whether data approximate a Normal distribu-

tion. One such method is to produce a graph called a **Normal plot** in which the horizontal axis represents the ordered numerical values of the variable, and the vertical axis represents the corresponding Standardized Normal Deviates. If the data are Normally distributed then the plot will be a straight line; if the data are not Normally distributed then the plot will deviate from the straight line so that a curve is produced. Often, we find it easier to judge whether the data follow a straight line than whether the histogram of the raw data is symmetrical. Hence, although this technique is also subjective, the Normal plot is commonly produced, usually on a computer, in an attempt to verify the assumption of Normality. We show an example in Fig. 3.6 in which the distribution of the sheep mechanical threshold data is not Normal (Fig. 3.6(a)) but the log transformed data is more nearly Normal (Fig. 3.6(b)).

- Occasionally, an objective test for Normality is required. The **Shapiro–Wilk W test** is available in many computer packages, as is the Lilliefors modification of the **Kolmogorov–Smirnov test**, both of which are extremely tedious to perform by hand. We can also derive measures of **skewness** (describing symmetry) and **kurtosis** (describing peakedness) for the observed data set and determine how these measures deviate from what would be expected if the data were Normally distributed.

(f) The Lognormal distribution

Many biological variables, such as parasite infestation data, display a distribution with a long tail to the right. When data are skewed to the right, we can generally Normalize the data by taking the logarithm (either to base 10 or to base e) of each observation (see Sections 2.6.1(c) and 11.2.2). The distribution of the resulting transformed variable will often be approximately Normal (see Fig. 3.6). The original variable is then said to have a **Lognormal distribution**, approximating the theoretical distribution of the same name.

(a)

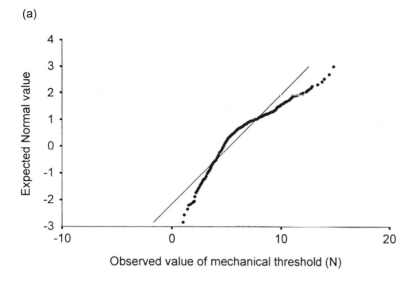

(b)

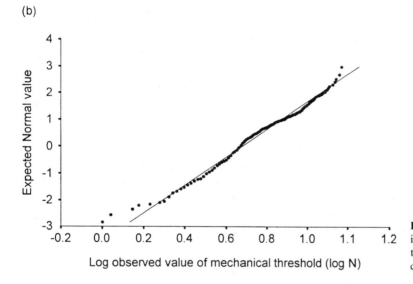

Fig. 3.6 Normal plots of the data shown in Fig. 2.10: (a) Normal plot of mechanical threshold, (b) Normal plot of log mechanical threshold.

The advantage of transforming data in this way so as to produce a transformed variable which is Normally distributed is that the properties of the Normal distribution are relevant to the transformed variable. In particular:

- We can use the probabilities (areas) of the Standard Normal curve to evaluate particular

population limits. So, 95% of the distribution of the logarithmic values lie in the interval defined by their mean ± 1.96 times their standard deviation. For example, for the sheep threshold data in Fig. 2.10, 95% of the log transformed threshold values would be expected to fall between $0.6778 \pm 1.96 \times 01927$, i.e. between 0.3001 and 1.0555 log newtons. Hence, by finding the antilogs of these values,

Box 3.6 Properties of the *t*-distribution.

- The *t*-distribution is symmetrical about the mean and is bell-shaped.
- It is completely characterized by what are called the degrees of freedom (*df*) so that knowledge of the degrees of freedom allows the probabilities of the *t*-distribution to be computed. We consider the degrees of freedom more fully in Section 6.3.6. For the moment, it is sufficient to note that they have a close affinity to sample size.
- The *t*-distribution is indistinguishable from the Standard Normal distribution when the degrees of freedom are large; as the degrees of freedom decrease, the *t*-distribution becomes more and more spread out compared to the Standard Normal distribution.

Box 3.7 Properties of the Chi-squared distribution.

- The Chi-squared distribution can only take positive values and is highly skewed.
- The degrees of freedom characterize this distribution, so that knowledge of them allows us to determine the relevant probabilities under the curve.
- As the degrees of freedom increase, the distribution becomes more and more symmetrical and eventually approaches Normality.

Box 3.8 Properties of the *F*-distribution and use of Table A.5.

- The *F*-distribution is the distribution of a ratio (see Section 3.6.2).
- It is characterized by two separate degrees of freedom: those attached to the numerator and those attached to the denominator of the ratio which defines it.
- Although the ratio could be either greater or less than 1, the tabulated probabilities of the *F*-distribution relate to a ratio which is always greater than 1, i.e. the numerator is greater than the denominator. Thus the tabulated values refer only to the upper tail of the distribution. Extra care has to be taken in evaluating the appropriate probabilities from Table A.5 (see Sections 8.3.1 and 8.3.3).

we would expect 95% of the threshold values in the population to lie between 1.20 newtons and 11.36 newtons.

- Furthermore, it is interesting to note that the antilog of the arithmetic mean of the logarithmic values is a sensible summary measure of location of the raw data; it is called the **geometric mean** (see Section 2.6.1(c)).

3.5.4 Other continuous probability distributions

There are numerous continuous probability distributions apart from the Normal distribution. Three particularly well-known and useful distributions are the *t*-, Chi-squared (χ^2) and *F*-distributions. You may find the discussions of these distributions too theoretical and laborious for comfort. You could skip them at this stage and refer to them only when (or if!) the need arises.

(a) Student's *t*-distribution

'Student', a pseudonym for W.S. Gossett, described the **t-distribution** in 1908 although it was perfected by R.A. Fisher in 1926. This distribution has revolutionized the statistical analysis of small samples. We

give the percentage points of the *t*-distribution in Table A.3, and summarize its properties in Box 3.6.

As we explain in Chapter 7, we use the *t*-distribution when we wish to test a hypothesis about a mean or a difference between two means.

(b) The Chi-squared distribution

We give the percentage points of the **Chi-squared (χ^2) distribution** in Table A.4, and summarize its properties in Box 3.7. We use the Chi-squared distribution when we analyse categorical data (see Chapter 9).

(c) The *F*-distribution

We give the percentage points of the **F-distribution** in Table A.5, and summarize its properties in Box 3.8. We may use the *F*-distribution to compare two variances if each is calculated from Normally distributed data (see Section 8.3). The main use of the *F*-distribution, however, is in comparing means using a technique called the analysis of variance which we discuss in Section 8.5. □

3.6 RELATIONSHIPS BETWEEN DISTRIBUTIONS

3.6.1 Normal approximations of the Binomial and Poisson distributions

The Binomial and Poisson distributions are skewed to the right when sample sizes are small, although they become more symmetrical as sample sizes increase. In fact, each distribution approaches Normality for large enough sample sizes when a smooth curve is drawn joining the discrete probability values.

(a) Consider a Binomial situation in which we observe a proportion, *p,* of successes in *n* trials. It is reasonable to use the Normal approximation of the Binomial distribution if both np and $n(1 - p)$ are greater than 5. The mean and variance of this Normal distribution are estimated by np and $np(1 - p)$, respectively. This approximation is particularly useful in statistical inference, for testing hypotheses about and calculating confidence intervals for proportions (see Chapter 9).

Example

Suppose that on a typical day, 18 cats are presented to a veterinary clinic, and 6 are seen to have fleas. The observed proportion of infested cats is 6/18 = 0.33. Hence, $np = 18 \times 0.33 = 6$, and $n(1 - p) = 18 \times 0.67 = 12$, and a Normal approximation is appropriate. The mean and variance of this Normal distribution are estimated by $np = 18 \times 0.33 = 6$ and $np(1 - p) = 18 \times 0.33 \times 0.67 = 3.98$. Thus, if we want to evaluate the probability that 10 or more cats will present with fleas, we determine $z_1 = (10 - 6)/\sqrt{3.98} = 2.01$, and refer this value to Table A.1. Dividing the tabulated probability by 2 because we are only interested in the upper tail of the distribution, we find that the required probability is approximately 0.02 (this is 0.0222 corrected to two decimal places). In fact, we should have applied the continuity correction (see the end of this Section).

(b) The Normal approximation of a Poisson distribution is acceptable if the average rate of occurrence of the event of interest, μ, is not too small (say, greater than 5). You will then find that the sample mean and variance are approximately equal to μ. This follows from the property of the Poisson distribution that the variance equals the mean. For example, we could analyse worm burden data using the Normal approximation to the Poisson distribution, providing that the average faecal egg counts per gram of wet weight faeces does not fall below five. □

These two Normal approximations are useful because we can use the tables of the Standard Normal distribution to evaluate probabilities for random variables which follow the Binomial or Poisson distributions. However, note the following:

- The Poisson and Binomial distributions both relate to discrete random variables.
- The Normal distribution relates to continuous random variables.

Therefore, if we use tables of the Normal distribution to provide approximations of the Binomial and Poisson distributions, we should apply a **continuity correction** to adjust for this discrepancy. We subtract 0.5 from the numerator of the Standardized Normal Deviate so our adjusted value is

$$z' = \frac{(x - \mu) - 0.5}{\sigma}$$

So, strictly, in the flea-infested cats example above, we should have applied the continuity correction to the determination of the probability that 10 or more cats will present with fleas, i.e. $z_1 = \{(10 - 6) - 0.5\}/\sqrt{3.98} = 1.75$. Referring to Table A.1, we find that the required probability is $(0.0801)/2 = 0.04$. We can see that for small numbers, the continuity correction makes a substantial difference.

3.6.2 Mathematical interrelationships

You may find these theoretical concepts difficult, immaterial or boring, in which case you should skip this section! Otherwise, you may find it interesting to note the following:

- The *t*-, Chi-squared (χ^2) and *F*- distributions each represent a specific function, expressed mathematically, of a Normally distributed variable.
- The Chi-squared distribution with *k* degrees of freedom is defined as the distribution of the sum of the squares of *k* independent variables, each of which has a Standard Normal distribution.
- If the degrees of freedom are 1, then the Chi-squared distribution is the square of the Standard Normal distribution.
- The distribution of a mean of a Normally distributed variable divided by its estimated standard error follows a *t*-distribution.
- The variance estimated from a sample of observations of a Normally distributed variable follows a Chi-squared distribution multiplied by σ^2, where σ^2 is the true variance of the variable in the population.
- The *F*-distribution is the distribution of the ratio of two independent variables, each with a Chi-squared distribution and each divided by its degrees of freedom.
- The ratio of two variances estimated from independent samples of observations of a Normally distributed variable follows the *F*-distribution.
- The *F*-distribution is related to both the *t*- and Chi-squared distributions. When the degrees of freedom of the numerator of the *F* ratio are 1, the tabulated values of the *F*-distribution correspond to those of the *t*-distribution on the same number of degrees of freedom as those in the denominator of the *F* ratio. When the degrees of freedom of the denominator are extremely large, tending to infinity, then the tabulated values of the *F*-distribution are the same as those of the Chi-squared distribution when the latter are divided by the degrees of freedom of the numerator of the *F* ratio. □

EXERCISES

The statements in questions 3.1–3.3 are either TRUE or FALSE.

3.1 The random variable, *x*, is Normally distributed. This implies that:
(a) Its distribution is skewed to the right.
(b) The mean and the median of its distribution are equal.
(c) The limits defined by the mean ± SD contain approximately 95% of the distribution.
(d) The distribution has a mean of 0 and a standard deviation of 1.
(e) All the animals on which this variable are measured are healthy.

3.2 The random variable, *z*, has a Standard Normal distribution. This implies that:
(a) *z* is a discrete random variable.
(b) The mean and standard deviation of its distribution are equal.
(c) The total area under its probability density function is 1.
(d) If $z = (x - \mu)/\sigma$, where *x* is a Normally distributed random variable, then *z* has a mean equal to μ and a standard deviation equal to σ.
(e) Approximately 68% of the distribution lies between the limits $z = -1$ and $z = +1$.

3.3 Indicate whether the following statements are true or false:
(a) A random variable which follows the Binomial distribution can take more than two values.
(b) The Binomial distribution is the most widely used theoretical distribution in biological statistics.
(c) If sample data approximate a Normal distribution then the data have been selected from a healthy population.
(d) The mean and variance of the Standard Normal distribution depend on the data set.
(e) The Lognormal distribution is obtained after we take logs of data which follow the Normal distribution.

3.4 A family is trying to decide whether to purchase a puppy bitch or a dog. Dad wants to have a bitch. Because they cannot agree on the pros and cons, Dad suggests that they roll dice to make the decision:
(a) He suggests that his youngest daughter has a go at rolling the two dice once; if she succeeds in getting a 'double' (i.e. two sixes, two fives, . . . , or two ones), then they will opt for a bitch, but if not they will have a dog. As she is about to roll, he does his calculations in his head of the probabilities involved and he has second thoughts.
(b) Instead, he proposes that his daughter rolls just one die, but five times. If she fails to get a 'six' in the five tries, then they will purchase a bitch. He believes that now he has the odds with him. Is he right?

Calculate the probability of getting a bitch in (a) and (b). Show how these dice rollings illustrate both the addition and the multiplication rules of probability. What type of probability approach is this (subjective, model, frequency)?

3.5 Do you think the data sets in (a) and (b) below are Normally distributed? If you conclude that either is not approximately Normal, would a log transformation achieve approximate Normality?

(a) The following data (based on the summary data in Coyne *et al.*, 1996) are oxytetracycline measurements from muscle samples from Atlantic salmon (*Salmo salar*). The antibiotic was added to the water over a ten-day period for therapeutic purposes; measurements were taken of muscle concentrations (μg/g of muscle tissue) at the eighth day to check effective levels after dosing.

1.3	1.6	1.5	0.5	1.8
1.9	2.5	1.4	0.0	2.1
2.1	0.4	0.3	0.7	0.8
1.2	0.1	1.2	0.8	1.9
0.6	1.7	2.5	2.5	2.4

(b) The following are alkaline phosphatase levels in serum of 12 normal adult dogs (IU/l) (International Units per litre).

5.4	7.3	20.3	17.5	35.9	16.8
28.6	54.3	10.0	14.0	11.7	24.3

3.6 The cell counts of erythrocytes in horse blood per small square of the counting chamber are determined. What theoretical distribution would these counts be expected to follow most closely? How can you check whether the counts follow this distribution?

3.7 The mean packed cell volume (PCV) of normal cats approximates a Normal distribution with mean 0.37 ml/ml and a standard deviation of 0.066 ml/ml.

(a) What percentage of cats have values above 0.40 ml/ml?
(b) What percentage of cats have values below 0.30 ml/ml?
(c) What percentage of cats have values between 0.30 ml/ml and 0.40 ml/ml?
(d) What is the range containing the central 90% of PCV values?

3.8 (a) What is the area of the Standard Normal curve:
    (i) Above 2.00?
    (ii) Below −1.00?
(b) What is the percentage point (i.e. z value) of the Standard Normal curves for which there is:
    (i) 5% of the total area in the upper tail?
    (ii) 2.5% of the total area in the lower tail?

Chapter 4

Sampling and Sampling Distributions

4.1 LEARNING OBJECTIVES

By the end of this chapter, you should be able to:

- Explain the need to distinguish between a sample and the population.
- Explain the concept of a sampling distribution.
- Give the formula for the standard error of the mean.
- Calculate the standard error of the mean.
- Distinguish between the standard deviation and the standard error of the mean.
- Give the applications of the standard deviation and the standard error of the mean.
- Outline the purpose of the confidence interval for the mean.
- Calculate a confidence interval for the mean when the population standard deviation is unknown.
- Interpret the confidence interval for the mean.
- Explain how the standard error of the proportion is calculated.
- Calculate a confidence interval for the proportion.

4.2 THE DISTINCTION BETWEEN THE SAMPLE AND THE POPULATION

It is a rare situation, indeed, when we are able to study a whole population of individuals. There may be constraints imposed by time and economic or practical considerations which preclude examination of the whole population. It would be most unusual, for example, to be able to investigate all the Thoroughbred mares in Great Britain. In this situation, we would be most likely to take what we would hope to be a representative sample of animals from the Thoroughbred population. We discuss, in Section 12.4, the principles of **sample surveys** and the methods by which we can select our sample. We then have to generalize the results from our sample to the larger population from which it was taken.

The price that we pay for sampling is that we cannot make statements of absolute certainty about the population; instead, we are able only to surmise about what we expect in the population, and there will always be some doubt associated with the conclusions that we draw about the population. We express this doubt as a probability (see Section 3.2). The larger the sample and the more representative it is of the population, the smaller our uncertainty and the more likely it is that our conclusions are correct.

4.3 STATISTICAL INFERENCE

4.3.1 Introduction

This process of generalizing to the population from the sample is called **statistical inference**. Statistical inference enables us to draw conclusions about certain features of a population when only a subgroup of that population, the sample, is available for investigation. It is very important that we are aware of the distinction between the sample and the population from which it is taken, as a major component of statistical theory is statistical inference.

There are two aspects of statistical inference which play an important role in statistical analysis: these are **estimation** and **hypothesis testing**. We discuss estimation in this chapter. Hypothesis testing is concerned with deciding whether the results we obtain from our sample enable us to discredit a particular hypothesis about the population or whether they lend support to it. We will introduce the concepts of hypothesis testing in Chapter 6.

4.3.2 Estimation of population parameters by sample statistics

The purpose of sampling is to learn something about the population. Usually, we want to know about various features, termed **parameters**, which characterize the population's distribution. We can describe the distribution if we know their values. The parameters which characterize the better-known discrete and continuous probability distributions are discussed in Sections 3.4 and 3.5. In particular, the parameters which characterize the Normal distribution are the arithmetic mean and the standard deviation.

It is impossible to determine the population mean exactly when we have selected only a sample of observations from that population. For example, we do not know the precise value for the mean number of races Thoroughbred mares have run when we only have the results of a selected sample. The best we can do is *estimate* its value from the sample, i.e. we have to calculate the *sample* **statistic** whose value is as close as possible to the true value of the parameter in the population. The population parameter and its sample statistic are usually calculated using the same formula, but the former uses population values and the latter uses sample values. For example, it can be shown that the sample mean is the best estimate of the population mean; the sample mean is the sum of all the observations *in the sample* divided by the number of observations *in the sample*; the population mean is the sum of all the observations *in the population* divided by the number of observations *in the population*. However, one noteworthy exception is that the population variance and its sample estimate are not calculated using exactly the same formula (see Section 2.6.2(c)).

4.3.3 Notation for population parameters and sample statistics

As it is important to maintain a distinction between the population parameters and the sample statistics which estimate them, it is helpful to use different notation for each. It is customary to use Greek letters for the population parameters and Roman letters for the sample statistics (see Glossary of Notation in Appendix D).

4.3.4 Sampling error

It is unlikely that the value of the sample statistic is exactly equal to the value of the population parameter that it is estimating. We have to recognize that there is always likely to be error in the estimate because we have sampled the population and are not looking at it in its entirety. We call this **sampling error**. We need to establish the precision (see Section 1.8) of the sample statistic as an estimate of the population parameter. For this purpose, we calculate the *standard error* of the estimate.

Suppose we want to know the average milk yield of Holstein-Friesian dairy cows. Milk yield is a *continuous* variable so we will use this example to develop the ideas of sampling error in relation to the mean in the following section (Section 4.4).

Furthermore, we might be interested in the proportion of cows that had been exposed to Leptospirosis. Either a cow has or does not have a positive titre for *Leptospira* (Little *et al.*, 1980), so this is a *binary* variable. We will use this example to explore sampling error in relation to a proportion (Section 4.6).

We will not discuss sampling error in relation to the variance as you are unlikely to need it in practice; you can obtain details in texts such as Armitage and Berry (1994).

4.4 THE SAMPLING DISTRIBUTION OF THE MEAN

4.4.1 Sampling error in relation to the sample mean

Let us suppose that we are interested in making inferences about the population mean of a quantitative variable, such as milk yield.

The first step is to take a representative sample of observations from the population. By 'representative' we mean, of course, that we have taken steps, such as random selection, to ensure that we have a sample which properly reflects the population. (Further details of sampling methods are given in Section 12.4.) We calculate the mean milk yield of this sample of observations to provide an estimate of the true mean milk yield in the population. Because of **sampling error** (see Section 4.3.4), it is unlikely that its value is exactly equal to the population mean. The extent to which a sample mean differs from the population mean depends on both:

- The size of the sample (the sampling error is greater for a smaller sample).
- The variability of the observations in the population (the sampling error is greater if the observations in the sample are more diverse).

4.4.2 The concept of the distribution of the sample means

The sample mean from one sample will probably be slightly different from that obtained if we were to take another sample of the same size from the population. Expressed in another way, there is **sampling variation** resulting from the fact that the value of the sample mean varies according to the particular sample chosen.

We can get some feel for this sampling variation by considering a *hypothetical* probability distribution; i.e. the distribution of sample means that we would obtain if we were to repeat the sampling procedure and take many different samples, each of the same size, from the population and calculate the sample mean from every sample. We must stress that this is a hypothetical

distribution because, in practice, we usually make inferences about the population mean from only a single sample from a population. However, by studying the properties of this theoretical distribution of the sample means, called the **sampling distribution of the mean**, we can evaluate the sampling error of the sample mean.

4.4.3 The properties of the sampling distribution of the mean

Figure 4.1 (b) and (c) is a diagrammatic representation of the distribution of the sample means. Just as with any other distribution, we can look at its shape, and obtain measures of location and spread as summary measures of its important features. We list the properties of the distribution of the sample means below:

- Its **distribution** is *Normal* if the distribution of the parent population is Normal. Furthermore, the sampling distribution is approximately Normal even if the distribution of the parent population is not Normal, provided the size of the samples, assumed constant, is large enough, say greater than about 30. This is expressed mathematically in the *central limit theorem*, and is a very useful result which contributes to the importance of the Normal distribution in statistical inference. The resemblance of the sampling distribution of the mean to a Normal distribution improves as the size of the samples increases.
- The **mean** of the sampling distribution of the mean is equal to the mean of the parent population. We say that the sample mean is an **unbiased** (free from **bias** – see also Section 5.4) estimate of the population mean; i.e. *it is unbiased because the mean of the sampling distribution of the sample statistic coincides with the parameter that the statistic is estimating.* Furthermore, we know that the sample means are distributed symmetrically around the true mean because of the Normality property.
- The **standard deviation** of the distribution of the sample means, each from a sample of size n, is given by $\sigma/\sqrt{n}$, where σ is the standard deviation of the observations in the popula-

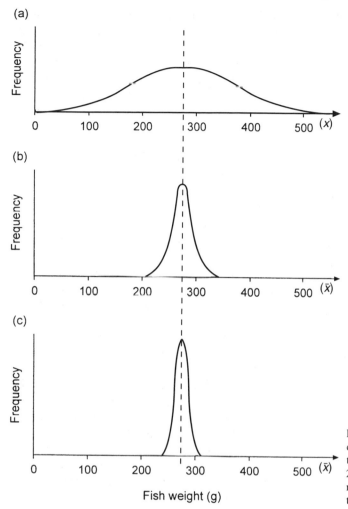

Fig. 4.1 The effect of sample size on the sampling distribution of the mean: (a) Normal distribution of the population values (x) of fish weights, with mean = 272 g and SD = 96.4 g, (b) sampling distribution of mean ($\bar{x}$) with sample size = 25, (c) sampling distribution of mean ($\bar{x}$) with sample size = 100.

tion. The standard deviation of the sampling distribution of the mean is a measure of the dispersion of the sample means. It is known as the **standard error of the mean**. When there is no ambiguity, it may be called simply the standard error, and is often abbreviated to SE, or SEM. So

$$SEM = \frac{\sigma}{\sqrt{n}}$$

From the formula, we can see that the standard error of the mean increases with increasing values of σ (i.e. as the variability of the parent population increases) and is smaller with larger samples; for example, for a given population with a fixed standard deviation, if we want to halve the standard error, we must quadruple the sample size. Therefore, we have a more precise estimate of the population mean if the sample size is large.

4.4.4 Estimation of the standard error using sample data

The SEM = $\sigma/\sqrt{n}$, where σ is the standard deviation of the observations in the population. If we are using our sample to estimate the population mean, it is very unlikely that we will have knowledge of σ. Hence we will have to replace σ in the formula for the SEM by its sample estimate, s. Thus, the estimate from the sample is

$$\text{SEM} = \frac{s}{\sqrt{n}}$$

where $s = \sqrt{\dfrac{\sum(x - \bar{x})^2}{n-1}}$

Example

The most recent standard lactations (305 days) of a random sample of 256 Holstein-Friesian cows, of mixed numbers of lactations, gave an estimated mean milk yield of 6414 kg with an estimated standard deviation of 2352 kg. The estimated standard error of the mean is therefore $2353/\sqrt{256} = 147$ kg.

4.4.5 The distinction between the standard deviation and the standard error of the mean

We have introduced you to the SD in Section 2.6.2(d) and the SEM in this chapter. But what are they for? They have very different applications; it is important that you have a clear understanding of the distinction between the standard deviation of the observations and the standard error of the mean. The two are frequently confused with the consequence that the wrong measure is used to describe the variability of interest; this may lead to a misinterpretation of the data.

- The **standard deviation** is a measure of the *scatter of the observations* (see Section 2.6.2(d)). It gives an indication of how close the observations are to their mean; it may be thought of as an average measure of the deviation of each observation from the mean. It may be used to construct a **reference interval** (see Section 2.7) which defines the *range of most of the observations* in a population.
- The **standard error of the mean** is a measure of the *precision of the sample mean* as an estimate of the population mean. It evaluates the sampling error by giving an indication of how close a sample mean is to the population mean it is estimating. As we show in Section 4.5, the

SEM may be used to construct a **confidence interval** which allows us to judge the *precision of our estimate of the population mean*.

4.5 THE CONFIDENCE INTERVAL FOR A MEAN

4.5.1 Understanding confidence intervals

We have stressed that the sampling distribution of the mean is a hypothetical distribution. In practice we do not take repeated samples from our population; we usually take just one sample and use the mean from this sample as an estimate of the population mean. However, we can exploit the properties of the sampling distribution of the mean to indicate how 'good' is our estimate.

The best way of establishing whether the estimate is good is to define the range of values within which we expect the true population mean to lie with a certain probability. This range of values, defined by its upper and lower limits (the **confidence limits**), is called the **confidence interval for the mean**.

- If the confidence interval is wide, then the sample mean is a poor estimate of the population mean.
- If the confidence interval is narrow, then the sample mean is a good estimate, i.e. it is a precise estimate of the population mean.

We are 95% certain that the population mean is contained in what is called the 95% confidence interval for the mean. Typically, we calculate the 95% confidence interval for a parameter but we may sometimes find that 90% or 99% confidence intervals are quoted. A 99% confidence interval will inevitably be wider than a 95% confidence interval because we need to be more confident that the parameter is contained in the interval.

The width of the confidence interval depends on:

- The degree of confidence required.
- The sample size (a larger sample provides a more precise estimate and therefore a narrower confidence interval).

- The variability of the characteristic under investigation (a more variable set of observations provides a less precise estimate and a wider confidence interval).

We develop the uses of confidence intervals in Section 6.6. We summarize the formulae for confidence intervals for frequently used parameters in the tables in Appendix B.

4.5.2 Calculating the confidence interval for the mean

The upper limit of a confidence interval for the mean is calculated by adding a multiple of the standard error to the sample mean; the lower limit is obtained by subtracting that multiple of the standard error from the sample mean. This is the general approach to calculating the confidence interval for most parameters. The difficulty is in deciding which multiple of the standard error to use to determine an interval of a particular confidence.

(a) Where σ is known

Provided we have knowledge of σ, the 95% confidence interval for the mean is $\bar{x} \pm 1.96 \times$ SEM, i.e.

$$\bar{x} \pm 1.96 \frac{\sigma}{\sqrt{n}} = \left(\bar{x} - 1.96 \frac{\sigma}{\sqrt{n}}, \ \bar{x} + 1.96 \frac{\sigma}{\sqrt{n}} \right)$$

The upper and lower limits of the confidence interval within the bracket are separated by the comma. For the 95% confidence interval, the multiple is 1.96 (often approximated by 2). The multiple is 2.58 for a 99% confidence interval; note that a multiple of 1.00 only gives a 68% confidence interval. The values for the multiples are obtained from Table A.2.

Justification
We know that the sampling distribution of the mean is approximately Normal, and that its mean is equal to the population mean, μ, and its standard deviation is equal to the SEM $= \sigma/\sqrt{n}$ (see Section 4.4.3). Thus, 95% of the sample means in the sampling distribution of the mean are contained in the interval, $\mu \pm 1.96$

SEM (see Box 3.5). An alternative way of saying this is that there is a 95% chance that a sample mean, $\bar{x}$, is contained in the interval $\mu \pm 1.96$ SEM. If we now interchange the μ and the $\bar{x}$, we can say that there is a 95% chance that μ is contained in the interval $\bar{x} \pm 1.96$ SEM, or that 95% of such confidence intervals on repeated sampling would contain μ. ☐

(b) Where *s* is unknown

Usually we do not know the value of the population standard deviation, σ, so we replace it by the sample estimate

$$s = \sqrt{\frac{\sum (x - \bar{x})^2}{n-1}}$$

We can no longer use the Normal distribution to determine the multiple (e.g. 1.96) for the confidence interval; instead, we use the *t*-distribution. Then the 95% confidence interval for the mean is

$$\bar{x} \pm t_{0.05} \frac{s}{\sqrt{n}} = \left(\bar{x} - t_{0.05} \frac{s}{\sqrt{n}}, \ \bar{x} + t_{0.05} \frac{s}{\sqrt{n}} \right)$$

where the multiple, $t_{0.05}$, is the percentage point of the *t*-distribution (Table A.3) with $n - 1$ degrees of freedom; it gives a total tail area probability of 0.05.

Justification
The distribution of the sample mean divided by its estimated standard error follows the *t*-distribution, provided the observations come from a Normal distribution (see Section 3.6.2). The multiple is affected by the sample size and increases as the sample size decreases. ☐

We should be aware that the multiple of the standard error obtained from the *t*-distribution is a slightly larger number than that obtained from the Normal distribution unless *n* is extremely large. This means that if we need to estimate the standard deviation from the sample, we will obtain a wider confidence interval than if we have knowledge of σ. However, the two intervals are much the same when the sample size is large, because the *t*-distribution approaches Normality when the degrees of freedom are large (see Section 3.5.4).

Example

In Section 4.4.4, we summarized the results of the milk yields of a sample of 256 Holstein-Friesian cows; the sample mean was 6414 kg and the estimated SEM was 147 kg. From Table A.3, $t_{0.05}$ for $df = 255$ is approximately 1.96. The 95% confidence interval for the true mean milk yield is given by

$$\bar{x} \pm t_{0.05} \frac{s}{\sqrt{n}} = (6414 - 1.96 \times 147, \ 6414 + 1.96 \times 147)$$

$$= (6126.9, \ 6702.1) \text{kg}$$

Hence we are 95% certain that the mean milk yield for the population of Holstein-Friesian cows lies between 6127 and 6702 kg.

4.6 THE SAMPLING DISTRIBUTION OF THE PROPORTION

4.6.1 The concept of the distribution of sample proportions

The concept of the distribution of sample proportions is the same as that of the distribution of sample means. It is a *hypothetical* distribution whose properties are useful if we want to make statistical inferences about the population proportion.

Suppose we are interested in the **proportion** of individuals in a population, π, who possess a certain attribute. For example, we may want to know the proportion of cattle in an area which have been exposed to *Leptospira* infection. We select a random sample of size n from this population and observe the number, r, with the attribute in the sample. We then take the proportion with the attribute in the sample, $p = r/n$, as our estimate of π. The sampling distribution of the proportion is the distribution of sample proportions that we would obtain if we were to repeat the sampling procedure and take many different samples, each of the same size, from the population and calculate the proportion from each sample. It is a hypothetical distribution because, in reality, we only take a single sample from the population.

4.6.2 The properties of the sampling distribution of the proportion

The distribution of sample proportions has the following properties:

- Its **distribution** is approximately *Normal* if the sample size is large; in fact, the distribution of a proportion is really a Binomial distribution (see Section 3.4.2) but, as we explained, this is approximately a Normal distribution for large n.
- The **mean** of the sampling distribution of the proportion is the population proportion, π. Thus the sample proportion, p, determined from a single sample, is an unbiased estimate of the population proportion.
- The **standard deviation** of the sampling distribution of the proportion is $\sqrt{\pi(1 - \pi)/n}$. It is called the **standard error of the proportion** and is a measure of the precision of p as an estimate of π. It is estimated from the sample by

$$\text{SE}(p) = \sqrt{\frac{p(1-p)}{n}}$$

Even though we estimate π by p, the sampling distribution of the proportion is still approximately Normal for large n.

Note, that if we replace the estimated proportion (p) by a percentage ($p\%$), then the estimated standard error of the estimated percentage is

$$\text{SE}(p\%) = \sqrt{\frac{p\%(100 - p\%)}{n}}$$

4.7 THE CONFIDENCE INTERVAL FOR A PROPORTION

The confidence interval for the population proportion, π, is calculated by adding to, and subtracting from, the sample proportion, p, a multiple of its standard error. The multiple is obtained from Table A.2 because the sampling distribution of the proportion is approximately Normal (see Section 4.6). In practice, we use the estimated standard error.

The 95% confidence interval for the population proportion is estimated by

$$p \pm 1.96 \, \text{SE}(p) =$$

$$\left(p - 1.96\sqrt{\frac{p(1-p)}{n}}, \; p + 1.96\sqrt{\frac{p(1-p)}{n}} \right)$$

The interpretation of this confidence interval is that we are 95% certain that the true population proportion is contained in the interval which spans p by 1.96 times $\text{SE}(p)$. Alternatively, 95% of such confidence intervals contain π in repeated sampling.

Note that we can modify this formula if we are working with percentages, rather than proportions, by replacing each proportion by the appropriate percentage and replacing the 1 inside each square root by 100.

Example

A sample of 115 cattle is randomly selected from the population in the area. Blood samples from the cattle are tested for the presence of antisera to *Leptospira* and, according to the titres, are classified as either positive or negative. In this sample, there are 36 cattle with positive titres. The estimated proportion of cattle exposed to *Leptospira* is thus $36/115 = 0.31$ (corrected to two decimal places). The estimated standard error of this proportion is

$$\text{SE}(p) = \sqrt{\frac{p(1-p)}{n}} = \sqrt{\frac{0.313(1-0.313)}{115}} = 0.043$$

The 95% confidence interval for the true proportion exposed is given by

$$p \pm 1.96 \, \text{SE}(p)$$
$$= (0.313 - 1.96 \times 0.043, \; 0.313 + 1.96 \times 0.043)$$
$$= (0.228, 0.398)$$

Hence, we are 95% certain that the true proportion of cattle exposed to *Leptospira* lies between 0.23 and 0.40.

EXERCISES

The statements in questions 4.1–4.3 are either TRUE or FALSE.

4.1 The standard error of the mean:
(a) Measures the accuracy of each observation in the sample.
(b) Is a measure of spread of the observations in the sample.
(c) Is a measure of precision of the sample mean as an estimate of the population mean.
(d) Is always less than the estimated standard deviation of the population.
(e) Decreases as the size of the sample from a given population increases.

4.2 The 95% confidence interval for the mean:
(a) Contains the sample mean with 95% certainty.
(b) Is less likely to contain the population mean than the 99% confidence interval.
(c) Contains 95% of the observations in the population.
(d) Is approximately equal to the sample mean plus and minus two standard deviations.
(e) Can be used to give an indication of whether the sample mean is a precise estimate of the population mean.

4.3 A sample of 14 dogs shows they have a mean plasma potassium of 4.57 mmol/l (Section 2.6.1(a)), and an estimated SD of 0.32 mmol/l (Section 2.6.2(d)); the standard error of the mean is thus 0.085 mmol/l. The 95% confidence interval for the mean is 4.42 to 4.72 mmol/l. This means that:
(a) There is a 95% chance that a dog's plasma potassium lies between 4.42 and 4.72 mmol/l.
(b) We can be 95% certain that the mean plasma potassium of the population of dogs lies between 4.42 and 4.72 mmol/l.
(c) 95% of sample means of dogs' plasma potassium would lie between 4.42 and 4.72 mmol/l in repeated sampling.
(d) 95% of dogs have a plasma potassium which lies between 4.42 and 4.72 mmol/l.
(e) There is a 5% chance that the sample mean of the dogs' plasma potassium lies outside the interval 4.42 to 4.72 mmol/l.

4.4 Calculate the 95% and the 99% confidence intervals for the population means, given the following information:

(a) Analysis of 100 grass samples gave a mean magnesium content of 2.35 mg/kg dry matter with a known population variance of 0.16 $(mg/kg)^2$.

(b) Milk progesterone values in 25 cows taken 24 days after insemination had a sample mean of 34.8 ng/ml and a sample SD of 13.0 ng/ml.

4.5 A representative sample of 60 sows from piggeries in Suffolk showed that 5 animals had joint lameness.

(a) Calculate the 95% confidence interval for the true proportion of joint lameness in the population of Suffolk sows.

(b) Would you expect the 99% confidence interval for this proportion to be wider or narrower than the 95% confidence interval?

(c) If you had a larger sample of sows, would your 95% confidence interval be wider or narrower than the one you have calculated?

Chapter 5

Experimental Design and Clinical Trials

5.1 LEARNING OBJECTIVES

By the end of this chapter, you should be able to:

- Describe what is meant by an observational study, clinical trial, longitudinal study, cohort study and case-control study.
- Explain the need for a 'control' group in a clinical trial.
- Explain the importance of randomization and describe methods for ensuring appropriate random allocation of individuals or groups.
- Explain the importance of 'blinding'.
- Describe the value of replication and blocking in experimental design.
- Define the term 'outlier' and describe methods to deal correctly with them.

5.2 TYPES OF STUDY

A study of statistics in veterinary and animal science overlaps with **epidemiology**, the study of disease patterns and their determinants in the population. In this chapter, we introduce you to some of the important concepts in epidemiology; they can be explored more fully in specialist texts, such as that by Thrusfield (1995).

Usually, there are restrictions on the availability of cases in studies of clinical conditions in animal populations. This may be because the condition is rare, or the cost of animals is too high, or there are time restrictions in a busy practice or animal industry. In order to make the most of the material available, it is important to design the study in the most productive way. Several different approaches are available.

In the planning stage of your study you are faced with a number of choices which are dictated by the problem you are investigating. Do

you wish to intervene or are you simply going to observe what is there? Do you intend to study your animals at a single point in time or do you wish to follow them over time? Do you want to start with healthy animals and observe whether the disease occurs, or do you start with diseased animals and investigate the causes?

5.2.1 The distinction between observational and experimental studies

(a) Observational study

In an **observational study**, we merely observe the animals in the study and record the relevant measurements on those animals. We make no attempt to intervene, for example, by administering treatments or withholding factors which we feel may affect the course of the disease. Clearly, we *cannot* randomly allocate animals to treatment groups in an observational study. A particular type of observational study is a **survey** in which we examine an aggregate of animals in order to derive values for various parameters in the population. This may be one of the following:

- A **population survey** which includes the entire population, e.g. a census.
- A **sample survey** in which we examine a representative sample of animals so that we may draw conclusions about the whole population of animals, as discussed in Section 4.3.

Many sample surveys are descriptive in that they attempt only to provide estimates of the population parameters. Some, however, are analytical because they are concerned with investigating associations. An *epidemiological* study, a particular form of an analytical sample survey, is concerned with investigating the aetiology of a disease by determining whether various factors (termed *risk factors*) are associated with the occurrence and distribution of the disease. For example, the prevalence of Cushing's syndrome in dogs is greater in toy breeds, a fact established by epidemiological studies comparing breeds.

(b) Experimental study

In an **experimental study**, we intervene in the study by, for example, deliberately applying a preventative measure, such as a treatment, or reducing the exposure of the animal to a factor, such as temperature. We then observe the effect of our intervention on the response of interest, usually with a view to establishing whether a change in response may be directly attributable to our action. Random allocation is an essential design component of an experimental study. Two examples of different types of experimental studies are **laboratory experiments** and **clinical trials**.

5.2.2 The distinction between cross-sectional and longitudinal studies

Studies in veterinary science may be either cross-sectional or longitudinal.

(a) Cross-sectional study

A **cross-sectional study** is one in which we take all our measurements on the animals included in the study *at a given point in time*. In an epidemiological investigation, this means we observe both the values of the risk factors and the disease state on every animal at the same time, within the bounds of practicality. Cross-sectional studies provide only limited information because they do not take into account the temporal relationship between the risk factors and the disease state. However, cross-sectional studies are useful when the aims of the study are essentially descriptive; for example, if we are estimating the

Box 5.1 The distinction between prevalence and incidence.

The *prevalence* and *incidence* of a disease are two terms which are often confused.

- The **prevalence** of a disease is the number of cases of the disease that exist at a specific instant in time (point prevalence) or in a *defined interval* of time (period prevalence).
- The **incidence** of a disease is the number of new cases of the disease that *develop* in a defined time period.

Both prevalence and incidence can be expressed as proportions (percentages) of the population at risk (i.e. those individuals who could succumb to the disease) at the mid-point of the study period or at the specified instant in time, as relevant.

point prevalence of a particular disease from a sample survey, see Box 5.1.

(b) Longitudinal study

A **longitudinal** study is one in which we investigate changes over time. The clinical trial is an example of a longitudinal study; we administer a treatment at one point in time, and observe the effect of that treatment at a later time. There are two types of longitudinal studies which are defined according to whether the changes over time are investigated **prospectively** (as in most *cohort* studies) or **retrospectively** (as in the case-control study) – see Section 5.2.3.

5.2.3 The distinction between cohort and case-control observational studies

(a) Cohort study

In a **cohort study** of disease aetiology, we start by defining groups (cohorts) of animals according to the exposure of the animals in the groups to the factors of interest. Generally, we follow these groups forward in time to see which animals develop the disease under investigation. For example, in exploring the mode of transmission of bovine spongiform encephalopathy (BSE), Wilesmith *et al.* (1997) wanted to determine if BSE-positive cows were more likely to produce offspring who developed BSE than those dams who were BSE negative. He studied two cohorts of cows: those which had developed BSE and those which had not shown clinical signs of BSE within six years (matched for sex, age and herd). The offspring of the cows in these two cohorts were then followed until their seventh year of life, or until they developed clinical signs of the disease.

We usually analyse data from cohort studies by estimating the true risk of the disease in the populations of animals who have been 'exposed' and 'unexposed' to the factor. The true **risk of disease** is the proportion of animals in a population of susceptible animals who develop the disease in the time interval under consideration; it represents the probability that an animal will develop the disease in the time period. The risk of the disease in a particular exposure group is estimated as the proportion of animals in the relevant cohort who develop the disease during the study period.

- The **relative risk**, the *ratio* of the disease risks in the exposed and unexposed groups, provides a measure of the strength of the association between the disease and the exposure to the factor. If the relative risk is unity, then exposure to the factor does not affect the animal's chance of developing the disease. If the relative risk (taken as the risk in the exposed cohort, divided by the risk in the unexposed cohort, say) is substantially greater than unity, then an animal has an increased risk of developing the disease if it has been exposed to the factor. For example, Wilesmith *et al.* (1997) found that 42 (14%) offspring of the 301 animals born to BSE-positive dams developed BSE within the first seven years of their lives, compared to 13 (4.3%) offspring of the 301 born to BSE-negative dams. This represents an estimated relative risk of 42/13 = 3.2, i.e. those calves born to BSE-positive mothers had more than a threefold greater chance of developing BSE than those from BSE-negative mothers.
- It may be more appropriate in studies relating to public health, rather than those concerned with disease aetiology, to consider the *difference* in the disease risks, and evaluate the

attributable risk. This can be measured in various ways; for example, the population attributable risk per cent determines the percentage of the total risk for the individual which is due to the risk factor. It can be estimated as

$$\frac{Risk_{total} - Risk_{unexp}}{Risk_{total}} \times 100\%$$

where $Risk_{total}$ is the estimated proportion of individuals with the disease in the whole population, and $Risk_{unexp}$ is the estimated proportion with the disease in those unexposed to the factor. In the BSE example, $Risk_{total} = (42 + 13)/602 = 0.09$, and the population attributable risk per cent is estimated as $100 \times (0.09 - 0.043)/0.09 = 52\%$, indicating that 52% of the diseased offspring have BSE as a consequence of having a dam with the disease. However, these data do not distinguish a possible genetic component from true maternal transmission.

(b) Case-control study

In a **case-control study** of disease aetiology, we start by defining the groups of diseased and healthy (or control) animals. Then we assess whether the animals in the two groups have differences in past exposure to various risk factors. Case-control studies are often termed *retrospective* studies because we have to go back in time in order to determine an animal's exposure to the risk factor. There are two types of case-control design which depend on the way in which we select our controls. Either we choose the controls so that each control animal is individually matched with a case with respect to variables that may be likely to influence the development of disease, such as the animal's breed, sex and/or age; this leads to what is termed a *matched* design. On the other hand, we may have an *unmatched* design in which the disease-free or control animals are selected randomly from a suitable population, but without any attempt at individual matching.

We cannot estimate the relative risk directly in a case-control study since the relative risk is a ratio of the risks of the disease in the exposed (to the factor) and unexposed groups of animals. In a case-control study, we start with animals with and without the disease rather than with different exposure groups, so we can only estimate the relative risk indirectly. We do this by calculating what is called the **odds ratio** which is the ratio of two odds, usually the odds of exposure in the diseased group divided by the odds of exposure in the control group. The **odds of exposure** in a group of animals is the ratio of the probability of being exposed to the probability of being unexposed. The odds ratio is a reasonable estimate of the relative risk provided the incidence of the disease is low, and the cases and controls are truly random samples from the same population.

5.3 INTRODUCING CLINICAL TRIALS

We use the term **clinical trial** to describe any planned experiment which involves human or animal subjects, and is designed to assess the effectiveness of one or more treatments or preventive measures such as vaccines. The term has been expanded from human clinical medicine to include studies in veterinary clinical medicine and animal health sciences; for example, the testing of the efficacy of novel pharmacological agents to control ectoparasites in dogs and cats, or a formal study of a novel method of repair of the anterior cruciate ligament. You can obtain a full discussion of clinical trials in Pocock (1983).

In the course of the development of veterinary treatments, there is usually a stage of experiment using laboratory animals to establish safety and efficacy of the treatment. If this is a drug development, this stage would also include pharmacological studies. A treatment which passes these preliminary assessments would then be examined in a clinical trial in which the treatment is applied to the species of interest but with a narrow range of its potential variation, e.g. beagles or Labradors as 'model' dogs. Up to this point, all these trials would usually be carried out in the UK under the Animals (Scientific Procedures) Act 1986.

We should distinguish the clinical trial from the **clinical field trial**. The former is a trial which takes place in well-regulated conditions; the clinical field trial is a comparative study involving new treatments or preventive measures applied under natural, field or semi-field conditions. It is usually carried out in the UK under the Veterinary Surgeons Act 1966.

- The clinical field trial introduces elements of variation attributable to the involvement of the owners or stockmen, and these are important in assessing the final efficacy of a treatment in a pragmatic setting. The overall effectiveness of a drug treatment, for example, involves not just the pharmacological action of the drug but the ability of the owner/stockman to administer it correctly, e.g. the use of helminthological treatments under farm conditions.
- The clinical field trial also introduces the full range of variation in a species, e.g. chihuahuas to Great Danes.

5.4 THE IMPORTANCE OF DESIGN IN THE CLINICAL TRIAL

We undertake a clinical trial in order to evaluate the benefit to be derived from introducing a new therapy or intervention in given circumstances. Our interest is in projecting the results from the sample of animals studied in the trial to some future population of similar animals suffering from the same condition and treated in comparable circumstances. In order to ensure that this hypothetical future population receives what is truly the best treatment, it is essential that the trial is based on rigorous scientific principles and is free from **bias**, i.e. from an effect which deprives a statistical result of representativeness by systematically distorting it (see Section 4.4.3). To this end, we must consider how we may:

- Allocate the experimental animals to the treatment groups.
- Evaluate the response to treatment.

We can then contemplate ways in which we can optimize the quality of the estimate of response to treatment, most notably by attempting to maximize its precision.

In the sections which follow, we describe the important features of design which contribute to a worthwhile trial leading to useful and valid conclusions concerning the effectiveness of the treatments or interventions. Note that a competent trial is invariably:

- *Comparative* – comprising more than one treatment group. We are then able to make judgements about the response to the new therapy or intervention in relation to the response that is obtained in the absence of therapy or compared to a standard therapy (see Section 5.5).
- *Randomized* – we assign the animals to the treatment groups by some chance process to ensure that the comparison groups are alike with respect to any variables which may influence response (see Section 5.6).

Incorporating both of these features into a trial leads to a **randomized controlled trial**, often abbreviated to **RCT**.

5.5 THE CONTROL GROUP

5.5.1 Why do we need a control group?

Without some basis for comparison, we cannot establish, with any degree of certainty, that the new therapy under investigation is preferable to the standard therapy or even to no therapy at all. It may be, for example, that the condition of the animal is going to improve over a defined period, purely as a consequence of time and the natural curative and healing properties of the body, and irrespective of the treatment the animal receives. Thus, we cannot make an inference that the new therapy is beneficial if we do not have any information about the response to the standard therapy given over the same period to a similar group of animals. Similarly, we may doubt the effectiveness of a new vaccine on a given population if there is no comparable information on a similar population of animals who are not given the vaccine.

Furthermore, in the absence of a comparison or **control group**, we will have knowledge of the treatment each animal is receiving, and in our enthusiasm for the new treatment, we may compromise the results, particularly if the assessment of response is subjective. A clinical trial which is not comparative is likely to lead to over-optimistic and therefore biased results.

5.5.2 Positive or negative control?

A comparative clinical trial is often termed a **controlled clinical trial**. The choice of control group depends on the exact circumstances of the trial. If a standard therapy exists, then it is ethically unacceptable to conduct the trial without including the standard therapy as the control which may then be termed a **positive control**. (In laboratory studies, a positive control has a different connotation – it is a treatment inducing the maximum response.) If, however, there is no known effective treatment, or if the condition is not so serious that the absence of treatment does not pose an ethical dilemma, then it is justifiable to have a control group, sometimes described as a **negative control** group, in which the animals receive no active treatment.

5.5.3 Historical controls

A **historical control** group is one in which the animals have previously been exposed to the control conditions and their results obtained prior to the onset of the trial. Occasionally, we may be tempted to use historical controls instead of **contemporary controls** in an attempt to reduce the number of animals needed in the experiment or from a desire to administer the new treatment to all animals in the trial. The major disadvantage of using historical controls in this retrospective comparison is that the test and control groups may not be truly comparable, both with respect to the type, source and condition of the animal and also to the experimental environment, so that biases may result. The consequence of including historical controls in a clinical trial is, again, a tendency to exaggerate the benefits of the new treatment.

5.6 ASSIGNMENT OF ANIMALS TO THE TREATMENT GROUPS

5.6.1 The need for random assignment

One important potential source of bias in the conduct of a controlled clinical trial is in the allocation of experimental animals to the treatment (test and control) groups. This bias may arise, either consciously or subconsciously, if we exercise personal judgment when we allocate the animals to the treatment groups. If the composition of the test and control groups differs in a systematic fashion, (e.g. if one group comprises more severely affected animals) then it is impossible for us to attribute any differences in response to the effect of treatment. In order to do so, it is essential that the test and control groups are as similar as possible and so are balanced in the factors that influence response, known as **covariates**, *whether or not these are known*. Sometimes, we find that two or more covariates are related to each other so that it is impossible to separate the effects of these variables on the response of interest; the covariates are then called **confounders** and the process is called confounding.

The most appropriate method of removing allocation bias and achieving this balance is the process of **random allocation** or **randomization** of the animals to the test and control groups. In random allocation, we assign the animals to the treatment groups in such a way that:

- All animals have the same chance of receiving any treatment.
- The assigning of one animal to a particular treatment has no influence on the assigning of any other animal.
- We cannot know in advance the treatment that each animal is to receive.

Thus, assigning the animals to the treatment groups in a *systematic* fashion by, for example, alternating the allocation, i.e. test, control, test, control, etc., would *not* comply with this definition. Systematic allocation is more likely to lead to bias than is a strictly random process of alloca-

tion. The investigator's knowledge of the allocation sequence may influence the allocation of particular animals to certain treatments.

Randomization has the following advantages:

- It removes bias from the allocation procedure.
- We do not require prior knowledge of factors likely to influence response, as the procedure should result in treatment groups which are comparable in unknown, as well as known, factors (apart from the actual treatment being given).
- Statistical theory is based on the concept of random sampling. If we construct the treatment groups using random allocation, then the differences between treatment groups are akin to those between random samples. We can, therefore, utilize the process of statistical inference (see Section 1.9) to evaluate treatment differences.

As a practical tip, you may find it helpful to mask the allocation sequence by using *sealed envelopes* in the randomization process. These are numbered consecutively; each contains the specification of the treatment regimen (determined by random allocation) to be administered to the next available animal.

5.6.2 Methods of randomization

It is best if you avoid mechanical methods, such as tossing a coin or throwing a die, for allocating the experimental animals to the treatment groups. Although they are probabilistically acceptable procedures which adhere to the definition of randomization, these techniques are cumbersome and cannot be verified.

A common way of employing randomization in the allocation process is to utilize a table of random numbers (Table A.11). This comprises the digits 0–9 generated in a random manner such that each digit occurs the same number of times, and there is no discernible pattern in the arrangement of the digits. If we choose an appropriate allocation scheme, some of which are outlined below, we can use the table to randomly allocate equal numbers of animals to the different treatments. Alternatively, a random number sequence can be generated on many calculators and computers.

(a) Simple randomization

We may allocate approximately equal numbers of animals to the different treatment groups using **simple randomization** – this is the basic randomization procedure which does not involve any refinements or restrictions. Suppose we have two treatment groups: a test group (T) and a control group (C). We begin by choosing a random starting point, i.e. a digit, in the table of random numbers. Then we follow the row of that digit to the left or the right, or the column of that digit up or down the page. Every number in the sequence of digits obtained in this way is either odd or even (taking 0 as even), the chance of an odd or even number being equal. If the number is odd, we allocate the next experimental animal in the trial to T, say, and if the number is even, we allocate that animal to C. So the sequence 386674559670 would result in the allocation TCCCTCTTTCTC. We may modify the procedure to accommodate three or more treatments. For example, if there are three treatments, A, B and C, we allocate the animal to A if the digit is 1, 2 or 3; to B if the digit is 4, 5 or 6; to C if the digit is 7, 8 or 9; we ignore zeros. Then, the above sequence would result in the allocation ACBBCBBCBC. As you can see, with only 12 animals, the group sizes in this randomization are disparate (see Section 5.6.2(c) for a solution to this problem).

(b) Stratified randomization

You should be aware that simple randomization, relying as it does on chance, is not infallible, particularly when the sample size is relatively small. Sometimes, we want to ensure that the treatment groups are similar with respect to one or two key confounding variables, as it is easier to promote comparability at the allocation stage rather than attempting to make adjustments for the confounders in the statistical analysis. This may be achieved by **stratified randomization**.

We divide the population into different strata according to the categorization of the key confounding variables. So, for example, for a study of arthritis in dogs, we may create three strata, one for each of large, medium and toy breeds, since the animal's body mass is believed to affect the response to treatment. Then, within each stratum, we randomly allocate the dogs to each of the treatment groups; provided we assign approximately equal numbers of dogs to each treatment group within each stratum, the treatment groups should be comparable with regard to body mass.

(c) Restricted randomization

Generally, we aim to have approximately equal numbers of animals in the various treatment groups. We are likely to achieve this with simple randomization if our sample size is large enough, but we may have an undesirable imbalance with a relatively small number of animals. We demonstrated this in the simple randomization example (see Section 5.6.2(a)) in which the use of a sequence of only 12 digits resulted in one animal being allocated to treatment A, six animals to B and four animals to C. We may overcome this inequality problem by using **restricted** or **blocked randomization**.

We decide that we would like to have a trial in which we are assured of balance in every block of n (e.g. $n = 8$, 10 or 20) animals that enter the trial, perhaps, because of batch variation in the treatment material. Suppose we have two treatment groups, T and C, and that we choose n equal to 8. We follow the sequence of digits in the random number table and allocate the animal to T if the number is odd and to C if the number is even. Once we have allocated four animals to one treatment group, then we must allocate the remaining animals in that block of eight to the other treatment group. So, the same sequence as before, 386674559670, would result in TCCCTC after the first six digits, i.e. four animals on C, indicating that we would have to allocate the remaining two animals in that block to T. This procedure, if continued, ensures exact balance after every group of eight animals, and approximate balance when all animals have been entered into the trial if the trial size is not a multiple of eight. It has the added advantage of guarding against imbalances which may result from any time-trend in the type of animals admitted to the trial, as well as facilitating balance in any interim analyses (see Section 12.3.4). Stratified randomization usually incorporates restricted randomization within each stratum provided the overall sample size is large enough.

(d) Group randomization

The **experimental unit** is the smallest unit in an experiment to which a treatment can be assigned, and whose response is independent of the responses of the other units. Generally, in human medicine, clinical trials use the individual person as the experimental unit although, occasionally, clusters of individuals, such as households, are used. However, we often regard the **group** as the most appropriate experimental unit in the veterinary and animal sciences. This is because food, drugs and vaccines are often administered to a group of animals in a litter, pen, paddock or barn, or to a complete herd or to all the fish in a tank. In this case, we apply the randomization procedure to the groups (i.e. **group randomization**), so that all animals or fish within each group receive the same treatment. We have to combine the results on the groups in the appropriate manner to evaluate treatment effects.

A second circumstance which may suggest instituting group randomization is when we *cannot* regard the individual animals within a group (litter, pen, paddock etc.) as *independent* units. This is likely to arise when we are appraising a vaccine against a parasitic disease; herd immunity and the possibility of vaccine organisms spreading to and protecting the controls would tend to camouflage the effectiveness of the vaccine. If the experimental unit is the animal rather than the group, the protection afforded the vaccinated animals leads to a reduced prevalence of disease in the group environment, resulting in a reduced incidence of disease in the control animals; this is what is meant by **herd immunity**. A similar process may also be applicable when

dewormed and control animals are allowed to graze on the same pasture. Short but useful discussions of this problem are given by Altman and Bland (1997) and Bland and Kerry (1997).

In group randomization, you must remember:

- To base the *sample size calculations* at the planning stage of the investigation on the number of *groups* that are randomized to the different treatments, and not on the number of animals within the groups. In practical terms, you may find you cannot satisfy a requirement for a large number of groups, for example, pens or herds; suggestions for overcoming the problem are given by Haber *et al.* (1991) and by Halloran and Struchiner (1991). Another useful reference is that by Kerry and Bland (1998).
- To base the *statistical analyses of results* on the group as the experimental unit, perhaps using cluster sampling techniques which incorporate weighted measures when the clusters (groups) are of unequal size. Useful papers in this context are those by Donner *et al.* (1981), Donner (1987), and Hseih (1988).

If, incorrectly, you take the animal within the group as the experimental unit when you use group randomization, you will underestimate the variation between animals. The lack of independence between these animals will result in less variation, and hence narrower confidence intervals for the parameters of interest, than would be expected if the animals were truly independent. This, in turn, would be likely to lead you to conclude, over-optimistically and erroneously, that there was a statistically significant difference between treatments. Thus, by underestimating the variation between animals, you are likely to overestimate the magnitude of the difference between treatments.

5.7 THE AVOIDANCE OF BIAS IN THE ASSESSMENT PROCEDURE

We use the randomization process in a clinical trial to ensure that the trial is free from systematic errors of *allocation*. However, biases may arise in the *assessment of response* to treatment because of the preconceived notions of the carer of the animals and/or the assessors as to the benefits of treatment. These biases are most likely to occur when the response to treatment is subjective, such as the body condition score in sheep or the starkness of coat in cats, but may also be present when the response is objective. As an example, consider the situation when discriminator limits must be set by the operator on an objective computer-based sperm motility analyser which recognizes sperm cells in a video image; although objective results are obtainable, the values are dependent on the subjective setting of the grey limit discriminators (Knuth *et al.*, 1987). The presence of assessment bias invalidates any statistical conclusion based on the assumed random distribution of errors, and compromises the reliability of the results.

We ensure that our trial is free from assessment bias by making the trial 'blind'. There are two levels of 'blindness' – double-blind and single-blind.

- Ideally, we should design the trial to be **double-blind** so that neither the carer(s) of the animals nor the assessor of response to treatment (test or control) is aware of which treatment each animal is receiving. If the carers are ignorant of the treatment each animal is receiving (i.e. they are *blind*), it is possible for them to handle the animals impartially and removes from them the temptation to atone, either consciously or subconsciously, for the supposed inferior control regimen. It is essential to keep the assessor blind if the response to treatment is subjective, thus guarding against the tendency to favour or disfavour a particular treatment. Clinical trials should have the maximum attainable degree of blindness in order to remove potential bias in the assessment process. Double-blind trials are desirable but not always achievable.
- In some circumstances, the trial may be **single-blind** in that only one of these two parties, the carer or the assessor, is blind. If the response to treatment is objective then it may be sufficient to have only the carer blind; if it is possible to distinguish the test and control

regimens, perhaps because of experimental procedures, then it may not be feasible to make the carer blind. For example, in a single-blind fertility trial of semen diluent treatments when only one treatment contains egg yolk, the inseminator will be aware of which treatment is used; the assessment of fertility (pregnancy test) must then be performed blind.

In order for the carer to be blind, it is essential that the physical appearance of the test and control treatments, as well as the treatment regimens, should be exactly the same. This may be facilitated by using a **dummy** treatment or **placebo**, a pharmacologically inert substance which is identical in appearance to the test treatment. It forms the baseline against which the effect of the test treatment is measured. The response induced by suggestion on the part of the animal attendants or the animal investigator when the animal receives a placebo is called the **placebo effect**. Placebos are most often used in drug trials; they may, if ethical considerations permit, be used in invasive procedures, e.g. injections of the solvent base (vehicle) for the drug or in sham-operations. These are common in experiments which are conducted in the UK under the Animals (Scientific Procedures) Act 1986.

5.8 INCREASING THE PRECISION OF THE ESTIMATES

5.8.1 Introduction

Our primary concern is with designing a trial which is free from systematic errors of allocation and from biases in the assessment of response to treatment. Our secondary objective is to promote the reliability of our conclusions by maximizing the precision of the estimates of the parameters of interest. Extraneous variations resulting from the inherent variability in the experimental units and from a failure to standardize the experimental technique tend to mask the effects of treatments; we want both to quantify and to minimize these variations.

5.8.2 Replication

We generally choose our trial size to be as large as possible. The greater the number of experimental units in the trial, usually individual animals but sometimes groups of animals (see Section 5.6.2(d)), the greater the precision of the estimates and the greater our chance of detecting a treatment effect, if it exists. We provide a detailed explanation of how to determine the optimal sample size in a trial in Section 12.3.

In addition, we sometimes incorporate **replication** into the trial design so that we can increase the precision of our estimates, and improve the effectiveness of the trial to detect treatment differences. By replication, we mean repeating the number of measurements (i.e. obtain duplicates, triplicates, etc.) of the same type on each experimental unit, for example, on each animal. This allows us to segregate the within-animal variability from the variation which is due to biological or treatment differences; this will enhance the comparisons of interest, whilst giving us the opportunity to evaluate repeatability (see Section 13.3.1). We must take care when analysing such data; we have to recognize that k repeated measurements on n experimental units do not provide nk independent observations. For example, if we are observing the number of visits garden birds make to a feeding basket, we may not be sure we are observing different birds at each visit. If a pair of birds each pay 10 visits to the feeder in an hour, this is not the same as 20 birds each paying a single visit in the hour. We must not treat these two situations in the same way for statistical analysis, recognizing that they imply quite different behaviour of the bird population. One simple approach often used for the analysis of data which comprise replicate observations is to work with the means of the replicate observations for each animal.

Do not confuse this form of replication with the situation in which a certain response is measured on several occasions on each experimental unit *over a period of time*. This latter design needs to be analysed in a special way, as the time factor may well be of interest, and care must be taken to ensure that treatment comparisons are made within rather than between animals; we discuss this briefly in **repeated measures designs** in Section 13.4.2.

5.8.3 The concept of blocks

We can incorporate careful grouping of the experimental units in a trial as a supplementary technique to reduce the variability in the comparisons of interest. We deliberately select groups (**blocks**) of animals (e.g. breeds) which are more homogeneous than the animals in the population at large; thus, the random variability *within* each block is smaller than that *between* the blocks. We allocate treatments randomly within each of the blocks (stratified randomization). In the analysis, it is possible to separate the variability in the results due to blocks from that due to treatments, allowing us to obtain a more precise estimate of the treatment effect than if we had not made use of blocks.

We have a **complete randomized block** design when each block contains a complete set of treatments. Other designs called **incomplete blocks**, in which each block need not contain the entire treatment set, are possible but their complexity is beyond the scope of this book. We refer you to discussion in, for example, Cochran and Cox (1957).

You should be aware that, sometimes, the use of blocks is governed by practical considerations rather than being promoted as a tool for increasing precision. In some situations, we may find it necessary to assemble groups of animals situated on several farms or at several kennels or catteries. Again, these groups of animals are blocks, but here they introduce an additional source of variation, that attributable to the different locations.

5.8.4 'Between' and 'within' comparisons

For simplicity, suppose that we are comparing just two treatments. There are two basic forms of design:

1. We can randomly assign the animals (the observational units) to the two treatments to create two **independent** groups. There is no

relationship between the individual animals in one group and the individual animals in the second group, and the sample sizes may differ. This is a *parallel group design* (see Section 5.9.6) in which the treatment comparisons are made *between* animals. An example is a feeding trial which compares the average gain in weight over a time period in two groups of animals in which only one of the two groups is given a dietary supplement.

2. We can improve our comparison if we deliberately create related or dependent groups. If the observations in the two groups are **paired**, each observation in one group is paired or individually matched with an observation in the other group, and the groups are therefore necessarily of equal size. The treatment comparisons are then made *within* the pairs. There is less variation *within* paired individuals than *between* unpaired individuals, so the treatment effects can be estimated more precisely. Data sets which exhibit dependency in the form of pairing or individual matching should not be analysed as if the data sets were independent. If we ignore the dependency, we lose information, and this reduces the chance of detecting a treatment difference if one exists.

(a) The pair may comprise the same animal (**self-pairing**) in different circumstances (see *cross-over* trials in Section 5.9.6), e.g. when two treatments are administered to an animal in random order. An example of self-pairing is when we compare a horse's metabolism on a treadmill and on a normal track (e.g. Exercise 7.3).

You should beware of the common mistake of regarding before and after treatment comparisons on the same animal as suitable for a simple paired analysis; for example, in comparing the heart rate (beats/min) of dogs before and after dosing with a putative cardiac stimulant. Unless the design includes a group of animals for which measurements are made both before and after a control (e.g. placebo) treatment is administered, it is impossible to be sure if a difference in the before and after active treatment measurements can be attributed to the effect of treatment alone. The correct analysis for this form of design is to compare the two sets of differences, those in the group receiving the control and those in the group receiving the active treatment. Thus, although we pair the observations at the outset, the statistical analysis is a two-sample comparison of differences.

(b) Another form of pairing often occurs in animal experimentation when litter mates provide the experimental material (**natural pairing**), and the treatments are allocated in such a way that every animal in one group has a litter mate in the other group.

(c) A third form of pairing occurs when the pair comprises two different animals which have been *matched* with respect to any variables that may be thought to influence response (**artificial pairing**). An example is a case-control study in dogs involving the effect of a drug on haematology values, where animals have been paired for treatment and control on the basis of approximate similarity in age and body size to avoid the confounding influence of these factors. Bland and Altman (1994) discuss matching in a brief but informative paper.

5.8.5 Use of specific animals

Note that substantial reduction in variability can also be obtained by using microbiologically, genetically or environmentally defined animals. Nevertheless, sufficient animals must be included to give satisfactory estimates. However, the results are only strictly relevant to the type of animal in the trial and may differ from what is found in 'normal' animals. You must exercise care in drawing conclusions on this basis.

5.9 FURTHER CONSIDERATIONS

5.9.1 The protocol

The protocol is a written document which details all aspects of the rationale, design, conduct and the proposed analysis of the trial. Typically, it contains statements relating to the background and objectives of the study, ethical problems, the trial design including methods of randomization, selection of animals, sample size calculations, exclusion criteria, protocol deviations, the potential sources of bias, the variables which will be measured, the measurement techniques, methods of, and forms for, data collection, drug regimens and suppliers, the duration of the trial, the manpower requirements and responsibilities, the statistical analysis and costs.

It is prepared at the outset of the trial, and serves a number of useful functions. It is required for submissions to funding bodies and for ethical committee approval; it is a useful reference document for the study investigators during the progress of the trial; and it is helpful in the final write-up of a study.

5.9.2 Outliers

(a) Identifying the outlier(s)

An **outlier** is an extreme observation which is inconsistent with the main body of the data. We must always check our data at the initial stages of the analysis to determine whether they contain outliers. This is most easily achieved by plotting the data, e.g. by producing a histogram, stem-and-leaf plot or a box-and-whisker plot (see Section 2.5.2) for a single continuous variable, or a scatter diagram when we are investigating the relationship between two continuous variables in regression analysis (see Section 10.2). As an alternative strategy, we may look at the range of our sample data to see if any observation in our sample lies outside the range of plausible values. Some statistical software packages contain an automatic procedure for detecting outliers; for example, all values that are greater than three standard deviations away from the mean.

The problem with outliers is that they often distort the results and the conclusions drawn from the statistical analysis. This may happen even when there are only one or two outliers in a data set. The real difficulty is in knowing what to do with the outliers. There are four ways in which we can handle them. We can:

1. Include them and proceed as originally planned, recognising that the distribution assumptions of the analysis may not be met.
2. Include them in the analysis but adopt a procedure which is appropriate for the data. For example, if the distribution of the variable of interest is skewed (see Section 2.5) because of the presence of outliers, then the median is a better measure of central tendency than the arithmetic mean (see Section 2.6.1), and we may prefer non-parametric methods of statistical analysis (see Chapter 11) for statistical inference.
3. Analyse the data both with and without the outliers to determine the effect, if any, of removing them.
4. Exclude them from the analysis (this is a high risk strategy, and, before you do so, you should thoroughly investigate the reason for their presence, see Section 5.9.2(b)). Beware that some computer packages will automatically eliminate outliers from the analysis.

Which of these approaches we choose will depend on the magnitude and the cause of the outlier(s).

(b) The causes of outliers

- Sometimes, we obtain an outlier because the animal on which we are making the measurement is atypical of the population from which it was drawn. We should not exclude an outlier unless there is a justifiable reason for doing so. Consider the following situation. For example, occasionally one animal in a group cannot be caught without considerable vigorous activity; this may result in a physiological variable exhibiting an extreme value which could be excluded.
- Alternatively, it may be apparent, on subsequent *post-mortem* examination, that a particular animal suffered an intercurrent disease which may have caused an outlier during a

clinical trial. Again, it is reasonable to omit the outlier from the analysis.

- We may also obtain an outlier because we have made a mistake, perhaps in reading an instrument or in transcribing information. Then it may be possible to correct the mistake, and include the corrected value in the analysis.

5.9.3 Missing data

Despite our best intentions at the start of a study, we may find that our data set is incomplete when we are ready to analyse our data. For example, the carer may have inadvertently lost a reading on an animal, or an animal ear-tag has been lost making identity uncertain, or an animal has died in the course of our investigation. When entering the data into the computer, it is advisable to code the missing observations in some recognizable format, so as to be able to distinguish them from other types of observations. The choice is yours, but you must select a code which is unique and cannot be confused with a real observation. Typically, the numbers 9 (for a variable whose maximum value is less than 9), 9.9, 99, or 999 are chosen, although some computer programs are prepared to accept an asterisk (*) or a bullet (•) or some other symbol.

We should always investigate the reasons for the omissions, to ensure that no biases (see Section 5.4) are likely to arise because of them. For example, if an observation goes beyond the scale of the measuring instrument, it cannot be recorded and may be coded as 'missing'. The failure to record this observation is related to its magnitude, and a bias may well result.

Some statistical software packages handle missing observations by automatically excluding from the analysis any individual which has a missing observation on at least one variable. Others replace the missing observations by the average of the remaining observations in the data set. Occasionally, missing observations which are left as blanks in the data file may be taken as zeros in the analysis; be warned that this is likely to have a considerable effect on the conclusions. *Always make sure that you know how your software package deals with missing data.*

5.9.4 Analysis by intention to treat

One of the greatest problems in the analysis of clinical trials is knowing what to do with the results from animals which do not strictly adhere to the protocol, possibly because they prove too difficult to treat with the treatment that was originally assigned to them. Additionally, some animals may deviate from the original treatment schedule, perhaps because of side-effects, and are switched to an alternative treatment or treatment is stopped altogether. Such observations do not count as missing (see Section 5.9.3) if the results are known, but are called **withdrawals** from treatment.

- Provided we have results, the appropriate way of dealing with withdrawals is to analyse them as if they still belonged to the treatment group *to which the animals were originally randomly assigned*. At first glance, you may find this so-called **intention to treat** or *pragmatic* approach, aimed at eliciting the effect of treatment in a clinical scenario, difficult to comprehend. You may wonder how you can justify analysing a result as if the observation were made on one treatment when, in fact, it arises from the application of another treatment. Be assured, however, that this is the correct approach.

- The alternative is to analyse the results according to the treatment actually received; this *explanatory* approach is aimed at understanding the processes involved. We do not recommend the explanatory approach as it is more likely to distort the treatment comparisons and lead to a biased result than the pragmatic approach. Remember that one of the reasons for employing randomization is to ensure that the treatment groups are balanced in the factors that influence response (see Section 5.6). If we use the explanatory approach, then the animals are not analysed in the treatment groups to which they were randomly assigned, and we may disturb this balance of potentially influential factors.

You will find a full discussion in Schwartz *et al.* (1980).

5.9.5 Pilot studies

A **pilot study** is a small-scale preliminary investigation. We conduct pilot studies for a variety of reasons:

- To see whether there is merit in developing a full-scale trial.
- To provide us with an indication of the variability in the results. If we have some idea of the expected variability in the results, we can calculate minimum group sizes to permit detection of real treatment effects in the full-scale trial (see Section 12.3).
- To ensure that the dosing regimen we have chosen for a treatment is appropriate.
- To develop techniques and iron out any difficulties we may experience.

As you will appreciate, a pilot study is well worth the time and resources invested in it, and can save much frustration later, especially if the proposed study breaks entirely novel ground.

5.9.6 Cross-over trials

Most clinical trials are **parallel group designs**; each individual animal receives only one treatment, and treatment comparisons are made between rather than within animals (see also Section 5.8.4). Occasionally, we may conduct a **cross-over trial**. As its name suggests, we apply two or more treatments in succession to each individual animal. The aim is to compare the responses to treatment *within* the animals, rather than *between* animals, thereby enhancing the precision of the estimate of the difference between treatments and reducing the sample size. However, we cannot entirely eliminate individual variation since the treatments are not contemporaneous, and there may be a period effect (when there is a systematic difference in response between the two periods of administra-

tion). This may occur, say, when the animals become more accustomed to dosing in the second period and therefore have a different physiological baseline. To minimize the influence of the passage of time and the period effect, the order in which each animal receives the treatments is chosen at random.

This sort of trial is ideally suited to the comparison of palliative treatments of chronic diseases rather than to the comparison of cures, since the condition must return, and be of equal severity, after treatment ceases in order to investigate the other treatments. Suitable examples are the use of dietary restriction or insulin on the control of blood glucose in diabetic dogs, or the use of topical ointments or oral preparations on the control of eczema.

Because of a possible carry-over effect, it is important to establish the question of how long a rest or wash-out period is necessary before instigating the next treatment, since some treatments may have a long lag phase before the effects are eliminated.

The analysis of cross-over trials is a relatively complex subject, and is covered in detail in Senn (1993).

5.9.7 Ethical issues

(a) Responsibilities and duties of the investigator

Wherever we contemplate experimental approaches using animals, issues of animal welfare and ethics are present. Even the seemingly innocuous question of a control group may present an ethical dilemma. For example, can we justify failing to treat a random selection of diseased animals in order to compare the effect of a treatment protocol? The answer we give will depend on the severity of the condition, the effectiveness of existing treatments, and the degree of suffering involved. Perhaps, as we suggest in Section 5.5, it may be appropriate to compare a novel treatment with the best existing treatment, thereby offering the most effective available treatment to the control group. However, with a novel treatment it is possible that the treatment group itself is at risk, and we have every duty to ensure that the risk is minimal and assessed as far as is in our power to do so.

(b) Legislation controlling animal investigation

Any invasive act of veterinary surgery, such as obtaining a blood sample or a tissue biopsy, is prohibited except when carried out for diagnostic purposes, and is limited to being carried out under veterinary supervision, preventing exploitation of animals. Obtaining samples from healthy animals by a veterinary surgeon without causing any significant discomfort, pain, suffering, distress or lasting harm in order to support a diagnosis, or to provide information relating to animal husbandry or clinical management is permissible, providing it is done with the informed consent of the owner. The main exceptions to this in the UK are under the Animals (Scientific Procedures) Act 1986, when particular biological scientists are licensed by the Home Office to perform specific procedures after demonstrating adequate training. Even modifying the diet of an animal for experimental purposes is controlled under this Act and may not be carried out without a licence.

In fact, it is rather easier to obtain human volunteers for research than to assemble animals for a study. This is because the principle of informed consent is easier to apply, although the situation for animals is not dissimilar to the situation involving children too young to give their own informed consent, where the parent or guardian must give consent for a procedure to be performed.

(c) The principles of animal welfare

The sensible approach to these issues is always to keep animal welfare in the forefront. We must devise protocols which minimize the inconvenience and discomfort to animals and provide safety for humans, but in the last analysis, the animal welfare concern is primary. In medical establishments, it is widely recognized that an ethics committee, made up of experts and inter-ested and suitably qualified members of the general public, is required to oversee investigative studies carried out on human subjects. The veterinary profession is rather slower to develop this concept, but it is beginning to find favour.

Even under the Animals (Scientific Procedures) Act 1986, the experiments must be justified by the welfare benefit to the animal population at large or by the advantage to human medicine before they can be approved. Furthermore, the welfare concerns must be addressed by reducing the numbers of animals used and by minimizing the discomfort to be applied.

Statistical procedures are valuable here in that they provide a guide to the minimum number of animals that may be needed for a statistically sound result (see Section 12.3). This avoids wasted trials owing to inadequate group sizes, or using unnecessarily large numbers of animals.

EXERCISES

The statements in questions 5.1–5.3 are either TRUE or FALSE.

5.1 Animals are randomly allocated to the treatment groups in a clinical trial:
(a) To ensure that there is no assessment bias.
(b) To ensure that all animals have the same chance of receiving any treatment.
(c) So that a control group can be incorporated into the design.
(d) So that the treatment groups are comparable with respect to any variables that are likely to influence response.
(e) So that the trial can be single- or double-blind.

5.2 The wattle reaction of chicks to the injection of phytohaemaglutinin (PHA) is used as an indication of the immune responsiveness. Chicks (3–6 days old) were randomly assigned to four groups, a control and three different monoamine treatments which were suspected of interfering with the immune responses. Thirty minutes after treatment, birds were injected in the wattle with $100\,\mu g$ PHA-P and wattle thickness was measured prior to the injection and 24 h later (Lukacs *et al.*, 1987). This is an example of:

(a) An observational study.
(b) A cross-sectional study.
(c) A retrospective study.
(d) A clinical trial.
(e) A sample survey.

5.3 Sedative treatments were administered to ten ferrets in a cross-over trial, and sedative and cardiovascular responses evaluated (Ko *et al.*, 1998). Diazepam, acepromazine and xylazine were administered to each animal in a random order; a wash-out period was allowed between each treatment. Xylazine produced the longest duration of recumbency and was judged most satisfactory as a sedative for ferrets.

(a) The wash-out period allowed the trial to be blind.
(b) The randomization ensured that there was no carry-over effect.
(c) This was an example of a parallel group design.
(d) The treatment comparison was made within animals.
(e) A more precise treatment comparison would be achieved if each ferret received only one treatment, so that the three treatment groups comprised different animals.

5.4 A study was conducted into the influence of spaying of bitches on their subsequent development of urinary incontinence. Young adult bitches presenting for spaying were randomly allocated to immediate ovariohysterectomy or to a deferred operation six months later. The bitches were followed during the six-month period. Was this:

(a) A cross-sectional or a longitudinal study, and why?
(b) An experimental or an observational study, and why?
(c) A cohort study or a case-control study, and why?
(d) Can you propose any other study design to explore this condition and its aetiology?

5.5 In a study of the benefits of surgical intervention in the repair of congenital umbilical hernia, kittens with a visible herniation within 48 h of birth were randomly allocated to surgery or to a *laissez-faire* approach. At the time of weaning, kittens were assessed for survival rate and hernia resolution. Criticize the choice of control and suggest any improvements.

5.6 Describe an appropriate randomization (simple, stratified, restricted, or group) for the following investigations:

(a) Three dose levels (mg/kg) of an acaricide applied to dogs seen at an urban veterinary practice.
(b) The testing of the efficacy of a treatment for *Ostertagia* (lungworm) in a herd of cattle in two plots of worm-infested land.
(c) Testing of the efficacy of vaccination of kittens against common cat viral diseases by vaccinating litters of kittens at random with one of two different commercial preparations.
(d) The allocation to treatment groups of individual animals in four different farm locations for a study of the effects of lambing indoors in pens or outside in makeshift straw shelters. For an optimal design, equal numbers of animals should be in each treatment group at each location.

Chapter 6

An Introduction to Hypothesis Testing

6.1 LEARNING OBJECTIVES

By the end of this chapter, you should be able to:

- Elaborate the basic concept of hypothesis testing.
- Define the null hypothesis.
- Distinguish between one- and two-tailed tests and decide which is appropriate in any investigative trial.
- Define a test statistic.
- Explain in simple terms the meaning of the term 'degrees of freedom'.
- Interpret the *P*-value.
- Summarize the hypothesis testing procedure.
- Define Type I and Type II errors in hypothesis testing.
- Distinguish between the approaches to testing a hypothesis using a test statistic and a confidence interval, identifying the strengths and weaknesses of both.

6.2 INTRODUCTION

We can categorize statistical theory into two general areas.

1. Firstly, there is **descriptive statistics** which uses the appropriate tools, typically tables, diagrams and/or numerical measures, to describe a data set and provide a summary of its distribution (see Chapter 2).
2. In addition, there is **inferential statistics** which is concerned with drawing conclusions about a population using information obtained from a representative sample selected from it.
   (a) One aspect of statistical inference is the **estimation** of a population parameter by the appropriate sample statistic (for example, the population mean by the sample mean). The estimation process is complete only when the precision of the estimate, as determined by its standard error or indicated by the confidence interval, is included (see Section 4.5).
   (b) The second aspect of inferential statistics is **hypothesis testing**. In this case, we examine a hypothesis, framed in terms of the parameters in one or more populations. We want to know if the hypothesis about the population(s) is supported by the sample data.

Estimation is concerned with *description* whereas hypothesis testing is ultimately concerned with *decision*.

6.3 BASIC CONCEPTS OF HYPOTHESIS TESTING

Hypothesis testing is a process which is concerned with making inferences about the population using the information obtained from a sample. We have to recognize that it is impossible to be absolutely certain that our inferences about the population are correct. One randomly selected sample from the population is unlikely to be exactly the same as a second randomly selected sample, and in neither of these is the sample statistic likely to be exactly equal to the population parameter it is estimating and about which we are testing a hypothesis. Because we take a sample, there is an element of uncertainty involved and, therefore, we should accompany the conclusions we draw about the population with a **probability**. This gives an indication of the chance of getting the observed results if the hypothesis is true. We replace an absolute statement by a probabilistic statement, and this forms the crux of hypothesis testing.

Although the basic concepts of hypothesis testing are not too difficult to grasp, the whole process is shrouded in statistical jargon. It is helpful if you have a proper understanding of this jargon, particularly if you obtain your results from computer output which may vary in form depending on the particular software package that you are using.

6.3.1 The null hypothesis, H_0

We are concerned with investigating a particular theory or scientific hypothesis *about the population* which is usually comparative in nature, involving some numerical **effect** of interest. Often this comparison is of different treatments, the measure which compares their responses being termed the **treatment effect**. This treatment effect is specified by the relevant parameter values in the treatment groups, for example the difference in the treatment means. For statistical purposes, we investigate the theory of interest by testing the hypothesis that there is *no* treatment effect in the population. For example, suppose we are interested in investigating whether cattle on new spring grass are in danger of hypomagnesaemia (grass staggers). A lower level of plasma magnesium in the outdoor cattle compared with those kept indoors would suggest a risk of grass staggers. We formulate the null hypothesis that the true mean values of plasma magnesium do not differ in the two groups. This is called the **null hypothesis, H_0,** and its specification is the starting point in hypothesis testing. We examine the sample data to see whether they support or contradict this hypothesis.

Should the null hypothesis be untrue, an **alternative hypothesis** holds:

• Usually, the alternative hypothesis states that a difference exists between the parameter values but the direction of that difference is not known. It leads to a **two-sided** or a **two-tailed test**. Unless otherwise specified, we assume that a test is two-tailed. In our example, although we might anticipate that eating new

grass would reduce the plasma magnesium concentration, the alternative hypothesis is merely that the two means differ. We have no prior reason to anticipate that the indoor 'treatment' can *only* be better them the grass 'treatment'.

• Very occasionally, however, we have sound prior knowledge that any difference between the treatments, if it exists, can be in one direction only. This must not be based on hopes or expectations about a novel treatment, but on an absolute certainty that the difference can only be in that direction, if the difference is not zero. This gives rise to a **one-sided** or a **one-tailed test** in which the direction of the difference is specified in the alternative hypothesis.

We must specify both the null and the alternative hypotheses at the outset, before we collect the data. We stress that the alternative hypothesis must be specified *before* the data are collected, and is, therefore, independent of the data. You may be tempted to use a one-sided test because it is more likely than a two-sided test to show a difference! Remember, though, that the prior certainty required for a one-sided test *very rarely exists*.

6.3.2 Getting a feel for the data

Having specified the null and alternative hypotheses, we then **collect** our sample data. It is important that we **look** at the data at this stage and check the *assumptions* inherent in the test. With the advent of the computer and easy access to statistical computer software, it is all too easy to overlook the nature of the data, including a lack of awareness of outliers that may be distorting the results, and consequently to draw inappropriate conclusions. A careful, albeit simple, initial look at the data may forestall erroneous judgments.

6.3.3 The test statistic and the *P*-value

From the data we calculate the value of a **test statistic** (an algebraic expression particular to the hypothesis we are testing), usually using a computer or occasionally, by hand. Attached to each value of the test statistic is a **probability**, called a *P*-value. It describes the chance of getting the observed effect (or one more extreme) *if the null hypothesis is true*. The 'if the null hypothesis is true' is crucial to the correct interpretation of the *P*-value; a common mistake is to omit this phrase, leading to the erroneous belief that the *P*-value represents the probability of the sample data arising by chance.

6.3.4 Making a decision using the *P*-value

According to the evidence obtained from our sample, we make a judgment about whether the data are consistent with the null hypothesis; this leads to a **decision** whether or not to reject the null hypothesis.

- If the observed results are *not* consistent with what we would expect *if the null hypothesis were true*, we conclude that we have enough evidence to **reject** the null hypothesis. We say that the result of the test is **statistically significant**.
- If, however, the observed results *are* consistent with what we would expect if the null hypothesis were true, we **do not reject** the null hypothesis. We say that the result of the test is **non-significant**.

Although semantically they may appear to be the same, we should note that *not rejecting* the null hypothesis is not synonymous with *accepting* the null hypothesis. Either we have enough evidence to reject the null hypothesis or we do not have enough evidence to reject it; the latter case does not imply that there is necessarily enough evidence to *accept* H_0. This can be likened to the situation in a law court – an analogy is drawn between the presumption of innocence and the null hypothesis. If there is enough evidence, the defendant will be found 'guilty' of the charge against him. If there is not enough evidence, the defendant will be found 'not guilty'. This does not prove that he is 'innocent', only that there is insufficient evidence to establish his guilt.

The *P*-value allows us to determine whether we have enough evidence to reject the null hypothesis in favour of the alternative hypothesis.

- If the *P*-value is very small, then it is unlikely that we could have obtained the observed results if the null hypothesis were true, so we reject H_0.
- If the *P*-value is very large, then there is a high chance that we could have obtained the observed results if the null hypothesis were true, and we do not reject H_0.

Clearly, distinguishing between large and small *P*-values is crucial to the decision-making process. We have to decide, *before we collect the data*, what constitutes a large or a small *P*-value, i.e. we have to choose a cut-off value, termed the **significance level** of the test. The choice of significance level is dependent on the nature of the data and the circumstances of the investigation.

It makes sense to choose a very low value for the significance level, say 0.01, if we want to err on the side of caution in rejecting H_0. This means that if, from our sample, we obtain a *P*-value which is less than 0.01, we reject the null hypothesis; we say the result is *significant at the 1% level*. For example, in investigating a rather costly novel antibiotic treatment, we would want to be very confident of its benefits over existing, and cheaper, products before introducing it into clinical practice. We might choose a much higher value, say 0.10, in initial testing of the efficacy of a new potential vaccine against a presently incurable infectious disease which is causing great economic loss. This ensures that a marginal benefit is not overlooked.

An arbitrary cut-off point of 0.05 is often chosen for the significance level such that if $P < 0.05$ then H_0 is rejected, and if $P \geq 0.05$ then H_0 is not rejected. Further distinctions are sometimes made by using asterisks to distinguish between very highly significant (*** representing $P < 0.001$), highly significant (** representing $0.001 < P < 0.01$), significant (* representing $0.01 < P < 0.05$) and non-significant (NS representing $P > 0.05$). *We stress that these values are entirely arbitrary and should not be taken as definitive.* You should avoid the asterisks and, where possible, *quote the exact P-value* invariably provided in computer output for the relevant hypothesis test. Then, your decision whether or not to reject H_0 can be substantiated by the reader. Remember, the smaller the *P*-value, the greater the evidence against H_0.

6.3.5 Deriving the *P*-value

Naturally, a vital link in the whole hypothesis test procedure is the relationship between the value of the **test statistic** and the **P-value**. In the chapters which follow we give the relevant formula for each test statistic corresponding to a specific hypothesis test. It is particularly important, in the context of this general explanatory chapter, that you understand that each test statistic has a known theoretical distribution. This means that its value obtained from a particular set of sample data can be compared to its known distribution to determine the *P*-value (the probability of obtaining the observed value of the test statistic if the null hypothesis is true). Typically, the known distribution of the test statistic is Normal, t, F or χ^2.

If you are performing a computer analysis, you will find the *P*-value you need in the computer output. If necessary, you can obtain the *P*-value by referring the test statistic to the table of its distribution, usually using both tail areas (two-sided test), but occasionally, a single tail area (one-sided test – see Section 6.3.1). You may have to *interpolate* (estimate the value between two tabulated values) when you use the table if the required value is not contained in the table. For example, if the degrees of freedom of the test statistic (see Section 6.3.6) are 35, Table A.3 has tabulated percentage points for degrees of freedom of 30 and 40 only. You would estimate the required percentage point as being midway between that for 30 and that for 40 degrees of freedom.

6.3.6 The degrees of freedom of the test statistic

You will find that the term **degrees of freedom** (***df***) occurs frequently in statistical analysis. If we are using tables to relate the value of the test statistic to the *P*-value, we generally have to know the degrees of freedom of the relevant distribution of our test statistic. The degrees of freedom of a statistic are the number of independent observations contributing to that statistic, i.e. the number of observations available to evaluate that statistic minus the number of restrictions on those observations. The easiest way of calculating the degrees of freedom of any statistic is to take them as the difference between the number of observations we have in our sample and the number of parameters we have to estimate in order to evaluate that statistic.

So, for example, suppose we are estimating a population variance, σ^2, of a variable, x, in a sample of size n by its sample statistic, s^2, given by

$$s^2 = \frac{\sum (x - \bar{x})^2}{(n-1)}$$

We have to estimate the mean in order to evaluate the numerator, and so the degrees of freedom of s^2 are $(n-1)$.

6.3.7 Quoting a confidence interval

The use of a **confidence interval** diminishes, to some extent, the reliance on the *P*-value and the subsequent significance or non-significance of a test result. We measure the precision of a sample statistic as an estimate of the population parameter by its standard error. This is used in the calculation of the confidence interval for the parameter (see Section 4.5). A small sample leads to a less precise parameter estimate than a large sample, so that its standard error will also be larger. Consequently, the confidence interval for a parameter derived from a small sample will be wider than that derived from a large sample. When we have a wide confidence interval, we need to look at the limits carefully and consider their implications, whether or not the test is significant.

Thus, if we want a full statement of the result of a hypothesis test, we should supplement the P-value by an estimate of the effect of interest (for example, the estimated difference in means if H_0 states that two population means are equal) with the relevant confidence interval. Then we, and others, can make an informed judgment about the results obtained from the hypothesis test. We will have an understanding of what is happening, rather than simply deciding whether or not to reject the null hypothesis.

6.3.8 Summary of the hypothesis test procedure

We assimilate this whole hypothesis test procedure by generalizing it to a six-step procedure:

1. Specify the **null hypothesis, H_0** and the **alternative hypothesis** (by default, we adopt a two-sided test unless a different alternative hypothesis is specified).
2. **Collect** the data and **look** at it, diagrammatically if possible, to investigate its distribution. Many tests make distributional assumptions about the data: check the assumptions underlying the test.
3. On the computer, select the **appropriate test**, or, by hand, calculate the appropriate **test statistic** using the sample data.
4. Relate the calculated value of the test statistic to a ***P*-value**.
5. Consider the P-value to judge whether the data are consistent with the null hypothesis. Then **decide** whether or not to reject the null hypothesis.
6. If appropriate, calculate the **confidence interval** for the effect of interest, phrased in terms of the parameter specification in the null hypothesis.

We assign significance to the result in the course of this procedure, and therefore this is sometimes called a *significance test*.

As you will see, the choice of test is not always simple – it depends on the nature of the data, the null hypothesis and the assumptions underlying the test. It is a logical procedure, and the flow charts in Appendix C will guide you through the process.

6.4 TYPE I AND TYPE II ERRORS

6.4.1 Making the wrong decision in a hypothesis test

You must recognize that the final decision whether or not to reject the null hypothesis may be incorrect. As a frame of reference, we discuss the common situation in which we are interested in comparing two population means using independent samples selected from these populations (see Section 7.4.1). The null hypothesis is that the two population means are equal or, equivalently, that the difference between these two population means is zero. Consider the example introduced in Section 6.3.1; we have the plasma magnesium levels for two groups of cattle, one kept indoors and the other put out on spring grass for the past week. A lower level of plasma magnesium in the outdoor cattle would suggest a risk of grass staggers. Our null hypothesis is that the mean values of plasma magnesium do not differ in the two populations from which we have taken our samples.

- We may find that the result of the test is significant. In this case, we reject the null hypothesis at the stated level of significance, and infer that the two population means differ. If this inference is incorrect, and in reality the two means are equal, then we have rejected the null hypothesis when we should not have rejected it (i.e. when it is true). We are making a **Type I error** (see Table 6.1).
- Alternatively, we may find that the result of the test is not significant. Then, we do not reject the null hypothesis at the stated level of significance, so we cannot infer that the

Table 6.1 The errors in hypothesis testing.

Description	Reject H_0	Do not reject H_0
H_0 true	Type I error	Correct decision
H_0 false	Correct decision	Type II error

two population means are different. If this is incorrect, and in reality the two means differ, then we have not rejected the null hypothesis when we should have rejected it (i.e. when it is false). We are making a **Type II error** (see Table 6.1).

6.4.2 The probability of making a wrong decision

It is crucial that you understand the importance of these two errors and what each represents as they both play a role in determining the optimal size of an experiment (see Section 12.3) – a critical design consideration.

- The **probability of making a Type I error**, denoted by α (alpha), is the significance level of the test. It is the probability of incorrectly rejecting the null hypothesis. So if $\alpha = 0.05$, we have a 1 in 20 chance of rejecting the null hypothesis when it is true. It is easy to control the size of α because we choose, at the design stage, the level of α which will lead to rejection of H_0, i.e. we decide we will reject the null hypothesis if $P < \alpha$.
- The **probability of making a Type II error** is usually designated by β (beta). It is the probability of not rejecting the null hypothesis when the null hypothesis is false. We control β at the design stage of the experiment. By giving consideration to the factors which affect β (i.e. the probability of a Type I error, the sample size, the size of the effect of interest, and the variability in the data), we can design our experiment so that β is small and controlled at a particular level. We explain how these inter-relationships affect β in Section 12.3.

In fact, instead of thinking about β, we usually consider its complement, $1 - \beta$, (often multiplied by 100 and expressed as a percentage). This is called the **power** of the test. It is the probability of rejecting the null hypothesis when the null hypothesis is false. In an experiment investigating the difference between two treatment means, the power of the test is the chance of detecting a treatment effect if it exists. We gener-ally design our experiment so that the power of the test is as large as possible (recognizing that it can never be 100%), typically exceeding 80% (see Section 12.3). In general, larger experiments are more powerful, implying that they have a greater chance of correctly detecting a treatment difference.

6.5 THE DISTINCTION BETWEEN STATISTICAL AND BIOLOGICAL SIGNIFICANCE

We should never consider the result of a hypothesis test expressed by the *P*-value and the decision whether or not to reject the null hypothesis in isolation. We must relate the result to the biological or clinical implications of the conclusion drawn from the test. A result that is **statistically significant** is not necessarily **biologically** or **clinically important**, and vice versa. Biological/clinical importance is a matter of individual judgment, and this may be difficult to discern in borderline cases.

Note that the *power* of a test (representing the ability of the test to detect a real effect, e.g. a treatment difference) is proportional to the *sample size* (see Section 12.3). The larger the sample, the greater the power, so that a large sample has a greater chance of detecting a real treatment difference than a small one. Thus, we may find that even small treatment differences which are biologically unimportant are statistically significant in large samples, whereas we may find that large and biologically important differences in small samples are not statistically significant.

For example, in field trials of modifications of semen diluents for frozen semen it is not uncommon to measure improvements in conception of only a percentage point or two. For such improvements to be statistically significant, many thousands of inseminations must be carried out under controlled conditions. Even then, statistical significance may be borderline. Nevertheless, a consistent improvement in fertility of the order of a percentage point represents a very substantial economic return and may be worth pursuing if the new diluent is not expensive to prepare.

Here then, biological importance may outweigh statistical significance.

In contrast, many anaesthetics used in veterinary medicine are known to cause minor, but consistent, variations in blood pressure. If measured over a sufficiently large sample, these effects would clearly be statistically significant, but normally they are of little biological importance because the effects are slight, and have no practical implications in the healthy animal undergoing elective surgery.

6.6 THE CONFIDENCE INTERVAL APPROACH TO HYPOTHESIS TESTING

We can use a confidence interval alone to make a decision to reject the null hypothesis about an effect of interest rather than going through the hypothesis testing procedure outlined in Section 6.3.8.

If, for example, we are interested in investigating whether two population means are equal, we first formulate the null hypothesis (that the two means are equal) and the alternative hypothesis (generally, that they are not); we then calculate the appropriate (usually, the 95%) confidence interval for the difference in the two population means. The 95% confidence interval for the difference in two population means is the interval within which the true difference in means is contained with 95% certainty (see Section 4.5). It represents the plausible range of values for the difference in population means. Zero is an implausible value for the difference in means if it lies outside the 95% confidence interval. So, if the confidence interval does not span zero, we would conclude that it is unlikely (the chance is at most 5%) that the difference in population means could be zero, and we would reject the null hypothesis that the means are equal at the 5% level of significance.

To summarize, there are two approaches to testing a null hypothesis.

- We can calculate the appropriate test statistic and determine the associated *P*-value. This represents the probability of obtaining the observed value of the test statistic if the null hypothesis is true. We reject the null hypothesis if the *P*-value is small. The whole process is called a hypothesis test or a significance test.
- We can calculate the 95% (say) confidence interval for the appropriate parameter expression (e.g. the difference in population means, $\mu_1 - \mu_2$, if we are testing $H_0: \mu_1 = \mu_2$); we reject the null hypothesis at the 5% level if the value of the parameter expression under the null hypothesis lies outside the confidence limits. The value of the parameter expression under H_0 is usually zero if we are investigating differences; the value is usually unity if we are investigating ratios such as the odds ratio or relative risk (see Section 5.2.3).

The confidence interval approach to hypothesis testing has the advantage that it is more informative than the corresponding significance test; it provides an interval estimate of the effect of interest as well as allowing us to make a decision to reject the null hypothesis. However, it is more restrictive than the significance test because we are limited to making this decision by considering only one level of significance, e.g. 5% for a 95% confidence interval. The corresponding significance test provides an exact *P*-value, which allows us to make a decision to reject the null hypothesis, as well as indicating the strength of belief we have in the truth of the null hypothesis.

6.7 COLLECTING OUR THOUGHTS ON CONFIDENCE INTERVALS

We have now introduced you to the three different uses of a confidence interval:

1. It is an indicator of the precision of the parameter estimate (see Section 4.5). A wide confidence interval indicates poor precision.
2. It provides a means of distinguishing between biological importance and statistical significance (see Section 6.5). The result of a hypothesis test that two means are equal may be significant, whilst the confidence interval for the difference in the two means is very narrow

and its limits only just greater than zero; here we may have statistical significance but it may not be biologically important. Alternatively, the result of the test may be non-significant, whilst the confidence interval is very wide, with the upper limit being very much greater than zero; here there is the potential for a biologically important difference although there is no statistical significance.

3. It can be used to test a null hypothesis about the parameter of interest (see Section 6.6). For example, the null hypothesis that there is no difference between two treatment means can be rejected if the confidence interval for the difference excludes zero.

A summary of the calculations of confidence intervals is given in Appendix B. A full discussion of confidence intervals appears in Gardner and Altman (1989). An accompanying computer program (Confidence Interval Analysis) is available for the calculations of confidence intervals for commonly used parameters.

EXERCISES

The statements in questions 6.1–6.5 are either TRUE or FALSE.

6.1 The null hypothesis for a test to compare two means states that:
(a) The sample means are equal.
(b) There is no difference between the population means.
(c) There is no significant difference between the population means.
(d) The probability of there being a difference between the means is zero.
(e) A difference between the means is not expected.

6.2 A one-tailed test:
(a) Refers only to the right-hand side of a distribution.
(b) Is more powerful than a two-tailed test.
(c) Is the more usual test.

(d) Requires knowledge, independent of the results, that the treatment effect, if it exists, can be in one direction only.
(e) Is used when group sizes are small.

6.3 The P-value gives the probability of:
(a) Obtaining a result as, or more, extreme than the one observed.
(b) The null hypothesis arising by chance alone.
(c) The null hypothesis being true.
(d) The observed results arising if the null hypothesis is true.
(e) The discrepancy between the observed values and those under the null hypothesis being due to chance.

6.4 $P < 0.01$ means that:
(a) There is less than a 1/100 chance that the null hypothesis is true.
(b) There is a greater than 99% chance that the alternative hypothesis is true.
(c) The probability of obtaining the observed results if the null hypothesis is true is less than 1%.
(d) The probability that the observed result has arisen by chance is less than 1%.
(e) There is a greater than 99% chance that the null hypothesis is false.

6.5 A test statistic is:
(a) The mean.
(b) The difference between the means.
(c) Assumed to follow a theoretical distribution.
(d) Less than 0.05 if the result of the test is significant.
(e) Only useful if the sample size is large.

6.6 A novel antispasmodic drug is being tested for its effectiveness in preventing smooth muscle contractions (a quantitative variable measured as tension in grams) on pieces of gut in an organ bath. It is tested against a control which is the vehicle minus the drug. State an appropriate null hypothesis and the alternative hypothesis for the test. How would the null hypothesis and the alternative hypothesis change if the novel drug were to be tested against an existing drug?

6.7 Ponies from the Sales need to be broken in. A trainer has his own methods for doing this effectively and wants to demonstrate the advantage of his system. He randomly allocates 15 of his ponies to be trained by his new system, the remaining 12 ponies being trained in the traditional manner. The ponies are tested to see if they will accept a bit and bridle one month after starting training. Any animal which refuses the bit and bridle is regarded as failing the test. What is the null hypothesis that you would investigate if you wanted to decide whether to adopt the new system? What is the alternative hypothesis?

Chapter 7

Hypothesis Tests 1 – The *t*-Test Comparing One or Two Means

7.1 LEARNING OBJECTIVES

By the end of this chapter, you should be able to:

- Distinguish between one- and two-sample tests.
- Distinguish between the experimental designs which lead to either paired or two-sample *t*-tests.
- List and verify the assumptions that underlie the paired and two-sample *t*-tests.
- Explain what is meant by the treatment effect in the context of the *t*-test.
- Relate the value of the test statistic in the *t*-test to the *P*-value.
- Draw appropriate conclusions from the *t*-test.
- Estimate the magnitude of the treatment effect when comparing means and calculate the relevant confidence interval.

7.2 REQUIREMENTS FOR HYPOTHESIS TESTS FOR COMPARING MEANS

7.2.1 The nature of the data

The *arithmetic mean*, a summary measure of location for a quantitative variable (see Section 2.6.1), is the focus of the hypothesis tests in this chapter. Suppose, for example, we are interested in measuring the stress of transportation of cattle (Nanda *et al.*, 1990). Cortisol is released from the adrenal gland in response to stressful situations; it is of interest to determine whether the mean of plasma cortisol measurement (ng/ml) during transport of dairy cows is different from that of cows at rest.

Before applying the methods described in this chapter and in Chapter 8, we must consider the nature of the data.

- There can be only a *single variable* of interest (e.g. plasma cortisol concentration).
- It must be measured on a *quantitative* scale (cortisol measurements are made in ng/ml).
- A further common feature is the assumption that the variable under investigation is *Normally* distributed (see Section 3.5.3). This is not unreasonable for biological measurements such as plasma cortisol. Note that if the sample size is large, then the sample mean is approximately Normally distributed even if the variable does not follow a Normal distribution (see Section 4.4.3), and we do not have to concern ourselves with the Normality of the data. However, as it is often difficult to distinguish a small sample from a large one, you should *not* ignore this assumption (see also Section 7.2.2).

In fact, the tests we discuss in this chapter are **robust** against a violation of the assumption of Normality; this implies that they are hardly affected if the data show a moderate departure from Normality (this is particularly the case if the sample sizes are equal in the two-sample comparison of means). Thus, in practice, approximate Normality is sufficient. We can verify this with a perfunctory plot of the data, perhaps using a box-and-whisker plot which highlights the median, the interquartile range and the extreme values (see Section 2.5.2(d)). Seldom will you find it necessary to delve into the more formal tests of Normality (see Section 3.5.3(e)) such as the Shapiro–

Wilk W test which is available in many statistical packages.

However, if there is a marked departure from Normality, there are two courses of action. Either we can transform the data in an attempt to achieve approximate Normality (see Section 12.2), or we can proceed to a suitable non-parametric test which makes no distributional assumptions (see Chapter 11).

7.2.2 The implications of sample size

In many animal investigations, it is not possible to assemble large numbers of subjects either on the grounds of cost or because of low disease incidence. The question of **sample size** is an important consideration. This section is concerned with the implications of sample size on the choice of hypothesis test. You can find details of how to estimate the sample size you need in Section 12.3.

If sample size refers to the total number of observations in the investigation, then:

- The distribution of the variable is difficult to establish for *very small* samples, each comprising, perhaps, only five or six observations. We advocate the use of the alternative *non-parametric methods* (see Chapter 11) for very small sample sizes, although you should be aware of the danger that very small samples may be unrepresentative of the population.
- If the sample size is *small* (say, less than 30), the test statistic follows a Student's *t*-distribution (see Section 3.5.4) provided the data are approximately Normally distributed (and the variances are equal in the two-sample comparison).
- If the sample size is *large*, the distribution of the test statistic is approximately Normal. We can take 'large' to be greater than 30 if the data are Normally distributed; alternatively, 'large' may be in excess of 100 if the data are not Normally distributed, but the extent of the deviation from Normality will influence our definition of 'large'.

In all the *t*-tests we discuss in this chapter, we assume that we have to use the sample data to estimate any population variances of interest.

It is difficult to clarify the distinction between large and small samples in the context of the *t*-test. You will find that many statistics texts distinguish between small and large samples by relating the test statistic either to the *t*-distribution (for small samples, equal variances in two-sample comparison) or to the Normal distribution (for large samples, equal or unequal variances). Since the *t*-distribution approaches Normality for large sample sizes, the *P*-value is virtually identical using either approach when the sample size is large. We therefore recommend the simpler practice of:

- Checking the data for Normality, and transforming, if necessary to achieve Normality.
- Assuming the test statistic follows the *t*-distribution (an exception is the modified approach discussed in Section 7.4.5).

7.2.3 Study designs

A most important aspect of **design** in this chapter is the *grouping* of the data.

- Very occasionally, we find it necessary to investigate the parameter of interest – in this case, the mean – in a **single group** of observations. We may wish to determine whether the mean assumes a particular value in the population; for example, in an investigation of metabolic profiles (total protein, albumin, calcium, phosphate and lactate dehydrogenase) of cattle kept together in groups, we might sample representative animals to estimate their group mean for each variable which we could then compare to a known value from a larger population. Alternatively, the comparison might be made with a particular set of published values.
- More commonly, however, we are interested in comparing the means of **two groups** of observations, these groups comprising either *independent* or *paired* observations (see Section 5.8.4).
- Sometimes, we may wish to compare the observations in **more than two groups**. The

correct approach to analysing such data is an **analysis of variance** (see Section 8.5). The distinction between independent and dependent observations is retained in the analysis even when there are several groups.

7.3 ONE-SAMPLE *t*-TESTS

7.3.1 Introduction

Occasionally, we may be interested in investigating whether the mean of a single group of observations takes a specific value. For example, the pigs in a particular pen on a farm are showing what appears to be a low daily live weight gain compared to the usual growth rate for this farm. We perform a test to determine whether the mean live weight gain of the pigs in this pen supports the hypothesis that they are growing at the expected rate for pigs on this farm.

7.3.2 Assumptions

The one-sample *t*-test assumes that the sample data are randomly selected from a Normally distributed population of values. As we said earlier (see Section 7.2), the test is hardly affected if the data deviate from Normality except in extreme cases where the data are visibly non-Normal. Then we may be able to Normalize the data by an appropriate transformation (see Section 12.2), typically a logarithmic transformation, in which case the test statistic is calculated using the transformed data values. Naturally, we need to convert the confidence limits obtained by using the transformed data back to the original scale of measurement. Alternatively, we can use an appropriate *non-parametric* test such as the **sign test** (see Section 11.3), the **Kolmogorov–Smirnov test** or the **runs test**. We refer you to Siegel and Castellan (1988) for details.

7.3.3 The approach

We present the approach in general terms and illustrate it using the pig example in Section 7.3.4.

1. Specify the **null hypothesis**, H_0, that the true population mean of the variable of interest is equal to a defined value, μ_0. Generally, the **alternative hypothesis** is that the mean is not equal to the specified value and this leads to a *two-tailed* test.

2. **Collect** the data and **display** them by a line plot, a simple histogram, a stem-and-leaf plot or a box-and-whisker plot. From the diagram, check the *assumption* that the data are approximately Normally distributed.

3. Calculate the **test statistic** as the difference between the sample mean ($\bar{x}$) and the specified value of the population mean under test (μ_0), divided by the estimated standard error of the mean ($s/\sqrt{n}$), where s is the estimated standard deviation and n is the sample size. We denote the test statistic by $Test_1$ to distinguish it from the *t*-distribution which it approximates.

$$Test_1 = \frac{\bar{x} - \mu_0}{s/\sqrt{n}} \quad \text{with } n-1 \text{ degrees of freedom.}$$

4. Obtain the **P-value** by referring the calculated value of the test statistic to the table of the *t*-distribution (Table A.3).

5. Use the *P*-value to judge whether the data are consistent with the null hypothesis. Then **decide** whether or not to reject the null hypothesis. Usually, we reject the null hypothesis if $P < 0.05$.

6. Quote the **confidence interval** for the mean because it allows you to judge the importance of the finding (see Section 6.3.7). The 95% confidence interval is

$$\bar{x} - t_{0.05}\frac{s}{\sqrt{n}} \quad \text{to} \quad \bar{x} + t_{0.05}\frac{s}{\sqrt{n}}$$

where $t_{0.05}$ is the critical value obtained from the table of the *t*-distribution with $n - 1$ degrees of freedom; it gives a total tail area probability of 0.05.

7.3.4 Example

Table 7.1 shows the average daily live weight gains of a random sample of 36 growing pigs in a rearing unit. The rearing unit expects growth

577 596 594 612 600 584 618 627 588 601 606 559 615 607 608 591 565 586	**Table 7.1** Average daily live weight gains (g) of 36 growing pigs.
621 623 598 602 581 631 570 595 603 605 616 574 578 600 596 619 636 589	

Mean, $\bar{x} = 599.194\,g$
Standard deviation, $s = 18.656\,g$
Standard error, $s/\sqrt{n} = 18.66/\sqrt{36} = 3.109\,g$

Frequency	Stem and leaf
1	55 . 9
1	56 . 5
4	57 . 0478
5	58 . 14689
6	59 . 145668
9	60 . 001235678
5	61 . 25689
3	62 . 137
2	63 . 16

Stem width: 10.00
Each leaf: 1 case(s)

Fig. 7.1   Stem-and-leaf plot of average daily live weight gains (g) of pigs.

rates to average 607 g per day for this stage of growth based on current performance indicators. Are these values consistent with an average gain of around 607 g per day?

1. H_0 is that μ_0, the true mean daily live weight gain, is 607 g. The alternative hypothesis is that it is not.
2. The stem-and-leaf plot in Fig. 7.1 shows that the data are approximately Normally distributed.
3. The sample mean is 599.194 g/day and the estimated standard deviation is 18.656 g/day. The test statistic is

$$Test_1 = \frac{\bar{x} - \mu}{s/\sqrt{n}} = \frac{|599.194 - 607|}{3.109} = 2.51$$

with 35 degrees of freedom.

4. We can see from Table A.3 that $0.01 < P < 0.02$. If we had used the computer, we would have obtained $P = 0.017$; so we have a less than 2% chance of getting a mean live weight gain as low as 599.2 g/day if the null hypothesis is true.

5. The null hypothesis is therefore unlikely to be true. We reject H_0, and conclude that the data values are inconsistent with a daily mean gain in weight of 607 g.
6. The 95% confidence interval for the true mean daily live weight gain is $599.194 \pm 2.03(3.109) = (592.88, 605.51)\,g$, where 2.03 is the value in the t table (Table A.3) with 35 degrees of freedom, corresponding to a total tail area probability of 0.05.

We could test this hypothesis using only the confidence interval (see Section 6.6). We can see that the range of values, 592.9 to 605.5 g, within which we expect the true mean daily weight gain to lie with 95% certainty, does not include the value 607 g. Thus we conclude ($P < 0.05$) that the sample is not drawn from a population with a daily mean weight gain of 607 g.

The test reveals that the pigs have a significantly poorer growth rate than expected. The confidence interval indicates that the true average weight gain may even be as low as 593 g per day. There may be a cause for concern in the unit; an investigation of the causes, whether infectious or environmental, is indicated.

7.4 TWO-SAMPLE *t*-TESTS

7.4.1 Introduction

The **two-sample *t*-test** (**unpaired *t*-test**) is one of the most frequently used and, perhaps, misused tests in statistics. You risk misusing the test when you have not properly investigated the assumptions on which it is based. The two-sample *t*-test is used to compare the means in two *independent* groups of observations using representative samples.

7.4.2 Assumptions

The validity of the two-sample *t*-test depends on various assumptions being satisfied. In particular:

- Each animal must be *randomly* selected from the population.
- The two samples must be *independent*; in order to achieve this in an experimental study, we randomly allocate each animal to one of the groups.
- Furthermore, the variable of interest should be approximately *Normally* distributed in each population from which the samples are taken. A small departure from Normality is not crucial and leads to only a marginal loss in power, i.e. the test is *robust* against violations of this assumption.
- In addition, the variability of the observations in each group, as measured by the two *variances*, should be approximately *equal*, in statistical jargon said to be **homoscedastic**. This assumption is important; we may verify this casually by eye or, more formally, by a Levene's test (see Section 8.4) or an *F*-test (see Section 8.3). Be warned, however, that the *F*-test is particularly sensitive to non-Normality of the data, whatever the sample sizes. If the variances do not differ significantly (and the other assumptions are also valid), then we can proceed to the test described in Section 7.4.3. If, however, the variances in the two groups are not equal (i.e. we have heteroscedasticity) we may apply the modified *t*-test, explained in Section 7.4.5.

If we cannot find an appropriate transformation to satisfy the assumptions, there are alternative non-parametric tests to the two-sample *t*-test, such as the **Wilcoxon rank sum test** (see Section 11.5).

7.4.3 The approach – equal variances

1. Specify the **null hypothesis** that the two population means are equal. Generally, the **alternative hypothesis** is that these means are not equal and this leads to a two-tailed test.
2. **Collect** the data and **display** them in a diagram. If the sample size in each group is relatively small, produce a dot diagram (see Section 2.5.2(a)). If the sample size is large, then it may be easier to show the median, interquartile range and extreme values of the response variable for each group in a box-and-whisker plot (see Section 2.5.2(d)). Either way, by studying the diagram, we can assess the approximate distribution of the observations in each group, and check the Normality assumption. We can also make an appraisal of their variability from the diagram; we check the assumption of equal variance by performing an *F*-test (see Section 8.3) or Levene's test (see Section 8.4). Usually, one of these tests will be included in the computer output.
3. The **test statistic** is the difference in the sample means divided by its estimated standard error. The computer package will perform this calculation but it is useful to have its derivation. The test statistic follows the *t*-distribution. It is

$$Test_2 = \frac{\bar{x}_1 - \bar{x}_2}{\sqrt{s^2 \left(\dfrac{1}{n_1} + \dfrac{1}{n_2} \right)}}$$

with $n_1 + n_2 - 2$ degrees of freedom

where, for the *i*th sample ($i = 1, 2$):

n_i the number of observations,

$\bar{x}_i$ is the sample mean,

s_i is the estimated standard deviation, and

$$s^2 = \frac{(n_1 - 1)s_1^2 + (n_2 - 1)s_2^2}{n_1 + n_2 - 2}$$

is the pooled estimate of variance.

Note that the denominator of $Test_2$ is calculated assuming that the true variances in the two groups are approximately equal but unknown; we estimate them from the samples as s_1^2 and s_2^2. Sometimes, we find that the two variances are significantly different when we perform an *F*-test or Levene's test. Then we modify the test statistic (see Section 7.4.4).

4. Usually, we obtain the **P-value** from computer output. If you have calculated the test statistic by hand, you can derive the *P*-value by referring the calculated value of the test statistic to the table of the *t*-distribution (Table A.3).
5. Use the *P*-value to judge whether the data are consistent with the null hypothesis. Then **decide** whether or not to reject the null hypothesis. Usually, although not necessarily, we reject the null hypothesis if *P* < 0.05.
6. Calculate the relevant **confidence interval** (in this instance, for the difference in the two group means) in order to promote understanding (see Section 6.3.7). If the 95% confidence interval for the difference in two means is not included in the computer output, we can calculate it as

$$(\bar{x}_1 - \bar{x}_2) \pm t_{0.05} \mathrm{SE}(\bar{x}_1 - \bar{x}_2)$$
$$= (\bar{x}_1 - \bar{x}_2) \pm t_{0.05} \sqrt{s^2(1/n_1 + 1/n_2)}$$

where $t_{0.05}$ is the critical value obtained from the table of the *t*-distribution with $n_1 + n_2 - 2$ degrees of freedom, and s^2 is the combined estimate of variance (assuming the two variances are equal) used in *Test*$_2$.

As the *sample size increases*, the critical value in the table of the *t*-distribution (Table A.3) which corresponds to a given probability, approaches that in the table of the Standard Normal distribution (Table A.1). In particular, the tabulated critical value, $t_{0.05}$, in the table of the *t*-distribution for a two-tailed probability of 0.05, is close to or equal to 1.96 (often approximated by 2) when the degrees of freedom are very large, say greater than about 200.

7.4.4 Example

Consider the comparison of the mean body weights at the time of mating in one group of ewes which have been flushed (put on a high plane of nutrition for several weeks prior to mating) and the other which have not.

1. The null hypothesis is that the mean body weights in the populations of flushed and control ewes are equal; the two-sided alternative is that they are different.

Table 7.2 Body weights (kg) in a group of 24 flushed ewes and in a control group of 30 ewes.

Controls			Flushed		
62.5	63.9	69.2	70.7	67.8	69.8
66.8	65.7	62.6	71.8	66.8	68.1
69.5	67.2	61.1	64.9	67.0	66.0
64.1	65.2	61.8	68.2	67.1	69.4
65.3	63.5	69.6	69.4	67.6	69.8
65.6	65.3	71.1	64.4	66.1	67.9
66.4	65.1	67.0	66.9	62.7	66.2
66.1	64.8	67.5	69.4	64.6	64.2
68.6	67.4	68.2			
62.5	66.0	63.6			

2. Each ewe in a random sample of 54 ewes is randomly allocated to the flushed or control group. Table 7.2 shows the weights of two randomly selected samples of 24 flushed and 30 control ewes. We can see from the box-and-whisker plot in Fig. 7.2 that the observations in each sample are approximately Normally distributed since, in each case, the median is more or less centrally situated in the box designated by the 25th and 75th percentiles and between the 2.5 and 97.5 percentile values. Furthermore, the range of observations in each sample appears similar, although the distribution of weights of the flushed group is slightly higher than that of the controls. Display 7.1 shows a typical computer output for the results of the two-sample *t*-test. The Levene test (Section 8.4), a formal hypothesis test for the equality of the two variances, is included and shows that the two variances are not significantly different, $P = 0.62$.
3. The test statistic for the two-sample *t*-test is 2.4 (Display 7.1 – equal variances assumed). It is derived as

$$Test_2 = \frac{\text{Difference in means}}{\text{SE (difference in means)}} = \frac{1.5933}{0.655}$$
$$= 2.43 \quad \text{with } 24 + 30 - 2 = 52 \; df$$

where SE (difference in means)

$$= \sqrt{\frac{23(2.52)^2 + 29(2.497)^2}{24 + 30 - 2}\left(\frac{1}{24} + \frac{1}{30}\right)} \; \text{kg}$$

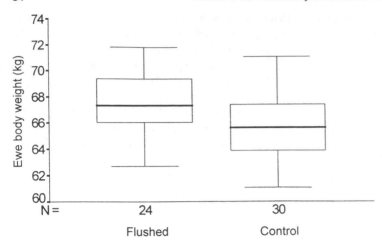

Fig. 7.2 Box-and-whisker plot of body weight (kg) in two groups of ewes.

Display 7.1 Typical computer output for the two-sample *t*-test: body weights (kg) of flushed and control ewes before mating (data of Table 7.2).

Group statistics

Group		N	Mean	Std. deviation	Std. error mean
Ewe body weight	Flushed	24	67.3667	2.2525	0.4598
	Control	30	65.7733	2.4972	0.4559

Independent samples test

		Levene's test for equality of variances		*t*-test for equality of means						95% confidence interval of the mean	
		F	Sig.	*t*	*df*	Sig. (2-tailed)	Mean difference	Std. error difference	Lower	Upper
Ewe body weight	Equal variances assumed	0.253	0.617	2.4	52	0.018	1.5933	0.6551	0.2788	2.9079
	Equal variances not assumed			2.5	51.2	0.017	1.5933	0.6475	0.2935	2.8931

N.B. The first line of the *t*-test result (equal variances assumed) is relevant in this instance because the result of Levene's test for the equality of variances indicates that the two variances are not significantly different (*P* = 0.617).

4. The *P*-value shown in Display 7.1 is *P* = 0.018, indicating that the chance of obtaining a difference in means as large as 1.59 kg is only 1.8% if the null hypothesis is true. Note that if relying on hand calculations, we would refer 2.43 to Table A.3 with 52 degrees of freedom, and find that $0.01 < P < 0.02$.

5. The null hypothesis, that there is no difference in the mean body weights in the two populations, is unlikely to be true. We therefore reject the null hypothesis in favour of the alternative hypothesis that there is a difference in the mean body weights. The mean ewe body weights are significantly different with the mean ewe body weight in the flushed ewes being, on average, 1.59 kg greater.

6. The 95% confidence interval for the true difference in means ranges between 0.28 and 2.91 kg. Note that these confidence limits are calculated as $1.59 \pm 2.007 \, (0.655)$ kg, where 2.007 is the value in the table of the *t*-distribution (Table A.3), corresponding to a two-sided *P* of 0.05 with 52 degrees of freedom. The significantly higher mean body weight of the flushed ewes implies an effect on metabolism and is expected to be associated with an optimal ovulation rate.

The confidence interval for the difference in means, 0.28 to 2.91 kg, excludes zero. Zero is the value of the parameter specification in the null hypothesis, i.e. H_0 is that the difference in means is zero. The fact that zero lies outside the 95% confidence limits provides an alternative approach to testing the hypothesis (see Section 6.6), resulting in the decision to reject H_0 at the 5% level of significance.

7.4.5 Modified *t*-test – unequal variances

If the variances in the two groups are *not* equal, then the pooled estimate of variance, s^2 used in the denominator of the test statistic, *Test₂*, described in Section 7.4.3, is not appropriate. Some computer packages offer an alternatively derived test statistic in the situations where the variances are not equal. If you have to resort to hand calculations, you should evaluate a modified test statistic, *Test₃*.

$$Test_3 = \frac{\bar{x}_1 - \bar{x}_2}{\sqrt{\dfrac{s_1^2}{n_1} + \dfrac{s_2^2}{n_2}}}$$

However, this test statistic does *not* follow the *t*-distribution, so that evaluation of the *P*-value is not straightforward. For large sample sizes (say, greater than 50), *Test₃* follows an approximately Normal distribution. We can then obtain the relevant *P*-value from the table of the Standard Normal distribution (Table A.1). If the sample sizes are not large, we must either transform the data to achieve equal variance or substitute an appropriate *non-parametric* method, such as the Wilcoxon rank sum test (see Section 11.5), for the two-sample *t*-test.

7.5 THE PAIRED *t*-TEST

7.5.1 Introduction

We use the **paired *t*-test** when two representative samples selected from the population comprise *dependent* or *paired* observations; for example, when we compare the preprandial serum glucose levels in dogs with insulin-dependent diabetes mellitus fed low- and high-fibre diets in a randomized cross-over trial (see Section 7.5.4).

7.5.2 Assumptions

The validity of the paired *t*-test is based on the assumptions that:

(a) There is *random* selection. The different circumstances are (see Section 5.8.4):
   - Self pairing: each animal is randomly selected from the population, and used as its own control.
   - Natural pairing: each pair of animals (e.g. litter mates) is randomly selected from the population of such pairs.
   - Matched pairing: each animal is randomly selected from the population, and is paired with a matched animal.

(b) In an experimental study, there is random allocation:
   - Self pairing: each animal is randomly allocated to receive one of the two treatments initially; it then receives the other treatment later.

- Natural and matched pairing: one member of the pair is randomly allocated to one of the two treatments; the other member receives the second treatment.

(c) The *differences* between the pairs of observations are approximately *Normally* distributed even though the original observations in the groups may not be.

If we suspect that the distribution of the differences is markedly not Normal, and the sample size is adequate, we may take an appropriate transformation of the observations before subtraction to Normalize the distribution of the differences (see Section 12.2). We perform the paired *t*-test on the differences of the transformed data.

If we cannot find a suitable transformation to Normalize the data, or if the sample size is small, we should use a *non-parametric test* such as the **Wilcoxon signed rank test** (see Section 11.4).

7.5.3 The approach

1. Specify the **null hypothesis** that the mean of the differences between the paired observations in the population is zero. As there is likely to be considerably less biological variation exhibited within pairs than between unmatched individuals, it is advantageous to focus the statistical analysis on the differences between the observations within each pair. Usually, the alternative hypothesis states that this mean difference is not zero, and this leads to a two-tailed test.

   Thus, we can see that the hypothesis test is reduced to a *one sample test of differences* in which the population mean (of differences), μ_0, equals zero. We employ the hypothesis test procedure used in Section 7.3 for the one-sample test on the differences between the pairs. These differences replace the raw data to create a new variable of interest. Consequently, the assumptions on which this test is based relate to the differences and not to the observations in each group.

2. **Collect** and **display** the data. Provided the sample size is manageable, we can display the data in a dot diagram, similar to that described for the two-sample *t*-test. In addition, we join each pair of points by a line. From the diagram, we are able to discern the average magnitude and direction of the differences. If most of the lines slope in the same direction, either mostly upwards or mostly downwards, then we can surmise that the effect of interest, the mean difference, is unlikely to be zero. If, however, the lines are approximately parallel to the horizontal axis or if they exhibit no consistency in their direction, then it is likely that the mean difference is zero. Furthermore, a simple dot plot or, if the sample size is large, a histogram, stem-and-leaf plot or a box-and-whisker plot of the differences will establish the approximate Normality, or otherwise, of their distribution.

3. When we are using a computer, we have to choose the appropriate test. The **test statistic** is similar in form to that used in the one-sample test. It follows the *t*-distribution, and is given by

$$Test_4 = \frac{\bar{d}}{\text{SE}(\bar{d})} = \frac{\bar{d}}{s_d / \sqrt{n}}$$

with $n - 1$ degrees of freedom

where

n is the number of pairs in the sample,
$\bar{d}$ is the mean of the differences in the sample,
$\text{SE}(\bar{d})$ is the estimated standard error of the differences, and
s_d is the estimated standard deviation of the differences.

4. Determine the **P-value** from the computer output. If you have calculated the test statistic by hand, you may obtain the *P*-value from the table of the *t*-distribution (Table A.3).

5. Use the *P*-value to judge whether the data are consistent with the null hypothesis. Then **decide** whether or not to reject the null hypothesis. Usually, we reject H_0 if $P < 0.05$.

6. Derive a **confidence interval** for the true mean difference. The 95% confidence interval is given by

$$\bar{d} \pm t_{0.05} \text{SE}(\bar{d}) = \bar{d} \pm t_{0.05}\left(s_d \ \sqrt{n}\right)$$

where $t_{0.05}$ is the entry in the table of the *t*-distribution (Table A.3) with $n - 1$ degrees of freedom, corresponding to a two-tailed probability of 0.05.

7.5.4 Example

Nelson *et al.* (1998) conducted a randomized cross-over trial of two diets in 11 insulin-dependent diabetic dogs; they measured serum glucose as the variable indicating the quality of diabetic control. The diets contained either low insoluble fibre (LF) or high insoluble fibre (HF). Each dog was randomly allocated to receive a particular diet first. The dogs were adapted to

the diet for two months and then fed on it for six months: evaluation was performed at six-week intervals. Table 7.3 has been developed from their summary results and gives the mean morning preprandial serum glucose concentrations (mmol/l) for each dog in each six-month period.

1. The null hypothesis states that the true mean difference in the preprandial serum glucose levels between the low-fibre and high-fibre diets is zero; the two-sided alternative is that it is not zero.
2. We can see from Fig. 7.3 that there is a tendency for the lines to slope downwards, indicating that the dogs' serum glucose concentration is lower on the high-fibre diet. For each dog, the difference (LF – HF) in serum glucose is calculated. Figure 7.4 is a dot diagram of these differences; it indicates that their distribution is approximately Normal.
3. Display 7.2 shows typical computer output for the paired *t*-test. The value of the test statistic, ignoring its sign, is $Test_4 = 4.37$ (which is the mean difference, 3.808 mmol/l, divided by its standard error, 0.872 mmol/l) which follows the *t*-distribution with 10 degrees of freedom.
4. The *P*-value is 0.0014 (it is called 2-tailed Sig. in Display 7.2). Hence, if the null hypothesis is true, we have only a 0.1% chance of observing a mean difference as large as 3.81 mmol/l. Note, referring 4.37 to Table A.3 gives $0.001 < P < 0.01$.
5. The data are not consistent with the null hypothesis which we therefore reject, $P =$

Table 7.3 Preprandial serum glucose levels (mmol/l) in dogs with insulin-dependent diabetes mellitus fed a low and high-fibre diet. (Based on summary data from Nelson *et al.*, 1998, with permission from the *Journal of the American Veterinary Medical Association.*)

Dog	Low-fibre diet (LF)	High-fibre diet (HF)
1	9.44	9.28
2	17.61	8.67
3	8.89	6.28
4	16.94	12.67
5	10.39	6.67
6	11.78	7.28
7	15.06	15.39
8	7.06	5.61
9	19.56	11.94
10	8.22	5.11
11	23.17	17.33

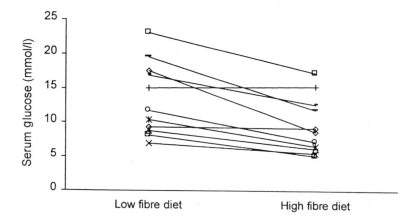

Fig. 7.3 Preprandial serum glucose concentration in 11 dogs with insulin-dependent diabetes mellitus on different diets. (Based on summary data from Nelson *et al.*, 1998.)

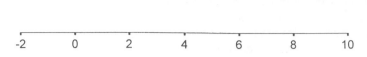

Difference (LF − HF) in serum glucose (mmol/l)

Fig. 7.4 Dot diagram of the differences in preprandial fasting serum glucose concentrations (mmol/l) in dogs fed low-fibre (LF) and high-fibre (HF) diets. (Based on summary data from Nelson *et al.*, 1998.)

Display 7.2 Typical computer output for the paired *t*-test: preprandial serum glucose (mmol/l) in dogs with insulin-dependent diabetes mellitus fed a low-fibre and a high-fibre diet (data of Table 7.3).

Paired samples statistics

		Mean	N	Std. deviation	Std. error mean
Pair 1	HF	9.657273	11	4.125271	1.243816
	LF	13.465455	11	5.301857	1.598570

Paired samples test

| | Paired differences | | | | | | | Sig. (2-tailed) |
	Mean	Std. deviation	Std. error mean	95% confidence interval of the difference Lower	95% confidence interval of the difference Upper	t	df	
Pair 1 LF − HF	3.808182	2.891563	0.871839	1.865603	5.750760	4.368	10	0.0014

0.001. The mean of the preprandial serum glucose differences (LF − HF), estimated as 3.81 mmol/l, is significantly different from zero, indicating that the high-fibre diet significantly reduces fasting blood sugar.

6. We can see from Display 7.2 that the 95% confidence interval for the true mean difference has limits equal to 1.87 and 5.75 mmol/l. Because the sample size is relatively small, this confidence interval is wide. If you are calculating the limits by hand, they are 3.8082 ± 2.228 × 0.872, where 2.228 is the value obtained from the table of the *t*-distribution (Table A.3) corresponding to a two-sided *P* of 0.05 with 11 − 1 = 10 degrees of freedom, and the standard error of the mean difference is 0.872 mmol/l.

Note that zero, the value against which the mean difference is tested in the specification of the null hypothesis, is smaller than the lower limit, 1.87 mmol/l, of the 95% confidence interval. This provides an alternative approach to testing H_0 (see Section 6.6) leading to the same conclusion to reject H_0.

EXERCISES

The statements in questions 7.1–7.2 are either TRUE or FALSE.

7.1 The two-sample *t*-test:
(a) Must have equally sized groups of observations.

(b) Is used on dependent groups of observations.
(c) Tests the null hypothesis that two sample means are equal.
(d) Assumes that the variances are not significantly different in the two groups.
(e) Is preferred to the paired *t*-test when the sample size is large.

7.2 The paired *t*-test:
(a) Tests the null hypothesis that the mean of the differences in the population is zero.
(b) Must have equally sized groups of observations.
(c) Can only be used if the sample size is large.
(d) Is appropriate for comparing independent groups of observations.
(e) Assumes that the data in each group are Normally distributed.

In questions 7.3–7.5, you should check that the assumptions underlying the tests that you choose are valid.

7.3 A study was made to compare the plasma lactate concentration (mmol/l) in Dutch warm-blood horses cantering at a constant speed either on a track or on an inclined treadmill. The speed was chosen as the horse's own comfortable speed on the track. Samples were taken after 5 minutes' cantering on track and treadmill, the order of which was randomized for the ten horses, and we show the plasma lactate concentrations (developed from data presented by Sloet van Oldruitenborgh-Oosterbaan and Barneveld, 1995).

Plasma lactate concentration (mmol/l)

Horse	1	2	3	4	5	6	7	8	9	10
Track	2.0	7.7	4.7	4.7	2.9	2.5	5.3	4.8	3.1	3.9
Treadmill	3.5	7.2	4.6	5.7	5.5	4.4	5.6	4.6	3.5	4.9

(a) What design is this?
(b) State the hypothesis you would test to investigate whether the exercise exerted by the horses can be considered to be of similar metabolic demand in both situations.
(c) Conduct a test of this hypothesis.
(d) What conclusion do you draw?

7.4 Observe the sperm numbers obtained either by electroejaculation (EE) or artificial vagina (AV) from 23 adult tom cats. The tom cats were randomly assigned to one of the two methods.

Sperm numbers ($\times 10^6$)
AV 61, 19, 51, 108, 34, 44, 57, 58, 73, 74, 85, 94, 67
EE 41, 11, 76, 23, 39, 34, 45, 49, 55, 66

(a) What design is this?
(b) State the hypothesis you would test to investigate whether the sperm numbers obtained from the two methods are similar.
(c) Conduct a test of this hypothesis.
(d) What conclusion do you draw?

7.5 Plasma urea and creatinine are routinely measured to evaluate renal function and, in healthy cats, the mean urea value in a given pathology laboratory is 7.5 mmol/l. Plasma urea values in a random sample of 140 healthy cats in January were measured to verify the assay. The data were approximately Normally distributed with a mean urea content of 9.7 mmol/l and an estimated standard error of 0.22 mmol/l. Is there any evidence to indicate that the assay performance in this laboratory changed in January?

7.6 Hiraga *et al.* (1997) performed cardiorespiratory tests on 12 Thoroughbred yearling horses before and after an eight-week breaking programme. Paired *t*-tests of a number of variables, comparing the effects before and after the breaking programme, showed that cardiopulmonary function was significantly higher after the breaking period. However, the authors conclude that whether this was due to the exercise during breaking or to physical growth of the horses is unclear. Criticize the experimental design, and provide a design which can separate the possible causes.

Chapter 8

Hypothesis Tests 2 – The *F*-Test Comparing Two Variances or More Than Two Means

8.1 LEARNING OBJECTIVES

By the end of this chapter, you should be able to:

- List and verify the assumptions that underlie the *F*-test.
- Explain the principles underlying the *F*-test for equality of variances.
- Elaborate the use of Levene's test.
- Explain the circumstances when an analysis of variance would be appropriate.
- List and verify the assumptions which underlie the one-way analysis of variance.
- Interpret the computer output of a one-way analysis of variance, and explain the result.

8.2 INTRODUCTION

In Chapter 7 we considered hypothesis tests, based on the *t*-distribution, that are used to compare means. For example, in Section 7.4, we performed a two-sample *t*-test to compare the mean body weights of flushed and control ewes. For this test to be valid, we needed to be sure that the two groups had similar variances.

In this chapter we review some tests whose test statistics follow the *F*-distribution (see Section 3.5.4), and which compare variances. These *F*-tests can be used in a wider context, as part of the analysis of variance, to compare two or more means – a not uncommon situation in veterinary and animal science.

Suppose, for example, we have four groups of observations to compare. Spurious *P*-values are likely to result if the difference in means (using a two-sample *t*-test) is investigated for every combination of pairs of groups. Four groups would result in six possible *t*-tests, and the more tests that we perform, the more likely it is that we will obtain a significant *P*-value on the basis of chance alone. If we perform 20 tests at the 5% level of significance, it is likely that one will be falsely significant and therefore lead to the erroneous conclusion that the means of these groups differ (see also Section 8.6.3). This is the Type I error discussed in Section 6.4.1. We can use the analysis of variance to address this problem.

As in the last chapter, the tests in this chapter apply to a single continuous quantitative variable which is assumed to follow a Normal distribution.

8.3 THE *F*-TEST FOR THE EQUALITY OF TWO VARIANCES

8.3.1 Rationale

The two-sample *t*-test and the analysis of variance (see Section 8.5) make the assumption of *homoscedasticity*, i.e. of equal variances in groups of data. The **F-test**, often called the **variance ratio test**, may be used to investigate the homoscedasticity of two data sets. **Levene's test** may be used for two or more variances (see Section 8.4).

Suppose we select two independent random samples of data from populations 1 and 2, and that we calculate s_1^2 and s_2^2 as estimates of the population variances, σ_1^2 and σ_2^2, respectively. We consider the ratio of these estimated variances and, by convention, we divide the larger by the smaller.

- If we find that the ratio is unity, or close to it, then we would conclude that the two population variances are probably equal.
- If, however, we find that the ratio of these estimated variances is much greater than 1, then it is unlikely that the populations, from which we have selected our samples, have equal variances. We have to make a decision whether or not the population variances are likely to be different. This means that we need a cut-off for the variance ratio; if the variance ratio exceeds this cut-off value, we will conclude that the variances are unequal.

We may determine this cut-off value formally, under the *null hypothesis* that the two population variances are equal, by referring to the table of the *F*-distribution (Table A.5). The *degrees of freedom* are n_1-1 in the numerator (the larger variance) and n_2-1 in the denominator (the smaller variance), where n_1 and n_2 represent the two sample sizes.

Note that this is actually a two-tailed test because the alternative hypothesis states that the two variances are not equal, rather than specifying which is the greater. However, the table of the *F*-distribution (Table A.5) shows tail area probabilities in only the upper tail, when the *F* ratio is greater than 1. For the required significance level in a two-tailed test, therefore, we must halve this tail area. So, for a two-tailed test at the 5% level of significance, we have to relate the test statistic to $P = 0.025$. For convenience, we give the upper percentage points corresponding to $P = 0.025$ and $P = 0.005$ (relating to two-tailed *P*-values of 0.05 and 0.01, respectively) in a separate table, Table A.5(b).

8.3.2 Assumptions

This hypothesis test is dependent on the assumptions that the independent samples are randomly selected from Normally distributed populations;

it is particularly sensitive to departures from Normality.

8.3.3 The approach

1. Specify the **null hypothesis** that the two population variances, σ_1^2 and σ_2^2, are equal, and specify the alternative hypothesis, usually, that the variances are not equal.
2. **Collect** and **examine** the data by constructing a dot plot, histogram or a box-and-whisker plot (see Section 2.5.2). Check the Normality assumption.
3. Select the appropriate test on the computer, or calculate by hand the **test statistic**. This is the ratio of the larger (s_1^2) to the smaller (s_2^2) estimated population variances derived from the samples. It follows the *F*-distribution and is given by

$$Test_5 = \frac{s_1^2}{s_2^2}$$

with n_1-1, n_2-1 degrees of freedom

The degrees of freedom for the *F*-test are, by convention, written in the order shown above, with the degrees of freedom for the numerator preceding those for the denominator. In this case, they are $n_1 - 1$ in the numerator (the larger variance) and $n_2 - 1$ in the denominator (the smaller variance), where n_1 and n_2 represent the two sample sizes.

4. Determine the **P-value**. You may find this in the computer output or, alternatively, you turn to the *F* table (Table A.5(b)). You will see that both Table A.5(a) and Table A.5(b) have columns and rows which correspond to the degrees of freedom for the numerator and the denominator, respectively, of the *F* ratio. The *P*-value for a two-sided *F*-test is obtained by consulting $P/2$ in Table A.5(b) (see Section 8.3.1), i.e. for a *P*-value of 0.05, consult $P = 0.025$ in Table A.5(b).
5. Use the *P*-value to judge whether the data are consistent with the null hypothesis. Then **decide** whether or not to reject the null hypothesis. Commonly, we reject the null hypothesis if $P < 0.05$.

Usually, we will be performing this test to establish the equality of the variances to satisfy that assumption in other tests, such as the two-sample t-test. It is, therefore, unlikely that we will need to consider the confidence interval for the ratio of the two variances. The confidence interval for a variance ratio is based on the F-distribution; you will find details in more advanced texts such as Armitage and Berry (1994).

8.3.4 Example

We illustrated the two-sample t-test by comparing the mean weights of two randomly selected samples of flushed and control ewes before mating (see Section 7.4.4).

1. One of the assumptions underlying the t-test is that the true variances of these two groups are equal. The null hypothesis for the test which follows is that the variances of the two populations from which the ewes are selected are equal. The alternative hypothesis is that they are unequal (direction unspecified), leading to a two-tailed test.
2. Figure 7.2 indicates that both samples are approximately Normally distributed.
3. We test the hypothesis of equal variances by finding the ratio of the two estimated variances. Display 7.1 shows that the two estimated standard deviations are 2.252 kg and 2.497 kg for the 24 flushed and 30 control ewes, respectively. The estimated variances are thus $5.072\,kg^2$ and $6.235\,kg^2$, so that the ratio of the larger to the smaller estimated variance is $6.235/5.072 = 1.23$.
4. We refer this quotient to the table of the F-distribution (Table A.5(b)) with 29 (in the numerator) and 23 (in the denominator) degrees of freedom. There is no column for 29 df or row for 23 df. However, we can see that our value (1.23) is less than the tabulated value (2.09) for infinity df in the numerator and 20 df in the denominator for $P/2 = 0.025$. Thus, $P > 0.05$.

5. There is no evidence of inequality between the variances, and the homoscedasticity assumption underlying the t-test is valid.

8.4 LEVENE'S TEST FOR THE EQUALITY OF TWO OR MORE VARIANCES

When you use the computer, you may encounter an alternative test of homogeneity of variance, called **Levene's test**. It may be used to *compare two or more variances*, and has the considerable advantage that it is less dependent on the assumption that the data come from Normal populations than most homogeneity of variance tests. It is particularly useful in the context of the analysis of variance. A test statistic is calculated in Levene's test which has an F-distribution. Since it is most unlikely that you will use this test other than when you are doing a computer analysis, we omit details of the calculation.

Note that Display 7.1, an SPSS computer output for the two-sample t-test, includes Levene's test for the equality of variance. This test gives $P = 0.617$, and it therefore is in agreement with the result we obtained by calculating the ratio of the variances (see Section 8.3.4). Should Levene's test be significant, note that the SPSS computer output offers a modified t-test allowing a comparison of means even when the two groups have unequal variances.

8.5 THE ANALYSIS OF VARIANCE (ANOVA) FOR THE EQUALITY OF MEANS

8.5.1 Rationale

The analysis of variance (ANOVA) is an expression used to describe a set of techniques which compare the *means* of two or more groups by investigating relevant variances. The analysis is based on the variance ratio test, i.e. an F-test, which compares two variances by examining their ratio and relating it to the F-distribution (see Section 8.3).

The principle underlying the analysis of variance is that the total variability in a data set is partitioned into its component parts. Each component represents a different source of variation. The variation is expressed by its variance. The sources of variation comprise one or more **factors**, each resulting in variability which can be accounted for or *explained* by the **levels** of that factor (e.g. the two levels, 'male' and 'female', defining the factor 'sex', or three dose levels for a given drug factor), and also *unexplained* or *residual* variation which results from uncontrolled biological variation and technical error. We can assess the contribution of the different factors to the total variation by making the appropriate comparisons of these variances.

Consider the simple case in which there is only one factor of interest, the levels of this factor defining different groups to which, in the experimental situation, individuals are assigned at random (this leads to a one-way ANOVA – see Section 8.6). The null hypothesis is that all the observations come from a single population. If H_0 is true, the levels of each factor do not affect the variation (i.e. the variation between the group means would be the same as that of the observations within the groups), and we would not expect the group means to differ. If there appears to be significantly more variation between the groups than would be expected under the null hypothesis, we reject the null hypothesis in favour of the alternative hypothesis, and conclude that the group means are different. Thus, despite its name, the analysis of variance is a device for comparing two or more means. Note that the alternative hypothesis is that there is *more* variation between the group means than within the groups – i.e. it is a one-tailed test, so we look up the *P*-values directly in Table A.5(a) (because we are comparing variances using an *F*-test), without any adjustment.

8.5.2 The ANOVA table

Although the basic concepts of the analysis of variance can be expressed in relatively simple terms, the mathematical details are cumbersome

and best avoided. We refer you to books, such as Cochran and Cox (1957), Cox (1958) and Gardiner and Gettinby (1998) for the underlying theory. It is more relevant, in this day and age, that you understand the computer output resulting from the analysis of variance. This comprises an **analysis of variance table** which lists the various sources of variation, e.g. Display 8.1. For each source of variation, you will find values for the **sum of squares** and the **degrees of freedom** (see Section 6.3.6); the sum of squares divided by the degrees of freedom determines the **mean square** which provides an estimate of the relevant variance. Finally, the appropriate mean squares are compared using an *F*-test (see Section 8.3). For each factor (source of explained variation), the null hypothesis states that the population means of the groups defined by the levels of that factor are equal.

8.5.3 Particular forms of ANOVA

The considerations of ANOVA which underlie the experimental design and subsequent handling of the data can be exceedingly complicated. In this section, we outline some of the common designs to give you an indication of the potential of ANOVA. You can skip this section without loss of continuity if you find it difficult.

The analysis of variance encompasses a broad spectrum of experimental designs ranging from the simple to the complex. In each case, the appropriate mathematical model is constructed which is based on the structure or pattern of the experimental design. The essential forms of these designs are illustrated in Fig. 8.1.

- We may regard the **one-way analysis of variance** (the simplest form of ANOVA for one factor) as an extension of the *two-sample t-test* when we need to compare the means of more than two groups (see Section 8.6).

  For example, in order to determine whether the build-up of calculus on dogs' teeth is affected by diet, Stookey *et al.* (1995) randomly allocated 26 dogs to one of three diets. One-way ANOVA was used to test the null hypothesis that the mean calculus accumulation was equal in the three diet groups after four weeks on the diet. We give full details in Section 8.6.4.

- The **one-way repeated measures ANOVA** may be regarded as an extension of the *paired t-test* when, for example, the within-subject/animal comparison is between three or more treatments. We say that we have repeated

One-way ANOVA

Diet group		
Control	Diet 1	Diet 2
x	x	x
x	x	x
x	x	x
x	x	x
x	x	x
x		x
x		
x		

One-way repeated measures ANOVA

	Treatment groups		
Beagles	Control	Dose 1	Dose 2
1	x	x	x
2	x	x	x
3	x	x	x
.	.	.	.
.	.	.	.
.	.	.	.
.	.	.	.
k	x	x	x

Two-way ANOVA

	Daily feeding schedule		
	1 portion	2 portions	3 portions
Feed 1	x x x x / x x x x	x x x x / x x x x	x x x x / x x x x
Feed 2	x x x x / x x x x	x x x x / x x x x	x x x x / x x x x

Fig. 8.1 Diagrams of the most common forms of the experimental designs analysed by ANOVA.

measures on a particular factor if each individual has measurements at every level of that factor. We describe a simple approach to analysing repeated measures data (as an alternative to ANOVA) in Section 13.4.2.

As an example of this ANOVA approach, Burton *et al.* (1997) compared the effects of three treatments (control, and two dose levels of a sedative drug, medetomidine) on the insulin concentrations of healthy adult beagles in a trial in which each dog received all three treatments. Each dog was used as its own control in a randomly allocated sequence of treatments. The ANOVA showed that the mean serum insulin values in the three treatment groups were significantly different when measured 60 minutes after administration of treatment (further investigation indicated that both of the doses of medetomidine significantly decreased the serum insulin when compared to control).

- The **two-way analysis of variance** examines the effect of two factors on a response variable, when each of these factors possesses two or more levels. We create a two-way table in which the rows and the columns represent the levels of each of the two factors; every cell in the table represents a unique combination of particular levels of the two factors. Each individual is randomly assigned to one of the different levels of each factor. Providing there is no replication in any cell of the table, the design is often called a **randomized block**. If there is replication in the cells, then it is possible to study the **interaction** between the factors; this is when the differences in the levels of one

factor are not consistent for the various levels of the other factor.

Suppose, for example, two different feed formulations for optimal growth promotion of kittens are to be compared, with the daily ration administered in one, two or three divided portions. This gives six unique treatment combinations; 42 animals are randomly allocated to one of these feeding regimes with 7 animals in each cell of the table, and their weight gain (growth) is monitored over a three-month period. The ANOVA would allow us to investigate whether there is any difference in the mean weight gain between the two different feeds, and between the number of daily portions. An interaction between the factors would imply that the difference observed in the mean weight gain between the feed formulations is not consistent for each of the three forms of administration of the feed (1, 2 or 3 daily portions).

- More complex experimental designs may involve hierarchical (nested) or cross-classifications of a number of factors (each at various levels), perhaps with repeated measures. These include the *Latin square*, *split-plot* and the more general *factorial designs* which reflect the flexibility of ANOVA. Details of each design are to be found in books such as Cochran and Cox (1957), Cox (1958) and Gardiner and Gettinby (1998).

In Section 8.6, we use the one-way ANOVA to illustrate the general approach; the principles underlying more complicated ANOVA are similar.　□

8.6 ONE-WAY ANOVA

8.6.1 Assumptions underlying one-way ANOVA

We apply the analysis of variance when the variable of interest is quantitative; the results are reliable only if the assumptions on which it is based are satisfied. The one-way analysis of variance is concerned with several levels of a single factor, where each level defines a group of observations. For example, the levels may represent different treatments as in a comparison of, say, a dry feed formula, a formulated tinned feed, and a raw meat diet for dogs. Alternatively, they can be different treatment dose levels of a drug, one of which is a placebo representing simply the drug vehicle, while the others are, say, 50%, 100% and 200% of the presumed effective dose. Animals are selected randomly from the population and, in the experimental situation, randomly allocated to one of the levels of the factor, i.e. to one of the groups.

The assumptions of the one-way ANOVA, stated more formally, are that the samples representing the groups are drawn *randomly* and *independently* from a *Normally distributed* population with variance σ^2; this implies that the group variances are the same. Approximate Normality may be established by drawing a histogram; moderate departures from Normality have little effect on the result. Constant variance, the more important assumption, may be established by Levene's test (see Section 8.4).

If we are concerned about the assumptions, we can take an appropriate transformation of the data or use an alternative non-parametric method such as the **Kruskal–Wallis one-way ANOVA** (see Section 11.6.2). As a point of interest, we can use the **Friedman two-way ANOVA** as a non-parametric alternative to the two-way ANOVA (see Section 11.6.3).

8.6.2 The approach to one-way ANOVA

1. Specify the **null hypothesis** that the population group means do not differ, i.e. the groups represent a single population. Generally, the alternative hypothesis is that at least one of the group means is dissimilar.

2. **Collect** the data and **display** them in exactly the same way as for the two-sample *t*-test (see Section 7.4) except that here there are more than two groups. Check the assumptions of Normality and homogeneity of variance.

3. Use the computer to calculate the **test statistic** which is found in the ANOVA table. It is the ratio of the between groups to the within groups mean squares (*F* ratio). This *F* ratio follows the *F*-distribution with $k - 1$, $n - k$ degrees of freedom, where k = the number of groups and n = the total number of observations in the sample.

4. Look at the **P-value**; it is usually given in the ANOVA table of the computer output. If you want to determine it for yourself, you have to refer to the table of the *F*-distribution (Table A.5(a)). You can read the appropriate degrees of freedom that you need for Table A.5(a) from the ANOVA table: use $k - 1$ for the numerator (the between groups degrees of freedom); use $n - k$ for the denominator (the within groups (residual) degrees of freedom).

5. Use the *P*-value to judge whether the data are consistent with the null hypothesis. Then **decide** whether or not to reject the null hypothesis; usually, but not necessarily, we reject H_0 if $P < 0.05$. If we reject the null hypothesis, we may need to establish which group means differ (see Section 8.6.3).

6. Derive the **confidence intervals** for differences between group means, in the same way as for the two-sample *t*-test (see Section 7.4.3). However, the combined estimate of variance used in the calculation of the confidence interval is the within group (residual) mean square in the ANOVA table.

8.6.3 Multiple comparisons

If we reject the null hypothesis in the one-way ANOVA (see Section 8.6.2), then we need to establish which group means differ. This will involve conducting a number of tests, but the more tests that we perform, the more likely it is that we will obtain a significant *P*-value on the basis of chance alone. We have to approach this problem of **multiple comparisons** in such a way that we avoid spurious *P*-values. Formal multiple comparison techniques should be used, such as **Duncan's multiple range**, **Bonferroni's**, **Scheffe's or Newman–Keuls tests** which are commonly available in computer packages, often termed *post hoc* procedures.

The Bonferroni approach is relatively simple, even without the aid of a computer; we concentrate on comparing those groups that are of particular interest, and then employ Bonferroni's correction. The procedure involves modifying the *P*-value obtained from any one comparison by multiplying it by the number of tests (in this situation, the two-sample *t*-tests) or comparisons that are to be performed. So, if we plan to undertake three *t*-tests, we should multiply the *P*-value (p_1, say) obtained from a single *t*-test by 3 to produce an amended *P*-value of $3p_1$ which we can assess for significance in relation to 0.05, say. Ideally, we should modify the denominator of the test statistic by using the pooled estimate of variance from all the groups, i.e. the residual mean square (variance) in the ANOVA table, and we should use this, too, in any calculations of confidence intervals. This approach works reasonably well if the number of comparisons is less than about five, but for more comparisons it is too conservative.

You may be tempted to rely solely on these multiple comparison methods, but it is sensible to start your analysis with the ANOVA when there are three or more levels of any one factor and/or when more than two factors are to be investigated. The ANOVA may act as a buffer, precluding 'fishing' expeditions to discover treatment differences. It therefore precedes, and perhaps even obviates the need for, pairwise comparisons of groups. *We only proceed to investigate differences between pairs of means if the P-value for that factor in the ANOVA is significant.*

You should be aware that this problem of multiple testing also arises in other circumstances, not just in relation to the comparisons in this relatively simple ANOVA design. Examples are when we have multiple outcome measurements, and when we subdivide our sample into subsets and investigate differences in these subgroups. Another particular example arises when we have repeated measurements on the same individual; you will find more information to deal with this situation in Section 13.4.2. In all such cases, you should attempt to avoid spurious *P*-values. This may not be a simple process and we recommend that you seek the advice of a statistician.

Furthermore, remember never to compare P-values as a way of judging the magnitude of different effects. Instead, obtain quantitative measures of the effects of interest (e.g. the differences in the treatment means) and use these for comparative purposes. It is wrong to compare the *P*-values as they are dependent on considerations such as the sample size, the power of the test and the variability of the observations.

8.6.4 Example of one-way ANOVA

Dogs were fed a dry diet coated with different agents which were believed to affect the build-up of calculus on the teeth. Calculus accumulation was measured by an index which combined estimates of both the proportion of the teeth covered by the deposit and the thickness of the deposit. Twenty-six dogs were randomly allocated to three treatments which were: control; soluble pyrophosphate (P_2O_7); and sodium hexametaphosphate (HMP). The calculus accumulation index was measured on each dog four weeks after it received treatment. We present the data in Table 8.1; they are developed from the summary results presented by Stookey *et al.* (1995). Display 8.1 contains the ANOVA results.

1. The null hypothesis is that the true mean calculus index in the three treatment groups are equal; the alternative hypothesis is that they are not all equal.
2. We can see from Fig. 8.2 that the data are approximately Normally distributed; Levene's test (Display 8.1) indicates that the variances of the observations in the three groups are not significantly different ($P = 0.44$).

	Dog	Control	Dog	P$_2$O$_7$	Dog	HMP
	1	0.49	10	0.34	19	0.34
	2	1.05	11	0.76	20	0.05
	3	0.79	12	0.45	21	0.53
	4	1.35	13	0.69	22	0.19
	5	0.55	14	0.87	23	0.28
	6	1.36	15	0.94	24	0.45
	7	1.55	16	0.22	25	0.71
	8	1.66	17	1.07	26	0.95
	9	1.00	18	1.38		
Sample size	9		9		8	
Mean	1.09		0.75		0.44	
SD	0.42		0.37		0.29	
SEM	0.14		0.12		0.10	
95% CI*	(0.81, 1.37)		(0.46, 1.03)		(0.13, 0.74)	

Table 8.1 Index of calculus formation on the teeth of dogs fed a control diet or one supplemented with soluble pyrophosphate (P$_2$O$_7$) or sodium hexametaphosphate (HMP). (Based on summary data from Stookey *et al.*, 1995, with permission from the *Journal of the American Veterinary Medical Association*.)

*These are the 95% confidence intervals for each mean (calculated using the residual mean square = 0.1353 from the ANOVA table as the combined estimate of variance).

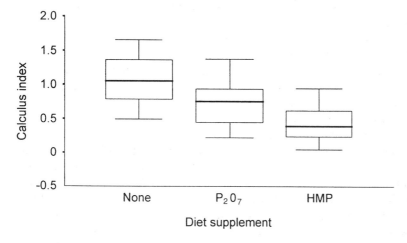

Fig. 8.2 Box-and-whisker plot of the calculus index of teeth in three groups of dogs. (Based on summary data from Stookey *et al.*, 1995.)

3. The *F*-ratio in the ANOVA table (Display 8.1) produces *P* = 0.005.
4. It is therefore unlikely that all the three means are equal and we reject the null hypothesis.
5. The means and their associated confidence intervals are shown in the Descriptives table in Table 8.1. Further examination by *post hoc* Bonferroni tests (see the multiple comparisons table in Display 8.1) indicate that the mean calculus index is significantly greater (*P* = 0.004) in the control group of dogs (mean index = 1.09; 95% confidence interval = 0.76, 1.41) than in the group of dogs receiving HMP (mean index = 0.44; 95% confidence interval = 0.19, 0.68). We estimate the difference between these means as 0.65; the 95% confidence interval for the true difference in means is (0.19, 1.11). The two other comparisons of means are not significant (*P* > 0.05); the relevant difference between these means and its associated confidence interval are given in Display 8.1.

Display 8.1 Typical computer output for analysis of variance of calculus data on three groups of dogs (data of Table 8.1).

Descriptives

		N	Mean calculus	Std. deviation	Std. error	95% confidence interval for mean	
						Lower bound	Upper bound
Treat group	None	9	1.0889	0.4225	0.1408	0.7641	1.4137
	P207	9	0.7467	0.3695	0.1232	0.4626	1.0307
	HMP	8	0.4375	0.2907	0.1028	0.1945	0.6805
	Total	26	0.7700	0.4435	8.697E-02	0.5909	0.9491

Note: E-02 means $\times 10^{-2}$.

Test of homogeneity of variances

	Levene statistic	$df1$	$df2$	Sig.
Calculus	0.855	2	23	0.438

ANOVA

		Sum of squares	df	Mean square	F	Sig.
Calculus	Between groups	1.805	2	0.902	6.668	0.005
	Within groups	3.112	23	0.135		
	Total	4.917	25			

Multiple comparisons

Dependent variable: Calculus
Bonferroni

(I) group	(J) group	Mean difference (I – J)	Std. error	Sig.	95% confidence interval	
					Lower bound	Upper bound
None	P207	0.3422	0.173	0.182	−0.1055	0.7899
	HMP	0.6514*	0.179	0.004	0.1899	1.1129
P207	None	−0.3422	0.173	0.182	−0.7899	0.1055
	HMP	0.3092	0.179	0.291	−0.1523	0.7707
HMP	None	−0.6514*	0.179	0.004	−1.1129	−0.1899
	P207	−0.3092	0.179	0.291	−0.7707	0.1523

* The mean difference is significant at the 0.05 level.

EXERCISES

The statements in questions 8.1–8.2 are either TRUE or FALSE.

8.1 In the one-way analysis of variance to compare the means of four groups of observations:
(a) The observations in each group should be Normally distributed.
(b) There should be the same number of observations in each group.
(c) The group variances should be equal.
(d) The groups should comprise matched individuals or the same individuals in different circumstances.
(e) The null hypothesis states that the sample means are all the same.

8.2 The *F*-test used on two groups of observations:
(a) Assumes that the means of the two groups are the same.

(b) Assumes that the data in each group are Normally distributed.
(c) Tests the null hypothesis that the two population variances are equal.
(d) Can be used instead of the paired *t*-test to investigate the mean difference.
(e) Should always be followed by a two-sample *t*-test.

In questions 8.3–8.4, you should check that the assumptions underlying the test that you choose are valid.

8.3 The following data show the liver weights (kg) taken from randomly selected cattle in two farms in south-west England during outbreaks of liver fluke disease. As a preliminary to testing the null hypothesis that the mean liver weights of the cattle in the two farms are the same, check that the variability of the observations in the two groups is similar.

Group 1: 18.0, 18.5, 18.9, 18.2, 17.9, 15.9, 16.8, 18.2, 17.3, 17.5, 17.7, 17.8, 17.1, 17.0, 16.3
Group 2: 14.3, 13.2, 17.3, 14.9, 16.4, 16.0, 18.6, 17.3, 15.5, 16.8, 15.7, 18.0, 15.2.

8.4 Look at the measurements of the mean fluorescence intensity of sperm cells stained with a fluorescent marker, 1-anilinonaphthalene-8-sulphonate (ANS), showing the effect of the presence of egg yolk in the diluent solution (Table 8.2). ANS fluoresces only when bound to the sperm membrane. Each value represents the mean of ten individual spermatozoa and is

Table 8.2   The effect of egg yolk in the medium on the fluorescence intensity of spermatozoa labelled with a fluorescent probe.

Egg yolk (%)		
1	5	25
0.944	0.865	0.811
1.048	1.000	0.862
1.026	1.001	0.910
1.007	0.900	0.799
0.933	0.923	0.837
0.998	0.876	0.854
1.035	1.046	
	0.990	

Display 8.2   ANOVA table of data in Table 8.2.

		Sum of squares	*df*	Mean square	*F*	Sig.
Fluoresc	Between groups	7.832E-02	2	3.916E-02	13.659	0.000*
	Within groups	5.160E-02	18	2.867E-03		
	Total	0.130	20			

Note: E-02 means $\times 10^{-2}$, E-03 means $\times 10^{-3}$.
*Implies $P < 0.001$.

estimated by a densitometer from photographic film. (The data are based on those of Watson, 1979.)

What evidence is there that the egg yolk affects the binding of the fluorophore to the sperm membrane? If you have the appropriate computer software, analyse the data yourself and see if you get the same ANOVA table as shown. If you do not have the software, you can use the ANOVA table to help you answer this question.

Chapter 9

Hypothesis Tests 3 – The Chi-squared Test Comparing Proportions

9.1 LEARNING OBJECTIVES

By the end of this chapter, you should be able to:

- Explain how to test a hypothesis about a single proportion.
- Outline the steps involved in comparing two proportions.
- Construct a 2×2 contingency table of observed frequencies.
- Explain the meaning of 'expected frequency' in a contingency table.
- Use the Chi-squared test to analyse data in a 2×2 contingency table.
- Analyse frequencies in an $r \times c$ contingency table.
- Describe the situations in which the Chi-squared test is not appropriate in the analysis of a contingency table.
- Describe the situation in which McNemar's test is appropriate.
- Compare two proportions using McNemar's test.
- Calculate the test statistic for a Chi-squared goodness-of-fit test.

9.2 INTRODUCTION

In Chapters 7 and 8 we discussed hypothesis tests for the *arithmetic mean*, a summary measure of location for a quantitative variable. In this chapter we describe some of the hypothesis tests for the *proportion*, a parameter that summarizes the observations of a binary variable. In addition, we explain how to analyse data when the qualitative variable has more than two categories.

You will recall that a **binary** variable is a qualitative (categorical) variable with only two cat-

egories of response, often termed *success* and *failure* (see Sections 1.5 and 3.4.2). For example, Little *et al.* (1980) investigated the influence of *Leptospira* infection on the incidence of abortion in cattle. The test which they used for the presence of leptospiral antibodies gives a binary response, either positive (success) or negative (failure). They compared the proportions of cows which were positive for *Leptospira* infection in two groups, those which aborted and those which calved normally.

In Section 7.2.3 we explained that when we test hypotheses about means, we improve our comparisons and measure our treatment effects more precisely if we give due consideration to the design of the study. Do we have a single group of observations, or do we have two or more groups of observations? Do these groups comprise independent or paired values? We should also be asking these questions when we test hypotheses about proportions.

9.3 TESTING A HYPOTHESIS ABOUT A SINGLE PROPORTION

9.3.1 The approach

In Section 4.6 we defined the properties of the sampling distribution of a proportion. We know that its distribution is approximately Normal if the sample size, n, is large; that the sample proportion, p, is an unbiased estimate of the population proportion, π; and that the standard error of the proportion is estimated in the sample by $\sqrt{p\,(1-p)/n}$. We use this information to test a hypothesis about the proportion of successes in a single population using the following approach:

1. Specify the **null hypothesis** that the proportion of successes in the population is equal to a specified value, π_1. Specify the alternative hypothesis – generally, that the population proportion is not equal to π_1.
2. **Collect** the data by selecting a random sample from the population, and classify each individual as a success or a failure.
3. Calculate the **test statistic** which approximates the Normal distribution. It is

$$Test_6 = \frac{|p - \pi_1| - \dfrac{1}{2n}}{\sqrt{\dfrac{\pi_1(1 - \pi_1)}{n}}}$$

where p is the observed proportion of successes and n is the number of individuals in the sample. The vertical lines to either side of the difference in proportions indicate that we ignore the sign of the difference. We subtract $1/(2n)$, called a **continuity correction**, from this difference to make an allowance for the fact that we are using the continuous Normal distribution to approximate the discrete Binomial distribution. The effect of the continuity correction is negligible when the sample size is large.

4. Determine the **P-value** by turning to the table of the Standard Normal distribution, Table A.1.
5. Make a **decision** whether or not to reject the null hypothesis according to the P-value. You may decide to reject the null hypothesis if $P < 0.05$.
6. Calculate the **confidence interval** for the proportion of successes. The 95% confidence interval for π is given by $p \pm 1.96 \sqrt{p(1 - p)/n}$ (see Section 4.7).

9.3.2 Example

Suppose we are investigating the sex ratio in wild rabbits. In the present season, we notice that the sex ratio of live births is distorted in favour of females. Our records show that in a random sample of 297 live births, 167 were female. Is this a chance deviation or do we have evidence of some

factor (e.g. a genetic mutation which predisposes to higher embryonic mortality in males) affecting the sex ratio?

1. The null hypothesis is that the proportions of female and male live births in this wild rabbit population are identical and equal to 0.5. The alternative hypothesis is that they are unequal.
2. The proportion of females in the random sample of 297 live births is $167/297 = 0.562$.
3. The test statistic is:

$$Test_6 = \frac{|0.562 - 0.5| - 1/(594)}{\sqrt{0.5(1 - 0.5)/(297)}} = 2.08$$

4. Referring to Table A.1, we find $P = 0.0375$ (corrected to two decimal places, $P = 0.04$).
5. There is evidence to reject the null hypothesis.
6. The 95% confidence interval for the true proportion of female live births is $0.562 \pm 1.96 \sqrt{0.562(1 - 0.562)/(297)} = 0.51$ to 0.62.

Although $P = 0.04$ leads us to reject the null hypothesis, the lower limit of the confidence interval only just exceeds 0.5, an equal proportion of males and females. We should be cautious in putting too much emphasis on the conclusion that some factor is affecting the sex ratio. This is an example where the confidence interval leads us to be more circumspect about the significance test's implications.

9.4 COMPARING TWO PROPORTIONS – INDEPENDENT GROUPS

9.4.1 Introduction

Hawkins *et al.* (1993) investigated the effect of neonatal castration on the prevalence of diabetes in mice. Mice were randomly allocated to receive either active (castration) or control (sham operation) treatment. They were interested in comparing, after a given time period, the proportions of diabetic animals ('successes') in these two independent groups of observations.

In an analysis of this sort, we regard these groups as samples from two populations, and use the sample proportions, p_1 and p_2, to estimate the population proportions, π_1 and π_2. We can test the hypothesis that the population proportions are the same in one of two ways.

- We can use the Chi-squared test, described in Section 9.4.3, which is based on the Chi-squared distribution (see Section 3.5.4).
- The other way of proceeding is to use the Normal approximation to the Binomial distribution (see Section 3.6.1), and derive a test statistic which approximates a Normal distribution.

As you will probably be using the computer to compare the two proportions, we do not feel that it is necessary to give details of both approaches. We expand on the Chi-squared test because it can be extended to compare more than two proportions (see Section 9.5) and other investigations of categorical data. In fact, the two tests produce identical results; the square of the test statistic approximating the Normal distribution is equal to the test statistic used in the Chi-squared test.

9.4.2 The 2 × 2 contingency table (the fourfold table)

We can summarize the results of the example introduced in Section 9.4.1 by presenting the *frequencies* in what is called a two-way **frequency** or **contingency table**. If each row (say) designates an outcome (success or failure), and each column (say) designates one of the two groups, then each of the four cells of the table contains the number or frequency of animals in a particular group who have the stated outcome. This type of contingency table is often called a **fourfold** or **two-by-two** (2 × 2) contingency table because it has two rows and two columns. The $r \times c$ contingency table has r rows and c columns. We show the general form of a 2 × 2 contingency table in Table 9.1(a) (a numerical example is shown in Table 9.2).

9.4.3 Comparing two proportions in a 2 × 2 table using the Chi-squared test

(a) Rationale

If there is no association between the outcome and the group, then we would expect the proportions of successes to be the same in the two groups. Thus we can compare the two proportions by investigating the association between the two factors which define the contingency table (see Table 9.1(a)). A **factor**, in this context, is a variable with one or more categories into which individuals can be classified. Our null hypothesis is that there is no association between the two factors (outcome, group), equivalent to the null hypothesis that the two population proportions are equal.

In order to calculate the test statistic using this approach, we have to compare the frequency we *observe* in each cell of the contingency table with the frequency we would *expect* in that cell *if the null hypothesis were true*. The null hypothesis is that the proportions of successes in the two populations are equal. If the null hypothesis is true, we would expect the overall proportion of successes, $(a + b)/n$, to apply to each of Groups 1 and 2. The expected successes under the null hypothesis are $(a + c) \times (a + b)/n$ in Group 1 and $(b + d) \times (a + b)/n$ in Group 2. The remaining numbers in each group are expected failures. Thus, we can build a table so that there is an expected frequency in each cell of the table corresponding to each observed frequency (see Table 9.1(b)).

If we find that the discrepancy between the observed and expected frequencies is large, we reject the null hypothesis. We decide whether the discrepancy is large by calculating the appropriate test statistic which approximates the Chi-squared distribution (see Section 3.5.4(b)); we refer the test statistic to Table A.4 to determine the P-value.

(b) Assumptions

In the Chi-squared test of association in a contingency table with two rows and two columns,

(a) Observed frequencies

Table 9.1   The 2×2 table of frequencies.

		Group		Row marginal total
		1	2	
Outcome	Success	a	b	$a + b$
	Failure	c	d	$c + d$
Column marginal total		$a + c$	$b + d$	Overall total $n = a + b + c + d$
Observed proportion of successes		$p_1 = \dfrac{a}{a + c}$	$p_2 = \dfrac{b}{b + d}$	$p = \dfrac{a + b}{a + b + c + d}$

(b) Expected frequencies in the four cells of the table

		Group	
		1	2
Outcome	Success	$\dfrac{(a + c)(a + b)}{n}$	$\dfrac{(b + d)(a + b)}{n}$
	Failure	$\dfrac{(a + c)(c + d)}{n}$	$\dfrac{(b + d)(c + d)}{n}$

we assume the individuals are randomly selected from the population. In the experimental situation, we have the responsibility of randomly allocating each individual to one of the two levels of the factor (e.g. to castrated or sham-operated). In the observational situation, the attribution of an individual to a group is determined for us (e.g. the *Leptospira* example in Section 9.2). The data are collected in the form of frequencies which indicate the number of successes and failures in each sample. The Chi-squared test of association in a 2×2 table is invalid if the *expected* frequency in any one of the four cells is less than 5. If this is the case, we employ **Fisher's exact test**; this involves calculating the exact probability of our particular table arising if we consider all possible 2×2 tables which have the same marginal totals as our observed table. These calculations are cumbersome and are best left to computer analysis.

(c) The approach

1. Specify the **null hypothesis** that the two population proportions are equal or, equivalently, that there is no association between the two factors of interest. Specify the alternative hypothesis, generally, that the two proportions are not equal or that there is an association between the two factors.
2. **Collect** the data. **Display** the observed frequencies in a 2×2 contingency table (see Table 9.1(a)).
3. Use the appropriate command(s) to select the **Chi-squared test** on the computer. If performing the test by hand, calculate the frequencies that you would *expect* in every cell of the table *if the null hypothesis is true*. Note, that the expected frequency for each cell is the product of the observed frequencies for the row marginal total and the column marginal total for that cell, divided by the observed overall

total (see Table 9.1(b)). Then calculate the **test statistic**, which approximates the Chi-squared distribution. It is

$$Test_7 = \sum \frac{(|O - E| - 0.5)^2}{E}$$

with one degree of freedom,

where O and E represent the observed and expected frequencies of a given cell, and the vertical lines surrounding them indicate that you take the absolute value of their difference, i.e. ignore its sign. The calculation $\{(|O - E| - 0.5)^2/E\}$ is computed for each cell of the table, and the summation is over all four cells of the table. The 0.5 in the numerator is known as **Yates' correction**, a continuity correction included to remove bias. This bias arises because we are assuming the test statistic approximates the continuous Chi-squared distribution although it has a discrete distribution.

A formula for calculating the test statistic which is identical to $Test_7$ when the contingency table has only two rows and two columns, but quicker to evaluate, is

$$Test_7' = \frac{n(|ad - bc| - 0.5n)^2}{(a + b)(c + d)(a + c)(b + d)}$$

4. Obtain a **P-value**, usually from computer output, but you can derive it by referring the calculated value of the test statistic to the table of the Chi-squared distribution, Table A.4. The test statistic has one degree of freedom – equivalent to the number of rows minus 1 (i.e. $2 - 1 = 1$), times the number of columns minus 1 (i.e. $2 - 1 = 1$).
5. Make a **decision** whether or not to reject the null hypothesis. Usually, we reject the null hypothesis of no association if $P < 0.05$. Remember, association does not necessarily imply causation, so that even if you reject the null hypothesis, you cannot infer that the effect on one factor is actually caused by a particular level of the other factor.
6. Calculate the relevant **confidence interval** for the difference in the two proportions. If the computer output does not provide this information, you can calculate the 95% confidence interval as $(p_1 - p_2) \pm 1.96 \, SE(p_1 - p_2)$, i.e.

$$(p_1 - p_2) \pm 1.96 \sqrt{\frac{p_1(1 - p_1)}{n_1} + \frac{p_2(1 - p_2)}{n_2}}$$

9.4.4 Example

The non-obese diabetic (NOD) mouse develops an autoimmune diabetes which is used as a model for human juvenile insulin-dependent diabetes. In the colony of Hawkins *et al.* (1993), the incidences for male and female NOD mice were 24% and 73%, respectively. Hawkins *et al.* investigated the causes of this sex difference by considering the effect of early castration on the incidence of diabetes in male NOD mice. (The following is based on their findings.) Fifty mice were randomly selected from 100 male mice and were castrated one day after birth; they were compared with the remaining 50 sham-operated mice. The mice were maintained for 140 days, and blood samples were collected bi-weekly starting at 42 days old. Diabetes was determined by three consecutive blood glucose levels greater than 200 mg/dl. It was shown that neonatal castration more than doubled the incidence of diabetes (52%) when compared with controls (24%) at day 112. But is this difference significant?

1. The null hypothesis is that the proportions of mice with diabetes are equal in the control and castrated populations. The alternative hypothesis is that they are not equal.
2. The data are displayed in Table 9.2(a).
3. Table 9.2(b) shows the expected frequency corresponding to each observed frequency for each of the four cells of the table.

$$
\begin{aligned}
Test_7 &= \sum \frac{(|O - E| - 0.5)^2}{E} \\
&= \frac{(|26 - 19| - 0.5)^2}{19} + \frac{(|12 - 19| - 0.5)^2}{19} \\
&\quad + \frac{(|24 - 31| - 0.5)^2}{31} + \frac{(|38 - 31| - 0.5)^2}{31} \\
&= 2.2237 + 2.2237 + 1.3629 + 1.3629 \\
&= 7.17
\end{aligned}
$$

Alternatively, we could have used the formula

$$Test'_7 = \frac{100(|26 \times 38 - 12 \times 24| - 50)^2}{38 \times 62 \times 50 \times 50} = 7.17$$

4. We refer the value 7.17 to Table A.4 with one degree of freedom, and find that $0.001 < P < 0.01$ (in fact, a computer analysis, the results of which are shown in Display 9.1, gives $P = 0.007$).
5. The data are not consistent with the null hypothesis that the true proportions of mice

Table 9.2 Frequencies of mice with and without diabetes.

(a) Observed frequencies (based on summary data from Hawkins *et al.*, 1993, with permission)

	Castrated mice	Control mice	Total
With diabetes	26	12	38
Without diabetes	24	38	62
Total	50	50	100

(b) Expected frequencies

	Castrated mice	Control mice
With diabetes	$\frac{50 \times 38}{100} = 19$	$\frac{50 \times 38}{100} = 19$
Without diabetes	$\frac{50 \times 62}{100} = 31$	$\frac{50 \times 62}{100} = 31$

N.B. Identical expected frequencies in the rows of Table (b) arise because the group sizes in Table (a) are equal.

with diabetes are equal in the control and castrated groups. There is evidence to indicate that neonatal castration is linked with the incidence of diabetes in NOD mice. This suggests that the difference in incidence of diabetes in male and female mice may be associated with the male hormone.

6. The 95% confidence interval for the true difference in the proportions of mice with diabetes in the two groups is

$$(p_1 - p_2) \pm 1.96\sqrt{\frac{p_1(1-p_1)}{n_1} + \frac{p_2(1-p_2)}{n_2}}$$
$$= (0.52 - 0.24)$$
$$\pm 1.96\sqrt{\frac{0.52 \times 0.48}{50} + \frac{0.24 \times 0.76}{50}}$$
$$= 0.28 \pm 1.96 \times 0.0929$$
$$= 0.098 \text{ to } 0.462$$

Thus, although castration is associated with an increased incidence of diabetes, estimated as 28%, the true effect could be as low as 10% or as high as 46%.

9.5 TESTING ASSOCIATIONS IN AN $r \times c$ CONTINGENCY TABLE

9.5.1 Introduction

We can extend the Chi-squared test of association in a 2×2 table to the larger contingency

Chi-square test

	Value	df	Asymp. sig. (2-sided)	Exact. sig. (2-sided)	Exact sig. (1-sided)
Pearson Chi-square	8.319*	1	0.004		
Continuity Correction[†]	7.173	1	0.007		
Fisher's exact test				0.007	0.004
N of valid cases	100				

* 0 cells (0.0%) have expected count less than 5. The minimum expected count is 19.00.
[†] Computed only for 2×2 table.

Display 9.1 Typical computer output for analysis of mice castration data in Table 9.2(a).

table which has r rows and c columns, where either r or c or both are greater than 2. We are interested in determining whether the two variables which determine the rows and columns of the table are related in some way. We test the null hypothesis of no association by calculating a Chi-squared test statistic.

9.5.2 Assumptions

We assume that the two variables are categorical, and that the data contained in the cells of the contingency table are frequencies. The data should be independent in that no animal/individual may be represented more than once in the table. No more than 20% of the cells of the table should have an expected frequency (calculated under the null hypothesis) whose value is less than 5. If necessary, we can reduce the contingency table in size by combining appropriate rows and/or columns to accommodate this latter assumption. Note that this requirement means that all cells must have expected frequencies that are at least 5 in a 2×2 table (see Section 9.4.3(b)).

9.5.3 The general approach

The approach to testing the null hypothesis, that there is no association in the population between the two categorical variables (i.e. factors) defining the $r \times c$ contingency table, is almost identical to that for the 2×2 table (see Section 9.4.3).

1. Specify the **null hypothesis** and the alternative hypothesis.
2. **Collect** the data and **present** them in a contingency table.
3. Select the **Chi-squared test** on the computer, or, by hand, calculate the **test statistic** which approximates the Chi-squared distribution. It is

$$Test_8 = \sum \frac{(O-E)^2}{E}$$

with $(r-1)(c-1)$ degrees of freedom,

where O and E represent the observed and expected frequencies of a given cell, and the summation is over all $r \times c$ cells of the table. Each expected frequency is evaluated under the assumption that the null hypothesis is true; for a given cell, it is calculated as the product of the marginal totals for that cell, divided by the overall total. You will note that this test statistic is almost identical to $Test_7$, the test statistic for the 2×2 table; the discrepancy is in the continuity correction (the subtraction of 0.5 in the numerator). The continuity correction has a negligible effect on the test statistic when the sample sizes are large, and is only necessary in the 2×2 table.

4. We determine the **P-value**, if it is not contained in the computer output, by referring the test statistic to the table of the Chi-squared distribution, Table A.4.
5. Make a **decision** whether or not to reject the null hypothesis by considering the P-value, often rejecting the null hypothesis if $P < 0.05$. Note that since we do not estimate an effect, we cannot calculate a confidence interval for it.

9.5.4 Example

Following training in insemination techniques in cattle, an artificial insemination centre compared three training methods whose success rates are given in Table 9.3. Is there any evidence for believing that the training methods show different rates of success?

1. The null hypothesis is that the true pregnancy rates are the same for the three methods. Another way of expressing this null hypothesis is that there is no association between the training methods and the pregnancy state of the cow. The alternative hypothesis is that the pregnancy rates are not equal.
2. The data are displayed in Table 9.3.
3. The expected frequencies which are required if the test is to be performed by hand are shown in brackets in Table 9.3. The expected number of pregnant cows for method I is (353 × 728)/(993) = 258.80, and so on for the other methods.

	Method I	Method II	Method III	Total
Pregnant	275 (258.8)	192 (187.7)	261 (281.5)	728
Not pregnant	78 (94.2)	64 (68.3)	123 (102.5)	265
Total	353	256	384	993
Proportion pregnant	0.78	0.75	0.68	0.73
95% CI for true proportion	0.73 to 0.82	0.69 to 0.80	0.63 to 0.73	

Table 9.3 Observed frequencies of pregnant and non-pregnant cows (expected frequencies in brackets).

CI = confidence interval.

The test statistic is

$$Test_8 = \frac{(275 - 258.80)^2}{258.80} + \frac{(78 - 94.20)^2}{94.20}$$
$$+ \frac{(192 - 187.68)^2}{187.68} + \frac{(64 - 68.32)^2}{68.32}$$
$$+ \frac{(261 - 281.52)^2}{281.52} + \frac{(123 - 102.48)^2}{102.48}$$
$$= 1.015 + 2.787 + 0.099 + 0.273$$
$$+ 1.496 + 4.110$$
$$= 9.78$$

4. Referring this value to the Chi-squared distribution (Table A.4) with $(3 - 1)(2 - 1) = 2$ degrees of freedom, we obtain $0.001 < P < 0.01$ (a computer analysis gives $P = 0.008$).
5. Hence we have evidence to reject the null hypothesis that the success rates are the same for the three methods. In this instance, because one of the variables is binary, we can estimate the proportion of successes for each of the methods, and evaluate the confidence interval for the true proportion (see Section 4.7) in each case. These quantities are shown in Table 9.3.

Further analysis by Chi-squared tests comparing the proportions of pregnancies obtained by any two methods shows that method III obtained a significantly lower pregnancy rate than method II (test statistic = 8.66, $P = 0.009$ after employing Bonferroni's correction for multiple comparisons – see Section 8.6.3) but no other comparisons are significant ($P > 0.05$).

9.5.5 Particular circumstances

We have explained the general approach to analysing $r \times c$ contingency tables in Section 9.5.3. There are, however, special considerations that we should afford the analysis when at least one of the categorical variables defining the table is **ordered** in some way (e.g. body condition score or age categories), or when we want to **combine** contingency tables. We only outline some of the approaches to the analyses in the different circumstances described below. You can obtain details in more advanced statistical texts, such as Armitage and Berry (1994).

- *The $2 \times c$ contingency table in which the variable defining the columns comprises c ordered categories.* We are interested in comparing the proportions of successes in c ordered groups, and would expect any differences in proportions, if they exist, to be related to the ordering. We can perform the **Chi-squared test for trend** to test the null hypothesis that there is no trend in the proportions.
- *The $r \times c$ contingency table in which one of the two variables defining the contingency table is ordered.* Firstly, we assign scores to the categories of the ordered variable. Then we can evaluate a test statistic, approximating the Chi-squared distribution, which tests whether the mean scores of the ordered variable are the same in the different categories of the other variable. Alternatively, we can apply the non-parametric Kruskal–Wallis test (see Section 11.6) to compare the categories of the unordered variable.
- *The $r \times c$ contingency table in which both of the variables defining the contingency table are ordered.* We assign scores to the categories of each of the two variables, and then regress one set of variables on the other (see Chapter 10). Alternatively, we can calculate the non-parametric Spearman's rank correlation coefficient (see Section 11.7) between the two variables.
- *Frequencies are available for various groups in a number of 2×2 contingency tables, each defined by the same two variables.* These groups may represent different subgroups or strata of the population (e.g. different sexes or different age groups); alternatively, they may represent different studies, each investigating the relationship between the

same two variables. We should like to know how best to use all the information to determine whether there is an association between the two variables. *Do not be tempted to pool the frequencies in the corresponding cells of the tables, and thereby obtain a single 2 × 2 table containing all the frequencies – you can come to quite the wrong conclusions.* Instead, analyse the data using the **Mantel–Haenszel** method which combines, in an appropriate manner, the information from each table. This approach can also be extended to combine a number of $r \times c$ tables.   □

9.6 COMPARING TWO PROPORTIONS – PAIRED OBSERVATIONS

9.6.1 Introduction

Sometimes we are interested in comparing two proportions when we have pairs of results on a binary variable. An analogy is the comparison of two means in dependent samples leading the paired *t*-test (see Section 7.5).

Suppose our random sample comprises m animals, each animal being investigated in two ways. We observe whether the response for each member of a pair results in a success or a failure – the two possible outcomes of the binary vari-

able of interest. For example, Schönmann *et al.* (1994) compared the efficiency of diagnosis of two methods to detect *Tritrichomonas foetus* in bulls. A sample was taken from each bull and classified by each of the two methods as positive (success) or negative (failure). They determined the number of pairs in which both methods yielded a success, both methods were a failure, and one was a success and the other a failure.

In Table 9.4(a) we use a general notation to show the frequencies of the four types of pair from two sample. We exhibit the same results in a slightly different format in Table 9.4(b). We use **McNemar's test** to test the null hypothesis that the true proportions of successes using the two methods are equal. These are estimated by $p_1 = (e + f)/m$ in method 1 and $p_2 = (e + g)/m$ in method 2. Their difference, $p_1 - p_2 = (f - g)/m$, focuses only on the discordant pairs, as does McNemar's test statistic; the frequencies relating to the concordant pairs are of no relevance in the analysis. McNemar's test is based on the observed frequencies, f and g, and their corresponding expected frequencies, calculated under the null hypothesis. These are incorporated into a test statistic, $\Sigma\{(O - E)^2/E\}$, which approximates a Chi-squared distribution.

(a) Observed frequencies

Type	Outcome using method 1	2	Frequency
1	Success	Success	e
2	Success	Failure	f
3	Failure	Success	g
4	Failure	Failure	h
Total			m

(b) Two-way contingency table of observed frequencies

		Method 2 Success	Failure	Total No. pairs
Method 1	Success	e	f	$e + f$
	Failure	g	h	$g + h$
Total No. pairs		$e + g$	$f + h$	$m = e + f + g + h$

Table 9.4 Two layouts to show the frequencies of the four types of pair in paired samples when there are two possible outcomes – success and failure.

9.6.2 Assumptions

We assume there are two possible outcomes (success and failure) to the variable of interest, and that we observe the outcome on each member of a randomly selected pair. The pair may comprise matched individuals, each assessed in one of two circumstances, or it may comprise the same individual assessed twice.

9.6.3 The approach

1. Specify the **null hypothesis** that the proportions of successes in the two populations are equal. Specify the alternative hypothesis, generally that the two proportions are unequal.
2. **Collect** the data and **display** them in a frequency table, as shown in Table 9.4(b).
3. Select *McNemar's test* on the computer or, by hand, calculate the **test statistic** which approximates the Chi-squared distribution. It is

$$Test_9 = \frac{(|f - g| - 1)^2}{f + g}$$

with one degree of freedom.

Sometimes, you may find that McNemar's test uses the related test statistic, $\sqrt{Test_9}$, which approximates the Standard Normal distribution. The 1 in the numerator of $Test_9$ is a continuity correction which is subtracted from the absolute difference (without regard to sign) between f and g to adjust for approximating a discrete distribution by the continuous Chi-squared distribution.

4. Obtain the **P-value**, either from computer output or by referring the test statistic to the table of the Chi-squared distribution, Table A.4, with one degree of freedom.
5. Make a **decision** whether or not to reject the null hypothesis by considering the P-value. Usually, we reject the null hypothesis if $P < 0.05$.
6. Calculate the **confidence interval** for the difference in the two proportions of successes,

estimated by $p_1 = (e + f)/m$ in sample 1 and $p_2 = (e + g)/m$ in sample 2. The approximate 95% confidence interval for the true difference in the proportions is given by

$$\frac{f - g}{m} \pm 1.96 \frac{1}{m} \sqrt{f + g - \frac{(f - g)^2}{m}}$$

9.6.4 Example

In the example introduced earlier, Schönmann *et al.* (1994) compared two methods of culture of *Tritrichomonas foetus* in the washings of the prepuce of infected beef bulls to determine the best method for detection of the organism. In comparing the methods of culture, Claussen's medium detected the organism in 61 of 83 samples whereas a commercial system detected the organism in 73 of the same 83 samples.

1. The null hypothesis is that the true proportions detected are the same using Claussen's medium and the commercial system. The alternative hypothesis is that the two proportions are different.
2. The full data are displayed in Table 9.5.
3. The test statistic is

$$Test_9 = \frac{(|14 - 2| - 1)^2}{14 + 2} = 7.56$$

This approximates the Chi-squared distribution with one degree of freedom.
4. Reference to Table A.4 gives $0.001 < P < 0.01$ (a computer analysis gives $P = 0.006$).
5. We have evidence to reject the null hypoth-

Table 9.5 Numbers of the organism, *Tritrichomonas foetus*, detected in bovine preputial washings using two different methods. (Data from Schönmann *et al.*, 1994, with permission.)

	Claussen's +ve	Claussen's −ve	Total
Commercial +ve	59	14	73
Commercial −ve	2	8	10
Total	61	22	83

esis; we conclude that the commercial system has the ability to detect the greater proportion of organisms.

6. We estimate the proportions of organisms detected by the Claussen's medium and the commercial system to be $61/83 = 0.735$ and $73/83 = 0.880$, respectively. The approximate confidence interval for the true difference in the proportions of organisms detected by the two methods, taking into account the pairings, is

$$\frac{14-2}{83} \pm 1.96 \frac{1}{83} \sqrt{14+2 - \frac{(14-2)^2}{83}}$$

$$= 0.1446 \pm 0.0892$$

$$= 0.055 \text{ to } 0.234$$

In other words, although Claussen's medium detected 74% of infected samples and the commercial system detected 88%, a difference of 14%, this difference could be as low as 6% or as high as 23%. We must judge, in the particular circumstances, whether 6% constitutes an important difference.

9.7 THE CHI-SQUARED GOODNESS-OF-FIT TEST

9.7.1 Introduction

We may be interested in establishing whether a set of observed data comes from a population which follows a particular theoretical distribution. The discrete or continuous distribution may be one of those to which we have already referred, such as the Binomial, Poisson or Normal (see Sections 3.4 and 3.5, but note that there are easier ways of establishing Normality, as discussed in Section 3.5.3(e)). Alternatively, it may reflect an expected distribution determined by the biological circumstances. Particular examples of these arise in genetics, where the assumed pattern of segregation of the alleles of a gene will lead to specific expectations of genotype (and perhaps phenotype) in the offspring.

The observed frequencies in each category of response (e.g. a genotypic class or an interval for a continuous variable) can then be compared to the number expected in that category if the data followed the theoretical distribution. This gives rise to a test statistic which approximates the Chi-squared distribution. Note that, in this text, we have not provided the equations for the Binomial or Poisson distributions from which expected numbers can be derived.

9.7.2 Assumptions

In the **goodness-of-fit test**, we assume that the sample is randomly selected from the population and the responses are independent and are categorized into distinct classes or intervals. The approximation to the Chi-squared distribution is poor if the expected frequency is less than 5 in more than 20% of the categories.

9.7.3 The approach

1. Specify the **null hypothesis** that the distribution of the variable in the population follows the specified theoretical distribution. The alternative hypothesis is that it does not.
2. **Collect** the data and **display** them in a frequency table.
3. Calculate the expected frequency in each category, and determine the **test statistic**, either by computer or by hand.

$$Test_8 = \sum \frac{(O-E)^2}{E}$$

where O and E represent the observed and expected frequencies in a given category, and the sum is over all categories. This test statistic approximates the Chi-squared distribution with degrees of freedom = (number of categories) – (number of parameters that have to be estimated in order to calculate the expected values) – 1. For example, the mean is the only parameter which has to be estimated in the Poisson distribution.
4. Obtain the **P-value** from the computer output or by looking at Table A.4.
5. Make a **decision** whether or not to reject the null hypothesis. Usually, but not necessarily, we reject the null hypothesis if $P < 0.05$. Note that, since the null hypothesis does not relate to an effect of interest, which we would estimate from the sample data, we do not calculate a confidence interval.

9.7.4 Example

The offspring of a random sample of roan Shorthorn cattle were classified according to coat colour: red 82, roan 209 and white 89. Is this distribution consistent with the hypothesis that coat colour is determined by a single pair of alleles with co-dominance? Co-dominance implies that neither allele is dominant, and the heterozygote exhibits the effect of both alleles.

1. The null hypothesis is that coat colour is determined by a single pair of alleles with co-dominance. If this is so, then the offspring would be expected to display coat colours in the ratio of $1:2:1$. The alternative hypothesis is that coat colour is not determined by a single pair of alleles with co-dominance.
2. The data are displayed in Table 9.6.

Table 9.6 Observed and expected frequencies of colour categories for Shorthorn cattle.

Colour	Observed frequency O	Expected frequency E	$O - E$
Red	82	380/4 = 95	−13
Roan	209	380/2 = 190	19
White	89	380/4 = 95	−6
Total	380	380	

3. The Chi-squared test statistic is

$$Test_8 = \frac{(-13)^2}{95} + \frac{(19)^2}{190} + \frac{(-6)^2}{95} = 4.06$$

This approximates the Chi-squared distribution on $(3 - 1)$ degrees of freedom. Note that, in this example, we have not had to estimate any parameters in order to calculate the expected frequencies.
4. Reference to Table A.4 gives $P > 0.05$ (computer analysis gives $P = 0.131$).
5. There is insufficient evidence to reject the null hypothesis, $P = 0.13$. These data are consistent with the hypothesis that coat colour is determined by a single pair of alleles with co-dominance.

It should be noted that, while this is a straightforward test of a simple segregation hypothesis, more complicated segregation involving multiple genes leads to complex hypotheses which are the domain of the trained geneticist. Moreover, corrections need to be built in, if the data are not a random selection due to biases in data collection. Nicholas (1987) covers these situations in more detail. ☐

EXERCISES

The statements in questions 9.1–9.2 are either TRUE or FALSE.

9.1 An investigator is interested in whether there is a breed-related basis for incidence of hip dysplasia in dogs. She selects samples of adult greyhounds and adult German shepherd dogs. From pelvic X-ray examination, the number of animals having shallow or abnormal coxo-femoral joints in each group is recorded. An appropriate test for the null hypothesis that there is no association between breed and the frequency of hip dysplasia in the population is the:
(a) Two-sample *t*-test.
(b) *F*-test.
(c) Chi-squared test for the difference in two proportions.
(d) McNemar's test.
(e) Chi-squared goodness-of-fit test.

9.2 In a study of the influence of artificial insemination on the occurrence of uterine infection in gilts, data were collected on the occurrence of bacteria in cervical swabs in two samples of gilts randomly allocated to either washing of the vulva or faecal contamination of the vulva before sham insemination. The results are presented in a 2 × 2 table; the proposed Chi-squared test for the difference in the proportions with uterine infection in the two groups:
(a) Is only valid if the observed frequency is greater than 5 in each cell of the table.
(b) Has degrees of freedom equal to 2.
(c) Tests the null hypothesis that there is no association in the population between uterine infection and the condition of the vulva.
(d) Tests the null hypothesis that there is a difference between the true proportions with uterine infection in the two groups.
(e) Is only valid if the data are Normally distributed.

9.3 The local National Farmers' Union Committee have just received the MAFF national figures for cattle numbers in England. They show that nationally the proportion of dairy cows in the national herd is 0.29. The committee express some surprise at this figure which they believe does not reflect their area, and they decide to do their own local survey. They take a random sample of the cattle holdings in their area, and in these 1375 cattle they discover there are 359 dairy cows. Is there evidence that the proportion of dairy cows in their area differs from the national figure?

9.4 Medroxyprogesterone (MPA) is administered to bitches to control the symptoms of oestrus. Stroving *et al.* (1997) investigated the effect of the administration of MPA to bitches on the chance of them subsequently developing mammary tumours. In a retrospective study they took 98 bitches, aged six to nine years, with mammary tumours and they chose a group of 98 bitches which were of a similar age but had no signs of mammary tumours. Thirty-eight bitches of the tumour-positive group and 21 bitches of the tumour-free group had previously received MPA. Is there evidence for there being a greater risk of mammary tumour in the event of being administered MPA?

Display the data in a frequency table. Formulate the null hypothesis, and calculate the expected frequency in each cell of the table. Conduct a suitable analysis to test this null hypothesis.

9.5 *Fasciola hepatica* (liver fluke) infestation in beef cattle is present if the animal sheds *F. hepatica* eggs. Welch *et al.* (1987) were interested in determining whether a positive reaction to an enzyme-linked immunosorbent assay (ELISA) could be used as an alternative test for liver fluke infestation. They investigated 143 calves from a number of beef cattle herds in central and southern Louisiana. Of 55 calves that were ELISA-positive, 39 were shedding eggs; of 53 calves that were shedding eggs, 14 were ELISA-negative. Present these results in a contingency table, and use them to test the null hypothesis that the two procedures are equally effective in detecting liver fluke infestation.

9.6 In a study to gauge the pregnancy rate in a large mob of sheep on an Australian sheep farm,

Table 9.7 Thirty-four groups of eight sheep sampled for pregnancy status from a large mob of sheep in Australia.

No. of pregnant ewes per sample	Observed No. of pregnant ewes	Expected No. for a Binomial distribution ($\pi = 0.64$, $n = 8$)
0	0	0.010
1	1	0.136
2	3	0.850
3	4	3.019
4	7	6.708
5	9	9.537
6	7	8.480
7	2	4.308
8	1	0.955

a sample of 272 sheep were taken for ultrasound scanning. For ease of handling, they were taken in groups of eight and the number of pregnant animals recorded for each group. The results of the ultrasound scanning are shown in Table 9.7. At lambing 64% of the mob gave birth to lambs. The table shows the numbers of pregnant ewes per group of eight expected if they followed a Binomial distribution with $\pi = 0.64$. Ignoring the difference in the proportions pregnant between ultrasound scanning and parturition and assuming that each ewe has the same chance of getting pregnant, use the Chi-squared analysis to assess whether the observed distribution conforms to the stated Binomial distribution.

Chapter 10

Linear Correlation and Regression

10.1 LEARNING OBJECTIVES

By the end of this chapter you should be able to:

- Recognize a linear relationship in a scatter diagram.
- Interpret Pearson's correlation coefficient.
- Explain the value of r^2.
- Test the null hypothesis that the correlation coefficient is zero.
- Elaborate circumstances when it would be improper to calculate the correlation coefficient.
- Identify data sets which are suited to linear regression analysis.
- Distinguish between the dependent and independent variables in regression analysis.
- Check the assumptions in linear regression analysis.
- Interpret the regression equation.
- Test the null hypothesis that the slope of the regression line is zero.
- Decide whether the regression line is a good fit to the data.
- Use the regression equation for prediction.
- Conduct a valid multiple linear regression analysis, given the appropriate computer software.
- Explain the circumstances in which a multiple logistic regression analysis is indicated.

10.2 INTRODUCING LINEAR CORRELATION AND REGRESSION

10.2.1 Types of variable

In Chapter 9 we examined the relationship between two *categorical* variables by considering the Chi-squared test of the null hypothesis that there is no association between the two variables. In this chapter, we describe the statistical techniques which we can use to investigate the association between two *continuous* variables, for example, the chest girth and live weight of sheep. The two techniques that we discuss are **linear correlation** and **linear regression**, each of which has a defined role.

10.2.2 The aims of linear correlation and regression

- In **linear correlation** we are concerned with determining whether there is a linear relationship between two continuous variables, and with measuring the degree of that relationship. We should like to know how well a straight line describes the linear association between the two variables. We derive a measure, called the correlation coefficient, which reflects the extent to which the points deviate from the straight line. In correlation analysis, we make no distinction between the two variables. We can interchange x and y, and we will still obtain the same value for the correlation coefficient.
- The purpose of **linear regression** is to describe the linear relationship between the two variables by determining the mathematical equation which relates the variables. We often use this equation to predict the value of one variable (called the dependent, response or outcome variable) from a value of the other variable (called the independent, explanatory or predictor variable). By convention, we take the y variable as the dependent variable, and the x variable as the independent variable. We assume that y is influenced by x (rather than

the other way round). *We cannot interchange x and y in regression analysis.* As an example, think about the standard curve prepared for a protein assay; the colour development (*y*) is plotted against the predetermined concentrations of protein (*x*), and the linear regression line is calculated as the line of best fit.

We give details of linear correlation and regression in the sections which follow. Note that the assumptions underlying the inferential procedures are different in correlation and regression.

10.2.3 The scatter diagram

The first stage, though, before we attempt any formal analysis, is to **plot** the data on a rectangular co-ordinate system so we can see what, if any, is the relationship between the two variables. If we represent the two variables under investigation by *x* and *y*, then each of the *n* animals in our random sample has a value for the *x* variable and a value for the *y* variable. Our sample data therefore consist of a series of *n* independent pairs of *x* and *y* values, $\{(x_1, y_1), (x_2, y_2), (x_3, y_3), \ldots (x_n, y_n)\}$.

Conventionally, we plot the data with the *x* values on the horizontal axis and the *y* values on the vertical axis (see Fig. 10.6 in which *x* = chest girth (cm) and *y* = live weight (kg) of sheep). Every pair of observations is marked by a point on the diagram, and once we have plotted all the observations, we have a scatter of points. Hence the term **scatter diagram** is used to describe the visual display of the data.

Before we are to proceed with either linear correlation or linear regression analysis, we must consider the 'curve' which approximates the data points. This line does not 'link' all the points, but is a line drawn through the midst of the points, illustrating the general 'drift'. If this is a straight line, then we can conclude that a linear relationship exists between the two variables, and can use the appropriate statistical technique to investigate that relationship. For example, we may be interested in using the linear relationship to predict the live weight of sheep from their chest girth. (Sometimes it is possible to linearize a non-linear relationship by transforming the data – see Section 12.2.)

10.3 LINEAR CORRELATION

10.3.1 The correlation coefficient

If we believe that there is a linear relationship between two quantitative variables with a change in one variable being associated with a change in the other, we may be interested in determining the strength of that relationship. We do not actually draw the line in correlation analysis (this is part of regression analysis), but we can imagine the line which approximates the data most closely. Are the points in the scatter diagram close to this line or are they widely dispersed around it? Provided a linear relationship exists between the two variables, the closer the points are to the line, the stronger the linear association between the two variables.

We measure the degree of association by calculating **Pearson's product moment correlation coefficient**, usually just called the **correlation coefficient**. It can take any value between −1 and +1.

- We say that we have *perfect correlation* if all the points lie on the line; in this case, the value of the correlation coefficient takes one of its extreme values, either +1 or −1 (see Fig. 10.1(a) and (b)).
- We have *positive correlation* if the sign of the correlation coefficient is positive; then there is a direct relationship between the two variables so that as one variable increases in value, so does the other variable (see Fig. 10.1(a) and (c)).
- We have *negative correlation* if the sign of the correlation coefficient is negative; then there is an inverse relationship between the two variables so that as one variable increases in value, the value of the other variable decreases (see Fig. 10.1(b) and (d)).
- We have no linear association (i.e. the variables are *uncorrelated*) if the correlation coefficient is zero; then there is a random scatter of

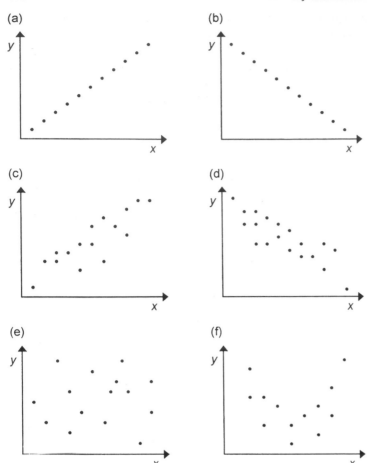

Fig. 10.1   Data with different correlation co-efficients: (a) perfect positive association, $r = +1$; (b) perfect negative association, $r = -1$; (c) positive association, $r = +0.86$; (d) negative association, $r = -0.85$; (e) no association, $r = 0$; (f) no linear association, $r = 0$.

points with no indication of a linear relation between the variables (see Fig. 10.1(e)). Note that a non-linear relationship between the variables can also give a correlation coefficient of zero (see Fig. 10.1(f))!

The closer the value of the correlation coefficient to either of its extreme values, the stronger the relationship between the variables, and the nearer the points are to the line.

We give the rather cumbersome formula for calculating the correlation coefficient, even though you will probably use the computer, or perhaps the appropriate function button on a hand-held calculator, to obtain its value. If we take a random sample of n independent pairs of observations $\{(x_1, y_1), (x_2, y_2), (x_3, y_3), \ldots (x_n, y_n)\}$

on two continuous variables, x and y, then we estimate the correlation coefficient, ρ (the Greek letter rho), in the population by the sample correlation coefficient

$$r = \frac{\sum (x - \bar{x})(y - \bar{y})}{\sqrt{\sum (x - \bar{x})^2 \sum (y - \bar{y})^2}}$$

Note that:

- The correlation coefficient is independent of the units of measurement of the two variables, i.e. it is dimensionless.
- We can interchange x and y without affecting the value of the correlation coefficient.
- The correlation coefficient is only valid within the limits of the data.

10.3.2 Testing a hypothesis that the correlation coefficient is zero

The correlation coefficient provides a measure of the strength of the linear association between two variables. There is no linear association between the variables if the correlation coefficient is zero, and so testing the hypothesis that $\rho = 0$ is a useful exercise in correlation analysis. Note, however, that even if the correlation coefficient is deemed significantly different from zero, this does *not* provide evidence of a *causal* relationship between the two variables; it merely indicates that they vary together.

(a) Assumptions

There are certain assumptions that have to be satisfied if we are to test a hypothesis about the correlation coefficient, or determine the confidence interval for it. In particular:

- The variables are measured on a random sample of individuals.
- Both of the variables, x and y, are quantitative.
- The hypothesis test that the true population correlation coefficient is zero only requires *at least one* of the two variables to be Normally distributed in the population (strictly, one variable is Normally distributed with constant variance for any given value of the other variable).
- If we calculate the confidence interval for the population correlation coefficient by taking a random sample of pairs of independent observations, $\{(x_1, y_1), (x_2, y_2), (x_3, y_3), \ldots (x_n, y_n)\}$ on two variables, x and y, then *both x and y* should be Normally distributed in the population (strictly, they should come from a bivariate Normal distribution, i.e. y is Normally distributed with constant variance for any given value of x, and x is Normally distributed with constant variance for any given value of y). If the data come from a bivariate Normal distribution, the scatter of points will be elliptical, although this will be difficult to discern if the correlation coefficient is close to either of its extremes.

If the data are measured on an ordinal scale or if we are concerned about the distributional assumptions in other circumstances, we should calculate **Spearman's rank correlation coefficient** (see Section 11.7), the non-parametric equivalent to Pearson's product moment correlation coefficient.

(b) The approach

1. Specify the **null hypothesis** that the population correlation coefficient, ρ, is equal to zero. Generally, we adopt the alternative hypothesis that the correlation coefficient is not equal to zero.
2. **Collect** the data and **display** them in a scatter diagram from which we can discern whether a linear relationship exists between the two variables. Check the assumption that at least one (or both if a confidence interval is to be calculated) of the variables is Normally distributed.
3. Calculate the sample correlation coefficient, preferably using a computer. You may find that the computer calculates a **test statistic** which has a t-distribution on $n - 2$ degrees of freedom. The test statistic is

$$Test_{10} = r\sqrt{\frac{(n-2)}{(1-r^2)}}$$

   where r is the sample correlation coefficient, and n is the number of pairs of observations in the sample.

   It is not difficult to calculate $Test_{10}$ by hand, but this is seldom required as there is a table (Table A.6) which relates the values of r directly to the P-values.
4. Obtain the **P-value**, generally from the computer output. You can refer r directly to Table A.6. Alternatively, you could refer $Test_{10}$ to the table of the t-distribution, Table A.3, with $n - 2$ degrees of freedom.
5. Make a **decision** whether or not to reject the null hypothesis by considering the P-value. Usually, although not necessarily, we reject the null hypothesis if $P < 0.05$.
6. Calculate the **confidence interval** for the true correlation coefficient. Although the

sampling distribution of r is not Normal, the distribution of a transformed variable, $z = 0.5\log_e\{(1 + r)/(1 - r)\}$, follows the Normal distribution, and we use this information to enable us to calculate the confidence interval for ρ.

It can be shown that the approximate 95% confidence limits for z are $z_1 = z - 1.96/\sqrt{n-3}$ and $z_2 = z + 1.96/\sqrt{n-3}$. We then back-transform, by taking exponentials, to get a confidence interval for ρ. Thus, the approximate 95% confidence interval for ρ is

$$\frac{e^{2z_1} - 1}{e^{2z_1} + 1} \text{ to } \frac{e^{2z_2} - 1}{e^{2z_2} + 1}$$

(c) Using the correlation coefficient as an aid to understanding

You should not rely solely on the magnitude of the correlation coefficient to judge the biological importance of the relationship between the two variables. You will see, if you look at Table A.6, that when the sample size is large, we reject the null hypothesis that the population correlation coefficient is zero, even though the value of the sample correlation coefficient is quite close to zero. For example, we reject the null hypothesis at the 5% level of significance if r is greater than 0.29, 0.20 and 0.16 for sample sizes of 45, 100 and 150, respectively. Furthermore, even when the sample size is much smaller (20, say), the result of the test is significant for quite low values of r ($P < 0.05$ if $r > 0.44$). A statistically significant result shows only that there is a linear relationship between the two variables. We need to gauge the importance of a significant result, and, clearly, we cannot do so by assessing the magnitude of the correlation coefficient.

Instead, we calculate the **square of the correlation coefficient, r^2**. It represents the proportion of the total variance in one variable that can be explained by or is attributed to its relationship with the other variable. It is usually multiplied by 100 and expressed as a percentage. So, if the correlation coefficient obtained from a sample of size 45 is 0.30, from which we can deduce that the true correlation coefficient is significantly

Table 10.1 Two measures of bone activity in 46 adult horses. (Based on summary data from Jackson *et al.*, 1996, with permission.)

wBAP (μgm/l)	PICP (U/l)	wBAP (μgm/l)	PICP (U/l)	wBAP (μgm/l)	PICP (U/l)
20	190	30	400	52	1005
31	186	36	380	61	1100
31	190	50	405	61	1070
22	205	54	370	57	810
18	210	31	490	59	720
16	290	35	470	63	740
18	306	39	470	65	700
55	1000	36	580	62	750
28	170	36	540	61	700
32	180	40	520	70	570
33	300	36	700	71	1300
38	303	34	800	88	1050
34	320	41	800	90	1100
21	360	48	850	90	1200
41	340	50	980	110	940
				34	360

different from zero ($P < 0.05$), its square is 0.09. Hence, even though the test of the correlation coefficient is significant, only 9% of the total variance of one variable is explained by its relationship with the other variable; the remaining 91% is unexplained by the relationship.

We advise you to calculate and interpret the value of r^2 routinely whenever you estimate the correlation coefficient. It is a great aid to understanding the strength of the underlying linear relationship between the two variables.

(d) Example

Jackson *et al.* (1996) developed a novel specific assay for measuring bone alkaline phosphatase acitivity, an enzyme which reflects bone metabolism. They were interested to know whether this measure, the wheatgerm lectin precipitated bone alkaline phosphatase activity (wBAP), was correlated with an independent marker of bone formation, the carboxy-terminal propeptide of Type I collagen (PICP). Table 10.1 is based on the results they obtained from a random sample of 46 adult horses. The data are plotted in Fig. 10.2, a scatter diagram in which both of the axes have logarithmic scales (this is an example of

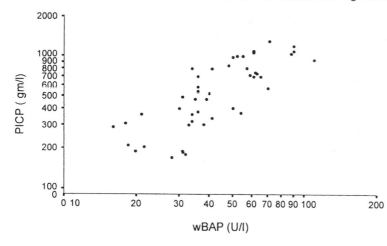

Fig. 10.2 Scatter diagram of the relationship between two measures of bone formation, bone alkaline phosphatase activity (wBAP) and Type I collagen concentration (PICP). Note that the variables are plotted on log scales. (Redrawn from Jackson *et al.*, 1996, with permission.)

data transformation – see Section 12.2.2 – the two variables being log transformed to Normalize the data). The relationship appears approximately linear, and the sample correlation coefficient is $r = 0.785$. Note that $r^2 = 0.62$, indicating that a substantial proportion, 62%, of the variance in log PICP is explained by its relationship with log wBAP. In order to test the null hypothesis that the true correlation coefficient is zero:

1. We specify H_0: there is no linear association between PICP and wBAP, i.e. $\rho = 0$; the alternative hypothesis is that $\rho \neq 0$.
2. The data are displayed in Fig. 10.2 which exhibits a positive linear relationship between the two variables when each is represented on a log scale. Separate histograms for log PICP and log wBAP reveal that each is approximately Normally distributed. Furthermore, the scatter of points suggests an ellipse, indicating that the data on the log scales are approximately bivariate Normal.
3. $r = 0.785$. Note that we could calculate $Test_{10} = 0.785 \sqrt{(44)/(0.3838)} = 8.41$.
4. When we refer 0.785 to Table A.6 with a sample size of 46, we find that $0.785 > 0.4742$ and that $0.785 > 0.4514$ (the entries in the table for sample sizes of 45 and 50), so $P < 0.001$. Note that we also obtain $P < 0.001$ if we refer $Test_{10}$ to Table A.3 with $46 - 2 = 44$ degrees of freedom.

5. We have strong evidence to reject the null hypothesis.
6. $z = 0.5\log_e(1.7846/0.2154) = 1.0572$. Hence $z_1 = 1.0572 - 1.96/\sqrt{43} = 0.7583$ and $z_2 = 1.0572 + 1.96/\sqrt{43} = 2.7122$. Thus the 95% confidence interval for ρ is:

$$\frac{e^{1.5166} - 1}{e^{1.5166} + 1} \quad \text{to} \quad \frac{e^{2.7122} - 1}{e^{2.7122} + 1}$$

$$= \frac{3.5567}{5.5567} \quad \text{to} \quad \frac{14.0624}{16.0623} = 0.64 \text{ to } 0.88.$$

The correlation coefficient is significantly different from zero, and even the lower limit of the confidence interval is indicative of a fairly strong linear association between the two measures; it would seem that the novel measurement of bone alkaline phosphatase activity indeed reflects the metabolic activity of bone tissue.

10.3.3 Misuse of the correlation coefficient

Unfortunately, the correlation coefficient is a frequently misused statistic. You must remember that a significant correlation coefficient does not provide evidence of a causal relationship between two variables. For example, just because the annual pet-food consumption in the UK is

(a)

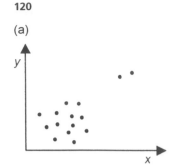

(b)

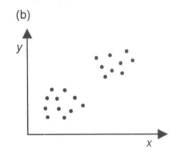

Fig. 10.3 Two circumstances in which the correlation coefficient should not be calculated.

correlated with the number of air-miles flown by UK residents, this does not suggest that pets are using food as a comfort substitute for absentee owners! Another example of misuse is when the correlation coefficient is relied upon to assess the repeatability of a technique or the agreement between two methods (see Section 13.3.1).

We have discussed the assumptions underlying the test of significance and the calculation of the confidence interval for the correlation coefficient (see Section 10.3.2(a)). Clearly, you must satisfy these assumptions in the relevant circumstances, but, remember that you *should not even calculate the correlation coefficient* when:

- There is an underlying relationship between the two variables, but it is not linear (see Fig. 10.1(f)).
- The observations are not independent; for example, when there is more than one observation on some or all of the experimental units.
- In the presence of outliers (see Section 5.9.2) when one or two extreme observations may distort the value of r (see Fig. 10.3(a)).
- The data consist of subgroups of animals, if these subgroups differ in their average response to one of the variables (see Fig. 10.3(b)).

10.4 SIMPLE LINEAR REGRESSION

10.4.1 The equation of the regression line

In simple linear regression analysis, we describe the relationship between two quantitative vari-

ables, x and y, by determining the straight line which approximates the data points on a scatter diagram most closely. We regard the x variable as one whose values can be measured without error or predetermined by the experimenter; so, for example, it may represent doses, ages, weights or concentrations at predetermined values. On the other hand, the y variable is a random variable which is subject to experimental variation, such as systolic blood pressure, haemoglobin concentration or colour intensity. We assume that y is *dependent* on x (rather than the other way round) so that if we change the value of x, this will lead to a change in the value of y, and not vice-versa.

- We call y the **dependent, response** or **outcome variable** and we represent this on the vertical axis of the scatter diagram.
- We call x the **independent, explanatory, regressor** or **predictor variable**, and we represent this on the horizontal axis.

We could draw 'by eye' what we believe to be the 'line of best fit' but this would be a subjective approach and not very satisfactory. Instead, we use an *equation* to describe the straight line relationship between x and y. If we imagine that, for each value of x, there is a *population* of y values, the equation would be:

$$Y_{pop} = \alpha + \beta x$$

where:

- Y_{pop} is the predicted or mean value of y for a given value of x.

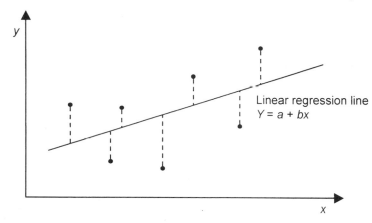

Fig. 10.4 Scatter diagram showing the fitted regression line and residuals (the dotted lines).

- α is the constant term which represents the *intercept* of the line; it is the value of y when x is equal to zero.
- β is the *slope* or *gradient* of the line and represents the average change in y for a unit change in x, i.e. it describes by how much y changes on average when x increases by one unit.

α and β are the parameters which define the line. They are both called **regression coefficients** although, frequently, you may find that this description is reserved only for β.

We have to *estimate* the two parameters α and β (by a and b, respectively) from our random sample of n pairs of observations, $\{(x_1, y_1), (x_2, y_2), (x_3, y_3), \ldots (x_n, y_n)\}$ in such a way that the line 'fits' the points as closely as possible.

- Generally, we approach the problem by requiring the deviations of the points from the line to be as small as possible. We take the deviation of a point from the line as the *vertical* distance of the point from the line, i.e. in the direction parallel to the y axis. We look at deviations in this direction because we believe that only the y variable is subject to experimental variation; we regard the x variable as measured without error. Each deviation, the difference between an *observed* value of y and its *predicted* or *fitted* value for a given value of x, is called a **residual** (see Fig. 10.4).
- Since some of the points are above the line and the corresponding residuals are positive,

and others are below the line with negative residuals, if we were to add the residuals, the positive and negative values would cancel each other out. We overcome this difficulty by determining a and b in such a way that the sum of the *squared* deviations is as small as possible (i.e. is minimized). Remember, the square of both negative and positive numbers is always positive. Hence the terminology, the **method of least squares**, to describe the technique for estimating α and β.

You do not need to concern yourself with the formulae for calculating a and b, since you will probably use the computer or the appropriate function buttons on a calculator. However, if you have to resort to hand calculations, the minimization procedure produces the following statistics

$$b = \frac{\sum (x - \bar{x})(y - \bar{y})}{\sum (x - \bar{x})^2} \quad \text{and} \quad a = \bar{y} - b\bar{x}$$

Then we estimate the best fitting line, called the **regression equation of y on x**, from our sample of observations as

$$Y = a + bx$$

where (see Fig. 10.5):

- Y is the predicted (fitted) value of y for a given value of x.
- a is the estimated intercept of the line.
- b is the estimated slope.

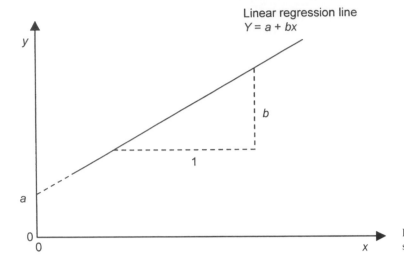

Fig. 10.5 Estimated linear regression line showing the intercept, *a*, and the slope, *b*.

Table 10.2 Live weight (LW) in kg and chest girth (CG) in cm of 66 sheep (data from Warriss and Edwards, 1995, with permission.)

LW	CG	LW	CG	LW	CG	LW	CG	LW	CG	LW	CG
30	76	20	63	28	77	29	73	18	62	19	67
24	71	28	70	25	71	30	74	28	70	27	69
20	63	22	65	27	72	21	64	27	71	31	74
25	69	28	72	28	74	28	74	30	73	23	67
25	67	25	67	25	65	48	89	28	72	22	63
19	62	20	62	20	64	17	60	22	69	35	75
35	77	35	78	35	78	46	86	48	90	44	84
37	84	43	81	32	73	43	84	31	73	31	73
39	78	36	81	33	80	44	82	39	80	45	86
43	88	41	87	36	82	43	80	33	79	35	78
38	78	36	76	35	74	39	81	34	74	39	76

We can *draw* the line on the scatter diagram by choosing two or, preferably (just to play safe), three values of *x* along the range of values of *x*. By substituting these values of *x* in the equation of the line, we can calculate the corresponding predicted *Y* values. We plot these points on the scatter diagram and join them by a straight line. The line must *not* be extrapolated beyond the limits of the data.

10.4.2 An example

It is necessary from time to time to estimate the body weight of sheep; for example, for accurate drug-dosing or for predicting market dates.

Unfortunately, weighing sheep is difficult, so it is helpful to be able to estimate the sheep's weight from some other, more easily obtained, measure. A study was conducted to investigate the relationship between the sheep's live weight and its chest girth. Table 10.2 shows the measurements of a random sample of 66 sheep studied whose chest girth lay between 60 cm and 90 cm (based on data from Warriss and Edwards, 1995). Figure 10.6(a) is a scatter diagram which shows the relationship between the live weight (kg) and chest girth (cm) in the 66 sheep. The estimated regression equation of live weight (*y*) on chest girth (*x*) is shown by a computer analysis (Display 10.1) to be

$$Y = -46.04 + 1.04x$$

(a)

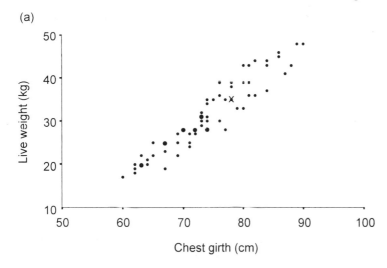

(b)

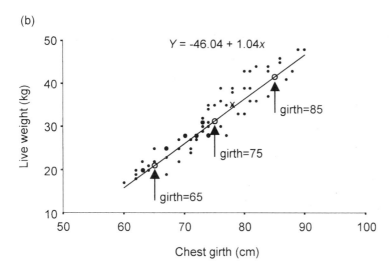

Fig. 10.6 Scatter diagrams of (a) sheep chest girth and live weight, and (b) the same data with fitted regression line as discussed in Section 10.4.2. A large solid circle (●) shows duplicate points, a cross (×) shows triplicate points and an open circle (○) shows a calculated point. (Data from Warriss and Edwards, 1995, with permission.)

The estimated slope indicates that a sheep's live weight increases on average by 1.04 kg as its chest girth increases by 1 cm. This estimated regression line is valid only in the specified range of values of chest girth (i.e. 60–90 cm) and should not be extrapolated beyond these limits. We have drawn the line by substituting three values of chest girth (65, 75 and 85 cm) into the equation to obtain the three corresponding values of live weight (21.56, 31.96 and 42.36 kg, respectively), plotting these points and joining them (see Fig. 10.6(b)).

10.4.3 Assumptions underlying linear regression

(a) What are they?

Before you go on to make inferences about the parameters which define the regression equation, or use the equation to predict values of y from x, you should be aware of the assumptions that underlie linear regression (see Fig. 10.7). They are that:

ANOVA

	Sum of squares	df	Mean square	F	Sig.
Regression	3972.930	1	3972.930	562.113	0.000
Residual	452.342	64	7.068		
Total	4425.272	65			

Predictors: (Constant), CHESTGTH.
Dependent variable: LIVEWT.

Display 10.1 Typical computer output for the simple linear regression analysis of the sheep girth data described in Table 10.2.

Coefficients

	Coefficients				95% confidence interval for β	
	b	Std Error	t	Sig.	Lower bound	Upper bound
(Constant)	−46.04	3.281	−14.03	0.000	−52.60	−39.48
CHESTGTH	1.04	0.044	23.64	0.000	0.95	1.13

Dependent variable: LIVEWT.

Note that the entry for b in the first row of the table represents the intercept or constant term, a, in the estimated regression equation. Coefficients (and CI) corrected to two decimal places.

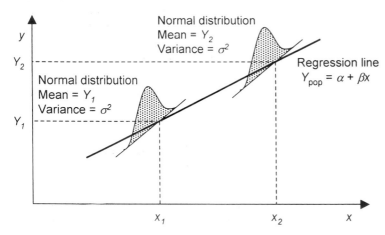

Fig. 10.7 Diagram illustrating assumptions underlying regression analysis.

- The relationship between x and y is linear.
- x is measured without error.
- For each value of x, the population values of y, from which we take a random sample, are Normally distributed.
- For each value of x, the population mean of the distribution of values of y lies on the line,

$Y_{pop} = \alpha + \beta x$.

- The population variance of the distribution of values of y is constant for each value of x.
- The observations are independent; this implies that each individual is represented once in the random sample.

(b) How do we check them?

It is essential to check these assumptions in linear regression analysis; this is an often over-looked process. Although we can sometimes get an indication of whether the assumptions are sat-isfied by plotting the data and drawing the best fitting line, the most efficient approach is to study the *residuals*. Remember, for each value of *x*, the residual is the difference between its observed and predicted values of *y*. We can only obtain the residuals once we have estimated the parameters of the line using the sample data. You may have to request the residuals from your computer package, although many packages produce them automatically.

If the assumptions underlying linear regres-sion are satisfied, then, in addition to the require-ments that *x is a variable measured without error* and the *observations are independent, the residuals are Normally distributed with a mean of zero, and their variability is constant throughout the range of the fitted values of y*. We can check the assumptions by producing appropriate plots of the residuals; in particular, using the sheep girth data discussed in Section 10.4.2 for illustra-tive purposes, we can verify that:

* *The relationship between x and y is linear* by plotting the residuals against the values of *x*. If the relationship between *x* and *y* is linear, the residuals should be randomly scattered around zero, and there should be no apparent trend in the residuals for increasing or de-creasing values of *x* (see Fig. 10.8(a)). Alterna-tively, we can simply plot *y* against *x* and observe whether the approximating curve is a straight line.
* *The residuals are Normally distributed* by pro-ducing either a histogram or a Normal plot (see Section 3.5.3(e)) of the residuals (see Fig. 10.8(b)).
* *The variability of the residuals is constant throughout the range of fitted values of y* by plotting the residuals against the fitted values. If the assumption is satisfied, we should expect a random scatter of residuals (see Fig. 10.8(c)). If we can discern a funnel effect, with the residuals appearing to increase (or decrease)

with increasing fitted values, then the constant variance assumption is not satisfied.

(c) What do we do if they are not satisfied?

The linearity and independence assumptions are the most crucial. Sometimes a simple transfor-mation of *x* or *y* will achieve linearity (see Section 12.2.2). If the linearity assumption is in doubt, we may decide that another form of rela-tionship, such as a quadratic, is more appropriate than a straight line (see Section 10.5.1(c)). A simple linear regression analysis would then be inappropriate.

If the residuals are not Normally distributed and/or do not have constant variance, we have two choices. Provided there are only moderate departures from the assumptions, we can pro-ceed with the analysis. We should be aware, how-ever, that the estimates of the standard errors and the *P*-values may be affected by a failure to satisfy the assumptions. Alternatively, and this is the only option if there are gross departures from the assumptions, we have to take an appropriate transformation (see Section 12.2), either of *x* or of *y* or of both of them. For example, we often find that a logarithmic transformation of the *y* variable is suitable. We then repeat the analysis by calculating another regression line of the transformed *y* on *x*, and check that the assump-tions underlying this new line are satisfied.

10.4.4 The residual variance and the ANOVA table

Corresponding to each observation is a residual which is the difference between the observed value of *y* and its predicted or fitted value, *Y*, where $Y = a + bx$. The variance of the residuals is estimated in a sample of size *n* by

$$s_{res}^2 = \frac{\sum (y - Y)^2}{(n - 2)}$$

and is usually called the **residual mean square** or the **residual variance**. We need the residual vari-ance if we want to test hypotheses about the

(a) Linearity

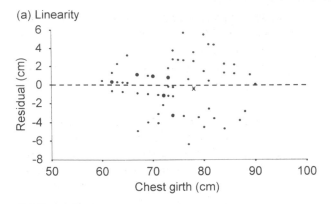

(b) Normality

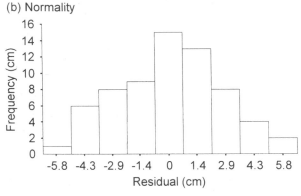

(c) Constant variance

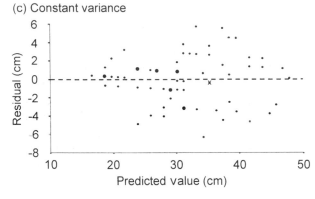

Fig. 10.8 Diagrams used to check the assumptions in a linear regression analysis of the sheep data discussed in Section 10.4.2. A large solid circle (•) shows duplicate points, a cross (x) shows triplicate to points.

parameters of the line or to calculate confidence intervals.

Instead of calculating the residual variance using the above formula, we can use the residual mean square in the computer generated **analysis of variance table** (see Section 8.5.2).

Justification

In the ANOVA table for linear regression analysis, the total variation of *y* is partitioned into two components: the variation which is *explained* by the linear relationship of *y* on *x*, and the *residual*

variation which is *unexplained* by the relationship. To understand this dichotomy, consider what happens if there is a perfect positive relationship between *x* and *y*; then every point lies on the line, and all the variation in *y* is explained by the relationship. This is an ideal circumstance; more usually, y tends to increase as *x* increases. Thus, only some of the variation in *y* is present because of the relationship between *y* and *x*, and this is the variation explained by the relationship. The remainder of the variation in *y*, that which is left over or residual, is unexplained by the relationship. Since the mean squares in an ANOVA table represent variances, the *residual variance is the mean square of the source of variation which is unexplained by the regression.*   □

The source of variation in the ANOVA table which is explained by the regression is sometimes called that which is *due to regression*, *explained by regression* or simply *regression*; the source of variation which is unexplained by the regression is sometimes called that which is *unexplained* or *residual*. We show the ANOVA results for the sheep girth data in the ANOVA table in Display 10.1. From this table, we can see that the residual variance is estimated as $7.068 \, \mathrm{kg}^2$.

10.4.5 Assessing goodness-of-fit

The usual way of establishing whether the line is a good fit is to determine the proportion of the total variation in y which is explained by the linear relationship of y on x; it is often denoted by R^2 and sometimes called the **coefficient of determination**. This proportion is the sum of squares explained by the regression divided by the total sum of squares, both sums of squares being obtained from the ANOVA table. *In simple linear regression, it is the square of the correlation coefficient, r^2 (see Section 10.3.2(c)).*

In the ANOVA table Display 10.1, the proportion of the variation explained by the regression is $(3972.930)/(4425.272) = 0.898$. Thus, approximately 90% of variation in the sheep's live weight is explained by its linear relationship with chest girth; this indicates that the line is a good fit in the specified range. Note that the estimated correlation coefficient between the sheep's live weight and chest girth is the square root of this quantity, i.e. $r = \sqrt{0.898} = 0.95$.

10.4.6 Investigating the slope

(a) The approach

Once we have determined the equation of the best fitting line, we usually proceed to investigate the parameters which define the line. Invariably, our primary interest lies with the slope of the line. The slope shows by how much y changes on average as we increase x by one unit. If there is no linear relationship between x and y, then as we increase x by one unit, the value of y is equally likely to increase or decrease, i.e. its average is zero. Thus, we can test the null hypothesis that the true slope, β, is zero, if we want to decide whether or not a linear relationship exists. The approach is:

1. Specify the **null hypothesis** that the true slope, β, is zero. Specify the alternative hypothesis, generally, that the slope is not equal to zero.
2. **Collect** the data and **display** them in a scatter diagram. Determine the best fitting line, $Y = a + bx$, where Y is the fitted value corresponding to a given value of x, and the statistics, a and b, estimate the parameters, α and β, respectively. Check the assumptions underlying linear regression by studying the residuals (see Section 10.4.3).
3. Select the **appropriate test** on the computer or calculate the **test statistic** by hand. This test statistic follows the t-distribution and is given by

$$Test_{11} = \frac{b}{\mathrm{SE}(b)} \quad \text{with } n - 2 \text{ degrees of freedom}$$

where $\mathrm{SE}(b) = \dfrac{s_{\mathrm{res}}}{\sqrt{\sum (x - \bar{x})^2}}$, and s_{res} is the standard deviation of the residuals.

The alternative approach is to refer to the ANOVA table in regression analysis (see Section 10.4.3) which is used to test the same null hypothesis, namely that β is zero. Then the test statistic is the F-ratio which is the 'due to regression' mean square divided by the residual mean square; it follows the F-distribution with one degree of freedom in the numerator and $(n - 2)$ degrees of freedom in the denominator. Note that the two tests produce identical results in that the square of $Test_{11}$ is equal to the statistic derived from the ANOVA table.

4. Determine the **P-value**. Usually the computer will do this for you. Alternatively, you can refer your test statistic to the table of the t- or F-distribution, as appropriate.
5. Make a **decision** whether or not to reject the null hypothesis; usually, but not necessarily, reject H_0 if $P < 0.05$. Note that when there is no linear relationship between the two vari-

ables, both the slope, β, and the correlation coefficient, ρ, are equal to zero.

6. Derive the **confidence interval** for the true slope, β. If the computer output does not contain this information, you can calculate the 95% confidence interval as

$$b \pm t_{0.05} \, \mathrm{SE}(b)$$

where $t_{0.05}$ is the critical value or percentage point (giving a tail area probability of 0.025 in each tail) obtained from the table of the t-distribution with $n - 2$ degrees of freedom,

and $\mathrm{SE}(b) = s_{\mathrm{res}} \Big/ \sqrt{\sum (x - \bar{x})^2}$.

(b) Example

In the sheep girth example of Section 10.4.2:

1. The null hypothesis is that the true slope, β, of the linear regression of live weight on chest girth is zero. The alternative hypothesis is that it is not zero.
2. The data are displayed in Fig. 10.6(b) in which the best fitting line, $Y = -46.04 + 1.04x$, is drawn. The assumptions underlying the regression analysis have been investigated in Section 10.4.3 by studying the residuals displayed in Fig. 10.8, and are valid.
3. A typical computer output which shows both the estimated regression coefficients and the test statistic (equal to $(1.043)/(0.044) = 23.70$), is shown in the Coefficients table in Display 10.1. Note that we could also use the F-ratio in the ANOVA table in Display 10.1, which has a value of 562.11, to test the null hypothesis. Apart from rounding errors, $t^2 = F$.
4. The P-value (i.e. Sig. $= 0.000$) from the computer output in both the ANOVA table and the Coefficients table in Display 10.1 indicates that $P < 0.001$. We could obtain this P-value by referring the value of 23.64 to Table A.3 of the t-distribution with 64 degrees of freedom (df), or the value of 562.11 to Table A.5(a) of the F-distribution with 1 df in the numerator and 64 df in the denominator.
5. The data do not appear to be consistent with the null hypothesis ($P < 0.001$), which we therefore reject. We have evidence which in-

dicates that the true slope of the line is not equal to zero.

6. The 95% confidence interval for the true slope, shown in Display 10.1, is between 0.95 and 1.13. We can calculate it as

$$1.04 \pm 2.00 \times 0.044$$

where the value 2.00 is the approximate percentage point from the t-distribution (Table A.3) with $66 - 2 = 64$ degrees of freedom.

10.4.7 Predicting *y* from a given *x*

We often use the regression line, once we have established that there is a linear relationship between x and y (i.e. that the slope is significantly different from zero), to **predict the mean value of y** that we expect for individuals or animals who have a specified value of x, say x_1. To obtain the predicted value is straightforward; we substitute the value of x in the equation, $Y = a + bx$, so that our mean predicted value is $Y_1 = a + bx_1$. In the sheep girth example of Section 10.4.2, we predict that sheep which have a chest girth of 73.2 cm would be expected on average to weigh 30.09 kg (i.e. if $x_1 = 73.2$, $Y_1 = -46.04 + 1.04 \times 73.2 = 30.09$).

We have to recognize, however, that because we only have a sample of observations, there is sampling error associated with this mean predicted value. It is possible to quantify it and therefore calculate a confidence interval for the mean predicted value. The formulae are not easy and we refer you to Armitage and Berry (1994) for details.

Sometimes we wish to determine a region, over the range of values of x, within which we expect the *true regression line* to lie with a certain probability (say, 0.95). This **confidence band region** or **interval for the line** is obtained, usually on the computer, by determining the 95% confidence intervals for the mean predicted values of y for various values of x. Each confidence interval has an upper limit above the regression line, and a lower limit below the regression line. The required band is obtained by connecting all the upper limits and, similarly, all the lower limits

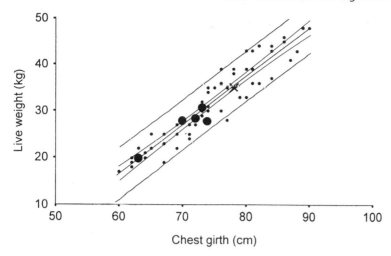

Fig. 10.9 Ninety-five percent confidence limits for the regression line (the inner limits on either side of the regression line) and the individual points (the outer limits). A large solid circle (●) shows duplicate points, a cross (x) shows triplicate points. (Data from Table 10.2.)

(see Fig. 10.9). The confidence band is narrower in the middle of the range of values of *x* than at the extremes, indicating that we have less confidence in the prediction of the mean of the *y* values as we move towards the extremes.

Occasionally, you may see a wider band illustrated (see Fig. 10.9). This relates to the scatter of the data points and is the region which contains approximately 95% of the *individual population values* (for a 95% confidence band).

10.5 MULTIPLE LINEAR REGRESSION

10.5.1 The multiple linear regression equation

(a) Explanation

Section 10.4 was concerned with the linear relationship of a dependent variable, *y*, and a *single* independent variable, *x*. Very often we are interested in investigating the *simultaneous* effect of a *number of factors* on a response variable when we believe these factors may be interrelated. For example, Pearson and Ouassat (1996) found that, by combining measurements of several variables rather than using just one variable, they could get an improved estimate of the body weight of donkeys (see Section 10.5.6). We can extend the simple linear regression equation, and form a **multiple regression equation**, to accommodate this situation. If there are

k independent, predictor or *explanatory* variables, sometimes called covariates, $x_1, x_2, x_3, \ldots, x_k$, which we believe may have an effect on a continuous *dependent* or *response* variable, *y*, the true regression model may be expressed as

$$Y_{pop} = \alpha + \beta_1 x_1 + \beta_2 x_2 + \beta_3 x_3 + \ldots + \beta_k x_k$$

where x_i is the *i*th predictor variable ($i = 1, 2, 3, \ldots, k$) measured on each individual; Y_{pop} is the predicted value of *y* in the population for the set of covariates; α is a constant term; and $\beta_1, \beta_2, \beta_3, \ldots, \beta_k$, are the **partial regression coefficients**, often simply called **regression coefficients**, corresponding to the *k* explanatory variables.

Then β_1 *represents the average change in y for a unit change in* x_1, *when the other explanatory* variables, $x_2, x_3, \ldots, x_k$, *are held constant.* A similar interpretation is afforded the other partial regression coefficients. The partial regression coefficients are obtained by mimimizing the sum of the squared residuals (a residual being the difference between an observed and a fitted value of *y*). The regression coefficients are estimated in the sample by $b_1, b_2, b_3, \ldots, b_k$ respectively, and α is estimated by *a*. The estimated regression line is thus

$$Y = a + b_1 x_1 + b_2 x_2 + b_3 x_3 + \ldots + b_k x_k$$

where *Y* is the fitted value of *y*.

We do not feel that it is necessary to give the formulae for estimating the coefficients or their standard errors since, invariably, you will use the computer to perform a multiple regression analysis. We outline the procedures involved, noting the similarity to simple linear regression and laying emphasis on the underlying concepts. You can obtain details of the analysis, and of the modifications to multiple regression described below, in more advanced texts such as Draper and Smith (1981), Schroeder *et al.* (1986) and Kleinbaum *et al.* (1988).

(b) Uses

The main reasons for performing a multiple regression analysis are:

- To predict the value of the dependent variable from the explanatory variables, using the optimal equation which relates y to the x values.
- To determine which explanatory variables are important predictors of the dependent variable, and the extent to which they influence the dependent variable.
- To be able to study the relationship between the dependent variable and each of the explanatory variables whilst controlling for the effect of the other explanatory variables in the equation.

(c) Modifications

- You should note that it is possible to include **interaction** terms in the multiple regression equation. An interaction occurs between two explanatory variables when the effect on the response variable of one of the explanatory variables is not the same for different values of the other explanatory variable. So, for example, we may find that if we are using a multiple regression equation to predict an animal's body weight (y) from a number of variables including its length (x_1), the relationship may be different for males ($x_2 = 0$, say) and females ($x_2 = 1$, say). We include an interaction term in the model by creating a new variable which is the product of the two explanatory variables, ($x_1 x_2$), and examine its coefficient in the same way as we would that of any explanatory variable.
- Sometimes, you may find that you have a non-linear (i.e. curved) relationship between y and x, e.g. quadratic or cubic, in which case a **polynomial** regression may be appropriate. Polynomial regression for the single explanatory variable, x, can be thought of as a special form of multiple regression, and can be analysed as such. Each explanatory variable in the multiple regression equation is replaced by successively higher powers of x. For example, the estimated cubic equation is of the form

$$Y = a + b_1 x + b_2 x^2 + b_3 x^3$$

10.5.2 Appropriateness of the model

(a) Assumptions underlying multiple regression

The assumptions underlying multiple linear regression are similar to those in simple linear regression (see Section 10.4.3).

- A linear relationship is stipulated between the predictor variable (which is a continuous random variable) and each of the explanatory variables (which are measured without error and do not need to be continuous; see Section 10.5.5).
- The residuals are independent – each individual is represented once in the sample.
- The residuals are Normally distributed with zero mean and constant variance.

We should produce appropriate plots of the residuals to verify the assumptions. These are illustrated in Fig. 10.10. In particular:

- Separate plots of the residuals against each of the explanatory variables will verify the linearity assumption providing no trend is apparent.
- A histogram or Normal plot of the residuals can verify the Normality assumption.
- A plot of the residuals against the fitted values of y will verify the constant variance assumption, providing there is no funnel effect.

(b) Relationship between explanatory variables

We expect some of the explanatory variables in a multiple regression to be related to one another. If this were not so, the multivariate analysis would be redundant; we could equally well perform a simple linear regression analysis between the response variable and each explanatory variable, and obtain the same regression coefficients as in the multiple regression incorporating all the variables. We can determine which variables are associated by calculating the correlation coefficients between every pair of explanatory variables, and observing which are significant. You should be aware that extremely highly correlated variables (i.e. those with correlation coefficients approximately equal to ± 1) often result in **collinearity** (sometimes called multicollinearity) in the multiple regression analysis. This may make it difficult to interpret the regression coefficients which, although individually non-significant in the multiple regression equation, may have a joint effect on the response of interest. You will find details of how to deal with collinearity in more advanced texts. Note, however, that using automatic selection procedures (see Section 10.5.4) may alleviate the problem.

10.5.3 Understanding the computer output in a multiple regression analysis

1. We can assess how well the model fits the data by calculating the proportion of the total variability that is explained by the relationship of y on the x values. This proportion is denoted by R^2; its square root is called the **multiple correlation coefficient**. We cannot use R^2 to compare the fit of different models as its value will be greater for models which include a larger number of explanatory variables.

To overcome this difficulty, an **adjusted R^2** is often calculated which affords a direct comparison of values to assess goodness-of-fit in models which contain different numbers of explanatory variables.

2. The computer output for a multiple regression analysis contains an **analysis of variance** table which separates the total variation of y into its two sources: that which is explained and that which is unexplained by the regression. The **F-test** in the table enables us to test the null hypothesis that *all* the partial regression coefficients are zero. If the result of the test is significant, we conclude that at least one of the explanatory variables is associated with the response variable.

3. Then we can determine which of the explanatory variables has a partial regression coefficient which is significantly different from zero by performing a **t-test** on each coefficient. Each test statistic is the estimated regression coefficient divided by its standard error, and has a t-distribution on $n - k - 1$ degrees of freedom, where k is the number of explanatory variables in the model. Computer output lists each estimated regression coefficient, usually with its standard error or a confidence interval, together with the test statistic and its P-value.

10.5.4 Choosing the explanatory variables to include in the analysis

Just because a computer program is available to perform a multiple regression analysis, this does *not* give you *carte blanche* to include, indiscriminately, a disproportionately large number of explanatory variables in the model. As a rule of thumb, remember that the sample size should *not* be less that ten times the number of explanatory variables. So, if you have 100 observations, you should include no more than 10 explanatory variables in the model. In any case, you should *only include those explanatory variables which you know are likely to have some relationship with the response variable.*

It is possible to use formal techniques for selecting the 'best' combination of variables in the multiple regression equation. These are particularly useful when some of the explanatory variables are very highly correlated. There is no single definition of 'best' but, usually, those variables are selected which optimize the amount of explained variation in y, so that it will not be significantly greater for a different selection.

- In **forward step-up selection**, we start with the single explanatory variable which contributes the most to the explained variation in y, and include more variables in the equation, progressively, until the addition of an extra variable does not significantly improve the situation.
- In **backward step-down selection**, we start with all the variables, and take them away sequentially, starting with the variable which contributes the least, until the deletion of a variable significantly reduces the amount of explained variation in y.
- **Stepwise selection** is essentially step-up selection, but it permits the elimination of variables at each step according

to defined statistical criteria specified by the computer package.

- In **all subsets selection**, we investigate all the possible combinations of variables and choose that one which is optimal in some sense, perhaps with the greatest adjusted R^2.

Unfortunately, the different approaches sometimes produce different combinations of variables! You alone can judge the *appropriate* combination to best explain your phenomenon.

10.5.5 Categorical explanatory variables

We can use multiple regression analysis when one or more of our explanatory variables is categorical. We tackle the problem by assigning codes to the variable so we are able to distinguish the different categories. In particular, we need to assign two codes to the variable if we have a **binary** explanatory variable. For example, we could assign the codes 0 and 1 to the variable representing 'sex', so that a male takes the value '0' and a female takes the value '1'.

We can use this approach to evaluate the effect of two different treatments on a response variable when we feel that it is necessary to take into account the effect of a number of explanatory variables on response. This is a particular example of an **analysis of covariance** problem (in ANCOVA – an extension of ANOVA (see Section 8.5) – we compare groups after adjusting for the effect of covariates) which can be analysed using a multiple regression approach. We assign a code to 'treatment', so that its value for animals on treatment A, say, is 0 and its value for animals on treatment B is 1. The 'treatment' regression coefficient is interpreted as the average difference in response between treatments A and B, adjusting for the other explanatory variables. If it is significantly different from zero, then the mean response on A is significantly different from the mean response on B, adjusting for the other explanatory variables. If it is positive then the average response is greater on B than on A (because of the coding of the treatment variable); if it is negative, then the reverse is true.

In the situation when a qualitative explanatory variable has more than two categories, we can create what are called *dummy* variables, but the approach is not straightforward. Within regression analysis, some computer programs have the capability to respond to instructions and create dummy variables. You need to understand how these dummy variables work, and you can find details in Armitage and Berry (1994).

10.5.6 Example

Another example of the problem of estimating body weight is the subject of a study by Pearson and Ouassat (1996), this time in Moroccan working donkeys. Here they were concerned to avoid overloading the draft donkeys, and needed to

Display 10.2　Typical computer output from the multiple linear regression analysis of the donkey data (six explanatory variables) discussed in Section 10.5.6.

Model summary

Model	R	R square	Adjusted R square	Std error of the estimate
1	0.927*	0.859	0.857	9.3812

*Predictors: (Const), UMBGIRTH, SEX, AGE, LENGTH, HEIGHT, HEARTGIR.

ANOVA*

Model		Sum of squares	df	Mean square	F	Sig.
1	Regression	203987.4	6	33997.899	386.305	0.000[†]
	Residual	33354.959	379	88.008		
	Total	237342.4	385			

*Dependent variable: BODYWT.
[†]Predictors: (Const), UMBGIRTH, SEX, AGE, LENGTH, HEIGHT, HEARTGIR.

Coefficients*

Model		Coefficients		t	Sig.	95% Confidence Interval for β	
		b	Std error			Lower bound	Upper bound
1	(Constant)	−216.3	7.667	−28.217	0.000	−231.403	−201.254
	AGE	0.262	0.184	1.422	0.156	−0.100	0.623
	HEARTGIR	1.770	0.115	15.390	0.000	1.544	1.996
	HEIGHT	0.157	0.110	1.433	0.153	−0.058	0.373
	LENGTH	0.893	0.117	7.605	0.000	0.662	1.123
	SEX	−2.293	1.015	−2.260	0.024	−4.289	−0.298
	UMBGIRTH	0.380	0.067	5.668	0.000	0.248	0.512

*Dependent variable: BODYWT.

be able to estimate body weight since weighing machines are a rarity! Rather than regress body weight on a single variable (as in our simple regression example on sheep), they chose a number of variables (the donkey's girth at the level of the heart (cm), girth at the umbilicus (cm), length from the olecranon to the tuber ischii (cm), height at the withers (cm), and the donkey's age (years) and sex (male = 0, female = 1)) to help them predict its body weight (kg). The variables were measured in a random sample of 400 adult donkeys. Many of these variables were interrelated but collinearity was absent since there was no extremely high correlation coefficient between any two explanatory variables. We performed a multiple linear regression analysis on a subset of these data

(excluding pregnant females) using body weight as the dependent variable, and all other variables as the explanatory variables. The results from a computer analysis are shown in Display 10.2.

We can regard the model as a good fit since the adjusted R square is 0.859, i.e. 86% of the variation in body weight is explained by its relationship with the explanatory variables. Apart from independence of the observations (which is not in doubt), the assumptions underlying the regression model can be assessed by studying the residuals. The plots of the residuals against the three predictor variables (heart girth, umbilical girth and length) in Fig. 10.10 show that the linearity assumption is satisfactory for these three variables. The plots

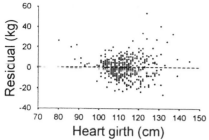

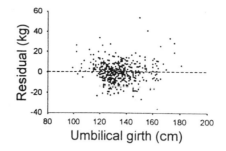

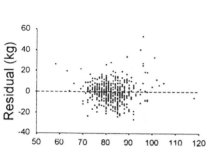

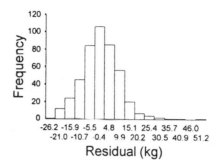

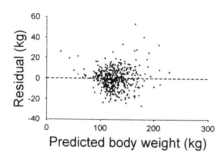

Fig. 10.10 Diagrams for checking the assumptions underlying the multiple regression analysis of the Moroccan donkey data. In the histogram the *x* axis labels relate to the midpoints of the intervals (from Pearson and Ouassat, 1996, with permission).

for the other independent variables are omitted for brevity, but they all accommodate the linearity assumption. We can see from Fig. 10.10 that the residuals are approximately Normally distributed, and, from the plot of the residuals against the predicted values, that they have constant variance and are centred around a mean of approximately zero.

The *F*-test in the ANOVA gives $P < 0.001$, indicating that at least one of the six partial regression coefficients is significantly different from zero.

In fact, as shown in the table of coefficients, four variables (heart girth, length, umbilical girth and sex) have partial regression coefficients which are significantly different from zero. We interpret these coefficients as follows: a donkey's body weight increases on average by 1.770 kg as its heart girth increases by 1 cm, adjusting for the other variables in the equation. Similarly, the body weight of a female donkey is 2.293 kg less, on average, than that of a male, after adjusting for the other variables, etc.

As there is no evidence that the height and age of the donkey are useful predictors of body weight, the multiple regression analysis was repeated using only the four variables

which had significant coefficients. The assumptions underlying this model were checked and found to be satisfactory. This second regression analysis (adjusted $R^2 = 0.856$) gives the following multiple regression equation:

$$\text{Bodywt} = -216.4 + 1.840\text{Heartgir} + 0.999\text{Length} - 2.917\text{Sex} + 0.396\text{Umbgirth}$$

which can be used to predict a Moroccan donkey's body weight. □

10.6 MULTIPLE LOGISTIC REGRESSION – A BINARY RESPONSE VARIABLE

10.6.1 Rationale

We can use a modification of the multiple regression equation to analyse data when we have a **binary response variable**.

Table 10.3 Results of the logistic regression analysis for the recumbency of cows during Caesarian section. (Data from Hoeben *et al.*, 1997, with permission.)

Variable, x_i	Numerical value of x_i	b_i	SE(b_i)	*P*-value	Odds ratio	95% CI for odds ratio
Type of animal	Dairy = 0, Beef = 1	−0.6599	0.2087	0.002	0.52	0.34–0.78
Parity	Heifer = 0, Mult. cow = 1	−0.6708	0.2106	0.002	0.51	0.24–0.77
Sedation	No = 0, Yes = 1	0.6683	0.1972	0.001	1.95	1.33–2.87
Exteriorization of uterus	Easy = 0, Difficult = 1	0.7049	0.2153	0.001	2.02	1.33–3.09

For example, we may wish to relate a number of explanatory variables to an outcome such as the presence or absence of an abnormality. We can define the response variable, y, so that $y = 1$ represents 'presence' and $y = 0$ represents 'absence'. However, we cannot use this variable directly in the multiple regression equation without an appropriate adjustment. This is because we would be unable to interpret any predicted values of it which are not exactly equal to 0 or 1. We therefore consider the *probability*, p, that this variable takes a particular value (say $y = 1$) as the response of interest. We then take a transformation of this probability to overcome the problem that we cannot interpret any predicted value outside the limits of 0 and 1, and we use this as the dependent variable in the equation. The transformation is called the *logistic* or *logit transformation* (see Section 12.2.2), leading to a **multiple linear logistic regression** equation, often simply called **logistic regression**. We cannot use ordinary multiple regression analysis to estimate the coefficients in the multiple logistic regression equation; instead, the computer estimates these logistic coefficients by an iterative method called maximum likelihood.

Each explanatory variable has a coefficient in the logistic equation which can be tested (the null hypothesis is that the true coefficient is zero) to determine whether that variable contributes significantly to an animal's chance of an abnormality, after adjusting for the possible confounding effects of the other variables. Because of the logistic transformation, the coefficients are interpreted in a different way from those in the ordinary multiple regression equation. The exponential of each logistic coefficient is the *odds ratio* or the estimated *relative risk* (see Section 5.2.3) of a particular outcome for a unit increase in the explanatory variable, keeping the values of the other variables constant. For example, if we have an explanatory variable, x_1, indicating which treatment an animal has received ($x_1 = 0$ for treatment A, and $x_1 = 1$ for treatment B), the exponential of its coefficient in the logistic regression equation, e^{b_1}, is the estimated risk of the presence of the abnormality on treatment B compared to that on treatment A, after adjusting for the other variables in the equation. A relative risk of unity indicates that the risk of the abnormality is the same for both treatments. The other coefficients in the logistic equation may be interpreted in a similar fashion. You can obtain details of logistic regression analysis in a number of texts such as that by Menard (1995).

10.6.2 Example

Hoeben *et al.* (1997) assessed 1000 Caesarian sections in standing cows performed under field conditions by veterinarians from the University of Ghent with a view to determining the factors which induce complications. This was in order to take some precautions to minimize the negative consequences, such as death of the cow or calf, placental retention, infection of the wound, etc. The most important complications are recumbency of the animal during the operation, exteriorization of the pregnant uterine horn, and increased contractility of the uterus.

Initially, a simple univariate analysis was performed to evaluate the effects of each of a number of variables on the occurrence of each of the three main complications. For each variable, the relative risk was estimated as the proportion of animals developing the complication if the factor was present divided by that if it was absent, and its significance from unity determined. Significant variables ($P < 0.05$) included experience of the surgeon, type of cow (dairy or beef), parity, use of the sedative xylazine (yes/no), quantity of sedative (ml), attempt to extract the calf (yes/no), use of epidural anaesthesia (yes/no), contractility of the uterus (relaxed/contracted), etc. For each of the three main complications, a multiple logistic regression analysis was then performed using only those variables which were shown to be significant in the univariate analysis.

In Table 10.3 we show the variables which had significant coefficients in the logistic regression analysis connected with recumbency of the animals during Caesarian section, after adjusting for the other prognostic variables. This table contains, for each variable, an estimate of the β coefficient in the logistic regression equation, with its standard error and *P*-value which results from the test of the null hypothesis that the coefficient is zero. The odds ratio estimates the relative risk; for example, the odds ratio of 1.95 for sedation implies that the risk of recumbency during the operation was 1.95 times more likely if the animal was sedated than if it was not, after adjusting for the other variables. The confidence interval for sedation tells us that we can be 95% certain that the true relative risk lies between 1.33 and 2.87. Note that this interval excludes unity; this is to be expected since we know that the coefficient is significant ($P = 0.001$).

From Table 10.3 we can see that there was approximately a twofold increase in the risk of recumbency of the animal during Caesarian section if the cow was sedated, or if the obstetrician met with difficulties when attempting to exteriorize the pregnant uterine horn; the risk of recumbency was approximately halved if the animal was a beef cow rather than a dairy cow, or if the cow was multiparous.

Similar analyses showed that attempts to extract the calf was the only factor that significantly increased uterine contractibility. The experience of the surgeon, the parity, the increased uterine contractibility, the position of the calf, and the presence of adhesions were associated with difficult exteriorization of the pregnant horn. ☐

10.7 REGRESSION TO THE MEAN

The concept of **regression to the mean** derives from Sir Francis Galton's studies of inheritance in 1889. He observed that in many instances, although one might expect that sons would inherit the characteristics of their fathers, the measurements on sons tend to be closer to those of the general population of men than to those of their fathers. This phenomenon can be demonstrated by considering the relationship between a man's height and his son's height. Although, as we would expect, tall fathers tend to have tall sons, when we look at the heights of the sons of tall fathers, they are, *on average*, less than those of their fathers. There is a regression, or going back, of the sons' heights towards the average heights of all men. The regression coefficient, when we regress the son's height on the father's height, is substantially less than 1. It is important to recognize that the regression to the mean height does not relate to a particular son, but rather to the whole group of sons.

Another instance in which regression to the mean can be demonstrated is when a variable is measured on two occasions on every animal in a group. For example, suppose we want to investigate the effects of a beta-blocking agent on tachycardia (elevated heart rate) in cats. We select for our trial a group of cats whose resting heart rates are all above the upper limit of normal, i.e. above 180 beats/min. Were we to record their heart rates a second time, *before* treatment, we should most likely find that their average heart rate was lower than before, perhaps even within the reference range; this is due to regres-

sion to the mean. However, if unaware of this phenomenon, we had treated the animals and then measured the heart rates, we could falsely attribute the decrease in heart rate to the action of the drug. Regression to the mean is therefore especially relevant in screening procedures.

EXERCISES

The statements in questions 10.1–10.4 are either TRUE or FALSE.

10.1 Pearson's correlation coefficient:
(a) Must always be positive.
(b) Cannot be calculated if at least one of the two variables is not Normally distributed.
(c) Measures how well a straight line describes the relationship between two variables.
(d) Is zero if there is no relationship between the two variables.
(e) Measures the average change in one variable for a unit increase in the other.

10.2 A simple linear regression equation:
(a) Measures the degree of the relationship between two variables.
(b) Predicts the dependent variable from the independent variable.
(c) Describes the straight line relationship between two variables.
(d) Assumes that both of the variables are Normally distributed.
(e) Makes no distinction between the two variables.

10.3 Multiple regression analysis:
(a) Requires all the independent variables to be Normally distributed.
(b) Requires the residuals to be Normally distributed.
(c) Can be used to determine whether the mean responses of animals on two treatments are significantly different.
(d) Can be performed with any number of independent variables.
(e) Is preferable to logistic regression analysis if the dependent variable has a binary response.

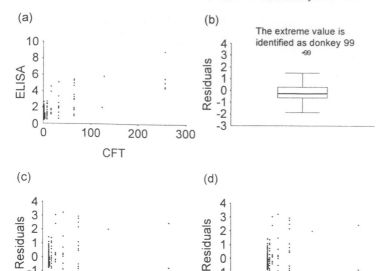

Fig. 10.11 Diagrams for checking the assumptions of linear regression analysis of data relating to a complement fixation test and an ELISA test for dourine infection. (Data from Lake *et al.*, unpublished.)

10.4 A partial regression coefficient in a multiple regression equation:
(a) Always lies between −1 and +1.
(b) Measures the degree of the relationship between its associated independent variable and the dependent variable, adjusting for the other independent variables.
(c) Measures the average change in the dependent variable for a unit increase in the associated independent variable, adjusting for the other independent variables.
(d) Describes the proportion of the variation in the dependent variable explained by its relationship with the associated independent variable.
(e) Is independent of the units of measurement.

10.5 Lake *et al.* (unpublished) obtained blood samples on a random sample of 124 donkeys in the Ngamiland area of Botswana, some of which were suffering from dourine, a venereal disease of Equidae caused by *Trypanosoma equiperda*. They were interested to know whether the ELISA and Complement Fixation Test (CFT) results on these donkeys were associated, and whether it would be possible to describe a linear relationship between them. High values of both

CFT and ELISA are indicative of dourine. The output for the regression analysis that they performed is shown in Fig. 10.11 and Display 10.3. Use this output to answer, with full explanations, the following questions.
(a) Do you think, by examining scatter plot (Fig. 10.11(a)), that it is reasonable to assume a linear relationship between CFT and ELISA?
(b) What is the estimated correlation coefficient between CFT and ELISA?
(c) What is the estimated linear regression line?
(d) Is it a good fit?
(e) Are the assumptions underlying the regression analysis satisfied (Fig. 10.11(b)–(d))?
(f) What can you conclude from the results of the ANOVA table?
(g) Interpret the slope of the linear regression line.
(h) Is it significantly different from zero?

10.6 Several disease states in dogs lead to alterations of the thickness of gastric rugal folds. However, there may be a relationship between rugal fold thickness and body size, and this must be investigated before rugal fold thickness can be used as a determinant of disease. Jakovljevic and

Model summary*

Model	R	R square	Adjusted R square	Std. error of the estimate
1	0.737[†]	0.543	0.539	0.974267

* Dependent variable: ELISA.
[†] Predictors: (Constant), CFT.

ANOVA*

Model	Sum of squares	df	Mean square	F	Sig.
1 Regression	137.467	1	137.467	144.824	0.000[†]
Residual	115.802	122	0.949		
Total	253.269	123			

* Dependent variable: ELISA.
[†] Predictors: (Constant), CFT.

Coefficients*

Model	Coefficients				95% confidence interval for β	
	b	Std Error	t	Sig.	Lower bound	Upper bound
1 (Constant)	1.207	0.096	12.513	0.000	1.016	1.398
CFT	1.982E-02	0.002	12.034	0.000	0.017	0.023

* Dependent variable: ELISA.

Display 10.3 Typical computer output of data described in Exercise 10.5 and Fig. 10.11(a).

Gibbs (1993) studied 29 dogs without known gastric lesions. The measurements (in mm) of the dogs' mucosal folds were determined radiographically and then related to their body weights (kg). The correlation coefficient between rugal fold thickness and body weight was 0.71 ($P < 0.001$).

(a) Explain what the correlation coefficient is measuring.
(b) What does the *P*-value tell you?
(c) The regression line was fitted to the data and estimated as

$$y = 2.064 + 0.069x$$

where y is the rugal fold thickness and x is the body weight. What additional information does the slope of the line give you?

(d) What fraction of the total variability of rugal fold thickness (y) is explained by the dog's body weight (x)?

(e) What do you conclude from your answer to (d)?

Chapter 11

Non-Parametric Statistical Tests

11.1 LEARNING OBJECTIVES

By the end of this chapter you should be able to:

- List the different approaches to adopt if the assumptions of the parametric test are not satisfied.
- Describe the differences between parametric and non-parametric tests.
- Recognize when it is advisable to apply a non-parametric test to a data set.
- Identify a data set to which the sign test is suited and conduct the test.
- Identify a data set to which the Wilcoxon signed rank test is suited and conduct the test.
- Identify a data set to which the Wilcoxon rank sum test is suited and conduct the test.
- Identify data sets to which the Kruskal–Wallis and Friedman ANOVAs are suited and interpret the results of such analyses.
- Calculate Spearman's rank correlation coefficient and test the hypothesis that its true value is zero.

11.2 PARAMETRIC AND NON-PARAMETRIC TESTS

11.2.1 The difference between parametric and non-parametric tests

The hypothesis tests that we discussed in Chapters 7–10 are **parametric tests** in that each makes certain assumptions about the underlying form of the distribution of the observations, and often the parameters (see Section 4.3.2) which define that distribution. For example, in the two-sample *t*-test (see Section 7.4) we assume the data are Normally distributed and the variances of the observations in the two groups are the same. Animal research often results in data sets which are less than perfect either in terms of numbers of observations, or the distribution of the data. Hence the assumptions of the tests may not be satisfied. The alternative type of test is a **non-parametric test** which does not make any distributional assumptions about the data. For this reason, they are often called **distribution-free tests**. The analyses in non-parametric tests are usually based on the **ranks** of the data, i.e. on the successive numbers assigned to the observations when they are arranged in increasing (or decreasing) order, rather than on the raw data.

11.2.2 What if the assumptions of the parametric test are not satisfied?

If the assumptions of the parametric test are *not* satisfied, then we have a number of choices. We can:

(a) Ignore the fact that the assumptions are not satisfied and proceed with the analysis. This approach may lead to an incorrect analysis in which the results of the test are distorted by its failure to adhere to the underlying assumptions. In particular, the *P*-value may not be the one which we believe we have evaluated. Some tests are **robust** against violations of certain assumptions (for example, the Normality assumptions in the two-sample and paired *t*-tests – see Sections 7.4.2 and 7.5.2) so that the *P*-value is hardly affected if the data depart from Normality.

(b) Take a particular **transformation** of every data value, and perform the analysis on the transformed observations. So, if the variable of interest is x, then we take a transformation of x to create a new variable, t_x, which is some function of x, for example, its logarithm, reciprocal or square root (see Section 12.2). There are a number of reasons for transforming data, the most common being:

- To achieve a Normal distribution of t_x when the distribution of x is skewed.
- To linearize a relationship; it is much easier to analyse data and investigate a relationship when that relationship can be described by a straight line.
- To stabilize variance; equal variance is assumed in the two-sample t-test (see Section 7.4.2) and in ANOVA (see Section 8.6.1), and statistical analyses often assume that the residuals (see Section 10.4.3) have constant variance in different circumstances.

(c) Perform an alternative **non-parametric test** which does not make distributional assumptions. The non-parametric analyses which we discuss in this chapter are shown, against their equivalent parametric procedures, in Box 11.1. You should be aware that a non-parametric test may not produce an identical result to its parametric equivalent, and the exact formulation of the null hypothesis may not be the same. The most usual approach is to use the parametric test provided its underlying assumptions are satisfied.

11.2.3 The advantages and disadvantages of using non-parametric tests

A non-parametric test can be used in the situation when the parametric equivalent is not appropriate for one or more of the following reasons:

- The sample size is very small comprising perhaps only five or six observations, and it is, therefore, difficult to establish that the data have a particular distributional form.

Box 11.1 Parametric tests and their non-parametric equivalents.

Parametric test	Non-parametric test
One-sample t-test	Sign test
Paired t-test	Sign test, Wilcoxon signed rank test
Two-sample t-test	Wilcoxon rank sum test
One-way ANOVA	Kruskal–Wallis one-way ANOVA
Two-way ANOVA	Friedman two-way ANOVA
Pearson correlation coefficient	Spearman rank correlation coefficient

- The distributional assumptions underlying the parametric test of interest are not satisfied.
- The data are measured on ordered or nominal scales.

However, if all the assumptions of the parametric test are satisfied, then the non-parametric test is less efficient because of the loss of information incurred by replacing the observations by their ranks. We can measure this loss of efficiency formally by evaluating the **power-efficiency** of the test: this is the extent (measured as a percentage) to which the sample size of the non-parametric test needs to be increased to make it as powerful as the parametric test for a fixed significance level. The power of a test, you will remember (see Section 6.4.2), is the chance of detecting a real treatment difference, and this is proportional to the sample size. So, for example, if the power-efficiency of a test is 90%, this implies that the sample sizes of the non-parametric to the parametric tests need to be in the ratio of $10:9$ if the two tests are to be equally powerful, provided all the assumptions underlying the parametric test are met. The power-efficiency of all the non-parametric tests discussed in this chapter is about 95%, with the exceptions of the sign test (falling eventually to 63% for very large sample sizes), the test for Spearman's rank correlation coefficient (91%) and the Friedman two-way analysis of variance (64–87%, depending on the number of groups). Details may be obtained from Siegel and Castellan (1988).

You should also be aware that non-parametric tests tend to be geared towards significance tests rather than to estimation. Although significance tests form an important part of statistical analysis, estimation of the effects of interest provide the necessary understanding of the biological processes involved. As the parametric counterparts of non-parametric tests usually incorporate parameter estimates in their calculation, parametric tests are preferred in many situations.

11.3 THE SIGN TEST

11.3.1 Introduction

If we are concerned about the assumption of Normality, the sign test can be used as an alternative to the one-sample *t*-test or the paired *t*-test. We would use the one-sample *t*-test if we wanted to test the null hypothesis that the mean value of a quantitative variable equals a specific value (see Section 7.3). Similarly, we can use the **sign test** to investigate whether a sample of values comes from a population with a specified median; we determine whether significantly more of the values in the sample are greater (or less) than this median.

We can also use the sign test when we want to establish whether the measurements of a single variable, measured on an ordinal (so they can be ranked) or quantitative scale, are similar in two groups of paired observations. The pairing may be achieved by matching the animals in a pair with respect to any variables that may be likely to influence the response, or each pair may represent the same animal on different occasions (see Section 5.8.4).

For example, in investigating a test diet which is believed may promote rapid growth in rats, each of a pair of age/sex matched litter-mates could be assigned to either the test diet or a control diet. The difference in weights (control v. test) between the litter-mates after a prescribed time, say 60 days, could be used to determine whether the test diet is effective. In particular, we can use the *signs* of the differences for this purpose.

11.3.2 Rationale

- *One-sample test.* If the median of a sample of observations is approximately equal to the value for the population median specified under the null hypothesis, then we would expect to find an equal number of observations both above and below this specified value. Expressed another way, we would expect half the observations in our sample to be greater than the specified value. This means that we test the hypothesis, framed in terms of the population, that half the observations are greater than the specified median. We are investigating a binary response (above or below a given value); we can therefore use the Binomial distribution (see Section 3.4.2), and the Normal approximation to it (see Section 3.6.1), to test this hypothesis.
- *Paired test.* We start by evaluating the difference, in a defined direction, in the responses for each pair. If the responses in the two groups of paired observations are equal, then we would expect there to be, on average, the same number of positive and negative differences. This means that we would expect about half of the differences to be positive if the null hypothesis – that there is no difference in the responses in the two groups – were true. Expressed another way, we test the null hypothesis that the true proportion of positive differences in the population, π, is 0.5. Because we have reduced the two-sample situation to a one-sample situation in which we are investigating a binary response variable (the difference, which can either be positive or negative), again we can use the Normal approximation to the Binomial distribution (see Section 3.6.1).

11.3.3 Assumptions

We assume that the variable under investigation is measured on an ordinal or quantitative scale, and that for the paired analysis, the observations in the two groups are matched. The data constitute a random sample from the population of interest.

11.3.4 Approach

We explain the approach in relation to the paired situation, but the same principles apply to the single-sample situation.

1. Specify the **null hypothesis, H_0**, that the true proportion of positive differences is 0.5. The alternative hypothesis is that this proportion is not equal to 0.5.
2. **Collect** the data and, if relevant, **display** them in the same way as for the paired *t*-test (see Section 7.5.3).
3. For a computer analysis, choose the *sign test* and proceed to step 4. Otherwise, **count** the numbers of positive and negative differences (ignore zero differences) and note the smaller number, k. (In a one-sample test we would count the numbers of observations above and below the specified median and note the smaller.)
   If $n \leq 20$, proceed to step 4.
   If $n > 20$, calculate the **test statistic**. It approximates the Standard Normal distribution and is given by

$$Test_{12} = \frac{|p - 0.5| - 1/(2n)}{\sqrt{0.5^2/n}}$$

where n is the number of non-zero differences – all tied pairs are excluded from the analysis; $p = k/n$ is the observed proportion of positive (or negative) pairs out of n untied pairs; and $1/(2n)$ is a continuity correction which makes an allowance for using the continuous Normal distribution as an approximation to the discrete Binomial distribution.

4. Determine the **P-value** from the computer output, or by either:
   If $n \leq 20$, referring k and n to Table A.8, or
   If $n > 20$, referring $Test_{12}$ to the table of the Standard Normal distribution (Table A.1).
5. Use the *P*-value to judge whether the data are consistent with the null hypothesis. Then **decide** whether or not to reject the null hypothesis. Usually, we reject H_0 if $P < 0.05$.

11.3.5 Example

It was claimed at a regional veterinary meeting that the mean time for a consultation was 12 minutes. A young graduate challenged this statement on the grounds that with such a skewed population (a few cases take considerably more than 12 minutes), the median would be a better estimate to quote. Further discussion led to a general agreement that the median consultation time was also around 12 minutes. The young graduate, being sceptical, decided to test his own practice and conducted a time-and-motion study during morning surgery for one week. A total of 43 cases were seen; the results are summarized in Table 11.1.

In order to determine whether the results are consistent with a median value of 12, we perform the sign test.

1. The null hypothesis is that the true median duration of a consultation is 12 minutes, or, equivalently, that the true proportion of consultations of duration greater than 12 minutes is 0.5. The alternative hypothesis is that this proportion is not equal to 0.5.
2. There is no useful way in which to display these data diagrammatically.
3. There were 15 consultations with duration greater than 12 minutes and 22 consultations with duration less than 12 minutes out of 37 consultations whose duration was not exactly 12 minutes.
4. Thus, in the notation of Table A.8, to which we now refer, $k = 15$ (the smaller number) and $n = 37$. This gives $P > 0.05$ (in fact, the computer gives $P = 0.39$).
5. Hence the data are consistent with the null hypothesis that the true median duration is 12 minutes, and there is no evidence to reject it.

Table 11.1 Duration of consultation times.

Duration of consultation	Number of cases
Less than 12 min	22
12 min	6
More than 12 min	15
Total	43

11.4 WILCOXON SIGNED RANK TEST

We can also use the **Wilcoxon signed rank** test as a non-parametric alternative to the paired *t*-test.

11.4.1 Assumptions

We assume that the variable under investigation is measured on an ordinal or quantitative scale, and that the observations in the two groups are paired. The data constitute a random sample from the population of interest.

11.4.2 Approach

1. Specify the **null hypothesis, H_0,** that the samples come from populations with identical distributions and the same median, or from the same population. Generally, the alternative hypothesis is that they do not.
2. **Collect** the data and **display** them in the same way as for the paired *t*-test (see Section 7.5.3).
3. Either select the *Wilcoxon signed rank test* on the computer and proceed to step 4, or:
   (a) Find the difference between each pair of observations, and indicate whether that difference is positive or negative.
   (b) Ignoring the signs of the differences, **rank** them in order of magnitude. This means that we have to assign successive numbers (the ranks), starting at unity, to the differences. The smallest difference (once we have ignored its sign) is given the rank 1, the next smallest difference gets the rank 2, etc. We ignore zero differences, and reduce the sample size accordingly, from n' to n, say. If two or more absolute differences (i.e. when we ignore their sign) have the same value, then these tied differences get the average of the ranks they would have received had they not been tied.
   (c) Affix to each rank the sign of its corresponding difference.
   (d) Find the **sum of the ranks** which have a positive sign, T_+, or the sum of the ranks which have a negative sign, T_-, usually,

whichever is the smaller. Let us assume here that $T_+ < T_-$.
If $n \leq 25$, proceed to step 4.
If $n > 25$, calculate the **test statistic**

$$Test_{13} = \frac{T_+ - n(n+1)/4}{\sqrt{n(n+1)(2n+1)/24}}$$

which approximates a Standard Normal distribution. If there are a large number of ties, then a correction factor should be applied to the denominator. Details may be obtained from Siegel and Castellan (1988).
4. Determine the **P-value**. You may find this in your computer output. Alternatively:
   If $n \leq 25$, refer T_+ to Table A.9.
   If $n > 25$, refer $Test_{13}$ to the table of the Standard Normal distribution (Table A.1).
5. Use the information to determine whether the data are consistent with the null hypothesis. Then **decide** whether or not to reject the null hypothesis. Usually, we reject H_0 if $P < 0.05$.
6. Your computer output may provide a **confidence interval** for the difference in the medians. We refer you to Gardner and Altman (1989) for details of the calculation. Usually it is sufficient to provide the *difference in the sample medians*, together with the interquartile range (see Section 2.6.2) or the range of values which encloses 95% (or 90%) of the observations, to give an indication of the magnitude of the effect of interest. Alternatively, you could show the *median of the differences* in the sample, together with an appropriate range of the differences.

11.4.3 Example

A novel diet for laboratory rats was tested to see if it had any potential to promote rapid growth. Several different strains were included in this preliminary trial, and weanling litter-mate rats, of the same sex, were used as the test unit. Eighteen pairs of litter mates were used; each rat in a pair was randomly allocated to test or control diets, the second rat then receiving the other

Table 11.2 Weights of litter-mate rats on two different diets.

Litter-mate pair	Weight on test diet (gm)	Weight on control diet (gm)	Difference (control − test) (gm)	Rank of difference
1	243	265	+22	15
2	161	165	+4	5.5
3	318	361	+43	16
4	270	270	0	–
5	214	235	+21	14
6	97	83	−14	11
7	189	170	−19	13
8	151	158	+7	9.5
9	143	143	0	–
10	117	121	+4	5.5
11	177	174	−3	3.5
12	204	211	+7	9.5
13	190	192	+2	1.5
14	134	131	−3	3.5
15	154	160	+6	8
16	273	291	+18	12
17	126	131	+5	7
18	188	190	+2	1.5

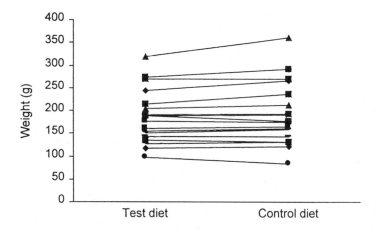

Fig. 11.1 Dot diagram showing weights of litter-mate rats on two different diets.

diet. At 60 days of age, the rats were weighed; these weights are shown in Table 11.2.

In order to investigate whether the test diet is effective, we go through the hypothesis testing procedure:

1. We are testing the null hypothesis that the rat's weight is unaffected by the novel diet, against the two-sided alternative that it is affected by the diet.
2. It is difficult to discern any obvious benefit of the diet from Fig. 11.1 which displays the data. The differences in the weights are skewed to the right (you should sketch them to check this), indicating that a non-parametric test is advocated.
3. Proceeding by hand, we rank the absolute differences (ignoring the two zero differences), as shown in Table 11.2. There are only 4 negative differences, whilst there are 12 positive differences. We therefore find the sum of the ranks of the negative differences = 11 + 13 + 3.5 + 3.5 = 31.
4. Referring this sum to Table A.9, we find that $0.05 < P < 0.10$. In fact, the exact P-value from a computer analysis is $P = 0.06$.

5. There is insufficient evidence to reject the null hypothesis. We have reason to doubt the claim that the novel diet is effective in promoting an increase in growth.
6. The median rat weight (with 25th and 75th percentiles) after 60 days is 183 (141, 221) gm on the novel diet and 175 (140, 243) gm on the control diet. The median of the differences in weight is 4.0 (−0.75, 9.75) gm.

11.4.4 Choosing between the sign test and the Wilcoxon signed rank test

The sign test is less powerful than the Wilcoxon signed rank test because it uses only the information about the *direction* of the differences; it ignores their *magnitude*.

Performing the sign test on the rats' weight example of Section 11.4.3, we refer 4 (the number of negative differences which is smaller than 12, the number of positive differences) to Table A.8. We find that $P = 0.076$, again having insufficient evidence to reject the null hypothesis.

11.5 WILCOXON RANK SUM TEST

11.5.1 Introduction

We can use the **Wilcoxon rank sum test** or the **Mann-Whitney U test** as an alternative to the two sample *t*-test if we are concerned that the underlying assumptions of the *t*-test (Normality and constant variance – see Section 7.4.2) are not satisfied. The two tests produce the same results; we shall explain the mechanics of the Wilcoxon rank sum test because its calculations are marginally simpler.

11.5.2 Assumptions

We assume that the variable under investigation is measured on an ordinal or quantitative scale. The two samples of observations are selected randomly and independently from the populations.

11.5.3 Approach

1. Specify the **null hypothesis, H_0,** that the two samples could have been selected from populations which have similar distributions with the same median or from the same population. Generally, the alternative hypothesis is that they have not been selected from such populations.
2. **Collect** the data and **display** them in the same way as for the two-sample *t*-test (see Section 7.4.3).
3. Using the computer, select the *Wilcoxon rank sum test* and proceed to step 4, or follow the sequence below:
   (a) Suppose there are n_1 observations in the first sample and n_2 observations in the second sample, and $n_1 < n_2$. Rank the observations in the two samples together (i.e. assign successive numbers from 1 to $n_1 + n_2$ to the observations after they have been arranged in increasing order of magnitude). If two or more observations have the same value, then these tied values get the average of the ranks they would have received had they not been tied.
   (b) Find the **sum of the ranks** of one sample (usually the smaller sample), T_1.
   If $n_1 \leq 10$ and $n_2 \leq 15$, proceed to step 4. Otherwise, calculate the **test statistic**

   $$Test_{14} = \frac{T_1 - n_1(n_1 + n_2 + 1)/2}{\sqrt{n_1 n_2 (n_1 + n_2 + 1)/12}}$$

   which approximates a Standard Normal distribution. If there are a large number of ties, the denominator should be modified (Armitage & Berry, 1994). Most computer packages adjust for tied ranks.
4. Determine the **P-value** from the computer output, or.
   If $n_1 \leq 10$ and $n_2 \leq 15$, refer T_1 to Table A.10. Otherwise, refer $Test_{14}$ to the table of the Standard Normal distribution (Table A.1).
5. Use the *P*-value to determine whether the data are consistent with the null hypothesis. Then **decide** whether or not to reject the null hypothesis. Usually, we reject H_0 if $P < 0.05$.
6. Your computer output may provide a **confidence interval** for the true difference in the

medians. The relevant formulae are given in Gardner and Altman (1989). Alternatively, you can provide an estimate of the median, together with the range (e.g. the interquartile range or that enclosing the central 95% of the observations) in each sample.

11.5.4 Example

Seventeen puppies were toilet-trained from weaning at six weeks of age by either positive reinforcement (praise and encouragement when defecating outdoors) or negative reinforcement (chastisement when defecating indoors). The time taken for establishment of the habit (seven consecutive days without defecating indoors) was recorded in days. The results are shown in Table 11.3(a). Are the two regimes equally effective?

1. The null hypothesis is that the two samples could have been selected from populations with the same median training time or from the same population. The alternative hypothesis is that the they are from populations with different median training times.
2. The data are plotted in Fig. 11.2; the sample sizes are small, and it would seem that the negative reinforcement training times are skewed to the right. Therefore, a non-parametric test is advocated.

3. The training times of the two samples are ranked together, as shown in Table 11.3(b). There are eight observations in the sample with positive reinforcement and nine in the

Table 11.3 Time taken (days) to establish toilet training in two groups of dogs.

(a) Results as they were obtained (time in days)

Positive reinforcement: 43, 41, 48, 44, 51, 48, 47, 35
Negative reinforcement: 42, 47, 57, 53, 74, 59, 65, 54, 46

(b) Results arranged in order (time in days)

Positive reinforcement	Negative reinforcement	Rank
35		1
41		2
	42	3
43		4
44		5
	46	6
	47	7.5
47		7.5
48		9.5
48		9.5
51		11
	53	12
	54	13
	57	14
	59	15
	65	16
	74	17

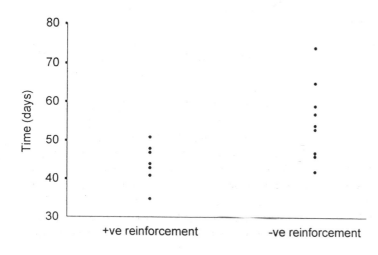

Fig. 11.2 Dot diagram showing time taken for puppies to become toilet-trained with positive or negative reinforcement.

sample with negative reinforcement. Hence we take T_1 to be the sum of the ranks of the sample with positive reinforcement = $1 + 2 + 4 + 5 + 7.5 + 9 + 10 + 11 = 49.5$.

4. We refer 49.5 to Table A.10 with $n_1 = 8$ and $n_2 = 9$, and find that $P < 0.05$ since 49.5 lies outside the limits in the table of 51–93, but $P > 0.01$ since the relevant tabulated limits are 45–99 (in fact, a computer analysis shows that $P = 0.03$).

5. The data are not consistent with the null hypothesis that the samples could have been selected from populations with the same median training time, and we have evidence to reject it. Hence we can conclude that there is evidence indicating that positive reinforcement is better than negative reinforcement.

6. The median training time (with the interquartile range) for the sample with positive reinforcement was 45.5 (41.5, 48.0) days, and for that with negative reinforcement was 54.0 (46.5, 62.0) days.

11.6 NON-PARAMETRIC ANALYSES OF VARIANCE

11.6.1 Introduction

In this section we indicate the approach used in two particular forms of non-parametric ANOVA – the **Kruskal–Wallis** and the **Friedman ANOVA**. It is unlikely that you will ever have to perform these analyses by hand, so we omit the details of the calculations. You will find them in Siegel and Castellan (1988). In both analyses, we assume the data are measured on an ordinal or a quantitative scale.

11.6.2 Kruskal–Wallis one-way ANOVA

(a) Procedure

In Section 8.6 we discussed the one-way ANOVA in some detail. You will recall that this may be regarded as an extension to the two-sample *t*-test if more than two independent groups of observations are to be compared. However, if either or both of the assumptions underlying the parametric ANOVA (namely, Normality and constant variance – see Section 8.6.1) are not satisfied, perhaps because the data are measured on an ordinal scale, then we may prefer to analyse the data using the equivalent non-parametric **Kruskal–Wallis one-way ANOVA**. It tests the null hypothesis that the $k \geq 3$ independent samples are selected from identical populations with the same median or from the same population.

The appropriate test statistic is determined by replacing the observations in the samples by their ranks. This means that the all the observations in the k samples are combined and are arranged in order of magnitude. The smallest observation receives the rank 1, the next smallest rank 2, etc. The test statistic is based on the sum of the ranks in each sample. It approximates the Chi-squared distribution with $k - 1$ degrees of freedom.

If the result of the Kruskal–Wallis test is significant, we reject the null hypothesis that all the samples are selected from identical populations with the same median. We infer that at least one of the samples comes from a population which is different from the others. We can then use the Wilcoxon rank sum test (see Section 11.5) to determine which pairs of groups differ. However, because of the potential for testing many combinations of groups (if we have k groups, we could make $k(k-1)/2$ comparisons), we are likely find spurious significant results unless we adjust for multiple comparisons (see Section 8.6.3).

(b) Example

Barber and Elliott (1998) investigated the aetiopathogenesis of renal secondary hyperparathyroidism (RHPTH) in a prospective study of 80 cats with chronic renal failure (CRF) using routine plasma biochemistry and assays of parathyroid hormone (PTH). The presence of RHPTH can only be diagnosed by the demonstration of elevated plasma PTH concentrations. A knowledge of the prevalence and aetiopathogenesis of RHPTH in naturally occurring feline CRF is imperative before the institution of correct treatment modalities to reduce RHPTH.

Cats presenting as first opinion cases over a three-year period and diagnosed with CRF were categorized subjectively into three groups (compensated, uraemic and endstage), according to the severity of clinical signs. Plasma concentrations were determined from blood samples by immunoradiometric assay. Their distributions in the three CRF groups are shown in Fig. 11.3. Note that here we have the common situation in which we perform a hypothesis test, in this case comparing the results of cats in three groups, which is not based on random allocation.

Because these distributions are skewed to the right, a Kruskal–Wallis one-way ANOVA is used to compare the medians. The sample medians (25th, 95th percentiles in brackets) for the compensated, uraemic and end-stage CRF groups are 25.1 (12.6, 40.0), 86.7 (35.1, 176.2) and 301.2 (148.7, 447.8) pg/ml, respectively. The null hypothesis is that the three population medians are equal. The result of the Kruskal–Wallis test is that $P < 0.001$, indicating that at least two of the medians differ. Wilcoxon rank sum tests, incorpo-

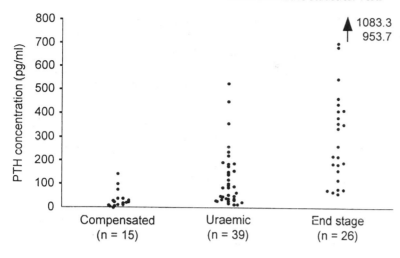

Fig. 11.3 Dot diagram showing distributions of plasma parathyroid hormone (PTH) concentration (pg/ml) in cats in three stages of chronic renal failure. (Redrawn from Barber and Elliott, 1998, with permission.)

rating the Bonferroni correction (i.e. multiplying each *P*-value by 3 because there are three two-sample tests) between each pair of groups shows that the median PTH is significantly greater in the end-stage CRF group than in the other two groups (*P* < 0.001) and that the median PTH is significantly greater in the uraemic CRF group than in the compensated group (*P* < 0.003).

11.6.3 Friedman two-way ANOVA

(a) Procedure

In Section 8.5.3 we gave an indication of the manner in which relatively complicated forms of designed experiments can be analysed by the ANOVA. In particular, we mentioned the one-way repeated measures ANOVA (often confusingly called a randomized block or, sometimes, a two-way ANOVA) which may be regarded as an extension to the paired *t*-test when more than two groups of dependent observations are to be compared. The non-parametric equivalent, called the **Friedman two-way ANOVA**, may be performed when the underlying assumptions (Normality, constant variance) of the parametric ANOVA are not satisfied. It tests the null hypothesis that the *k* ≥ 3 matched or dependent samples are selected from the same population or from populations with the same median.

The observed data are arranged in a two-way table, with the columns, say, representing the *k* samples (e.g. treatments) and each of the *r* rows representing a different individual (if each individual has an observation in each of the *k* samples) or matched individuals. The test statistic is determined by ranking the observations separately in each of the *r* rows. Thus, the observations in each row are replaced by the ranks 1, 2, . . . , *k* according to their positions in the ordered set within that row. The test statistic is based on the sum of the ranks in each sample (column), and approximates a chi-squared distribution with *k* − 1 degrees of freedom.

A significant test result implies that the *k* samples are not selected from populations with the same median. We can establish where the differences lie by performing the Wilcoxon signed rank test on pairs of samples, remembering, of course, to adjust for multiple comparisons (see Section 8.6.3).

(b) Example

Ketoprofen, a non-steroidal anti-inflammatory drug, was administered to horses rectally in three different bases to measure its bioavailability (%) by this route. One gram of drug was distributed in a fatty suppository suspension (A), as a polyethyleneglycol solution (B) and as an aqueous suspension (C). Each of the six horses in the study received Ketoprofen in the three different bases, with the order in which they received the 'treatments' being randomized. There was a wash-out period of one week between the adminstrations of the treatments. We show the results (derived from summary data presented by Corveleyn *et al.*, 1996) in Table 11.4. We can see that the variances in the treatment groups are quite different. Futhermore, it is difficult to establish Normality of the data since there are only six values in each treatment group. Hence we advocate a non-parametric analysis. The Friedman two-way ANOVA is appropriate because the samples are dependent, with each horse receiving all three treatments.

The null hypothesis is that the three repeated measures come from the same population or populations with the same medians. This null hypothesis implies that the bioavailabilities are the same in the three different treatment groups. The alternative hypothesis is that the three repeated measures do not come from populations with the same medians. A Friedman computer analysis gives *P* = 0.31. Thus, there is insufficient evidence to allow us to reject the null hypothesis; it appears that the formulation base makes little difference to the bioavailability. We show the summary

Table 11.4 Bioavailability (%) of Ketoprofen administered in three bases, A, B and C. (Based on summary data from Corveleyn *et al.*, 1996, with permission.)

Horses	Bases		
	A	B	C
1	22.5	28.2	37.5
2	11.5	43.8	25.1
3	16.7	36.8	28.9
4	32.1	48.6	33.3
5	36.7	2.1	40.0
6	27.5	12.9	22.9
Median (%)	25.0	32.5	31.1
Mean (%)	24.5	28.7	31.3
Variance (%^{2})	89.99	329.41	46.58
SD (%)	9.48	18.15	6.82
Range (%)	11.5–36.7	2.1–48.6	22.9–40.0

measures, including the medians, for each base formulation in Table 11.4.   ☐

11.7 SPEARMAN'S RANK CORRELATION COEFFICIENT

11.7.1 Introduction

The Pearson product moment correlation coefficient provides a measure of the strength of the linear association between two variables (see Section 10.3). Often we are interested in testing the null hypothesis that the true correlation coefficient in the population is zero, in which case there is no linear association between the two variables. In order to test this hypothesis, we assume that at least one of the two variables is Normally distributed. If we wish to calculate a confidence interval for the correlation coefficient, we assume that both of the variables are Normally distributed (see Section 10.3.2(a)). If we are concerned about these assumptions, we can calculate the **Spearman rank correlation coefficient** as a non-parametric equivalent to the Pearson correlation coefficient. You may also come across **Kendall's** τ (the Greek letter tau) which is another non-parametric correlation coefficient.

11.7.2 Calculation

To calculate the Spearman rank correlation coefficient:

- We start by replacing the observations on each of the two variables, x and y, by their ranks. If our random sample consists of a series of n pairs of x and y values, $\{(x_1, y_1), (x_2, y_2), (x_3, y_3), \ldots (x_n, y_n)\}$, we replace the $(x_1, x_2, x_3, \ldots, x_n)$ by the ranks from 1 to n according to the values of x in the ordered set (the smallest x gets rank 1, the largest x gets rank n), and we replace the $(y_1, y_2, y_3, \ldots, y_n)$ by the ranks from 1 to n according to the values of y in the ordered set. Tied values get the average of the ranks they would have received had they not been tied.
- The sample value of the Spearman rank correlation coefficient, r_s, is then equivalent to the Pearson product moment correlation coefficient calculated using the ranks instead of the observations themselves. This is the easiest approach to calculating the Spearman rank correlation coefficient if using computer software.
- Alternatively, we can calculate the Spearman rank correlation coefficient using the formula

$$r_s = 1 - \frac{6 \sum d^2}{n^3 - n}$$

where each d is the difference between the ranks for a pair. This formula should be modified if there are tied values in a data set, although the effect is slight if there are few ties. Siegel and Castellan (1988) give details.

11.7.3 Interpretation

The Spearman rank correlation coefficient provides a measure of the association (not necessarily linear) between two variables, but does not imply causality. Similarly to the Pearson product moment correlation coefficient, its limits are −1 and +1. If it takes the value +1, then the individuals have the same *ranks* for both variables; if it takes the value −1, then the *rank* order of one variable is the reverse of that of the other variable. If the Spearman rank correlation coefficient is zero, the two variables are not associated.

11.7.4 Hypothesis testing and calculation of confidence intervals

In order to test the null hypothesis that the two variables, x and y, are not associated (i.e. the true correlation coefficient in the population, ρ_s, is zero), we follow the procedure for testing the Pearson correlation coefficient (see Section 10.3.2(b)). If we have 15 or less pairs of observations, we should assess significance using Table A.7. When the number of pairs is greater than 15, we can use, as an approximation, Table A.6 or $Test_{10}$, to assess significance, as for the Pearson correlation coefficient.

We calculate the confidence interval for ρ_s in the same way as for the Pearson correlation coefficient replacing r by r_s (see Section 10.3.2(b)).

11.7.5 Example

At a recent dog show, two judges were asked to inspect the entrants, and give them a score out of ten (including half marks). In this particular class, there were 12 entrants. Unfortunately, judge B misunderstood the instructions, and ranked the dogs in order (rank one being the best in the class) instead of assigning a score. The results are shown in Table 11.5(a). Do the two judges agree in their assessment of the dogs?

The Spearman rank correlation coefficient is preferred to the Pearson correlation coefficient since one of the two assessments was recorded on a ranking scale. We rank the scores for judge A and determine the differences between the two sets of ranks, as shown in Table 11.5(b). Then the Spearman rank correlation is the Pearson correlation coefficient between the judges' ranks. This is estimated as 0.73. The alternative approach is to estimate it as

$$r_s = 1 - \frac{6\sum d^2}{n^3 - n} = 1 - \frac{6(74.5)}{1728 - 12} = 0.74$$

The small discrepancy between the two estimates is a consequence of there being three dogs tied at the same rank in the scores assigned by judge A.

We can then assess the significance of the true correlation coefficient in the population by adopting the following procedure:

1. The null hypothesis is that the true correlation coefficient is zero. The alternative hypothesis is that it is not.
2. The data have been collected and are displayed in a scatter diagram, see Fig. 11.4.
3. We refer $r_s = 0.73$ to Table A.7 with a sample size of 12.

Table 11.5 Two judges' assessments of 12 dogs.

(a) Scores given by judge A and ranks given by judge B

Dog	1	2	3	4	5	6	7	8	9	10	11	12
Judge A	7.0	5.5	8.5	8.0	7.0	3.0	7.5	9.0	7.5	9.5	6.0	7.5
Judge B	6	5	4	2	5	12	7	3	8	1	10	9

(b) Ranks accorded to the scores of judge A with the ranks of judge B (in each case Rank 1 is the best dog).

Dog	1	2	3	4	5	6	7	8	9	10	11	12
Judge A	8.5	11	3	4	8.5	12	6	2	6	1	10	6
Judge B	6	5	4	2	5	12	7	3	8	1	10	9
Diff. d	2.5	6	−1	2	3.5	0	−1	−1	−2	0	0	−3

4. Since 0.73 lies between the tabulated values of 0.7273 and 0.8182, $0.002 < P < 0.01$.
5. We have evidence to reject the null hypothesis. This indicates that there is an association between the two judges' assessments of the dogs, with reasonable agreement between the two.
6. The 95% confidence interval for the true correlation coefficient is

$$\frac{e^{2z_1} - 1}{e^{2z_1} + 1} \text{ to } \frac{e^{2z_2} - 1}{e^{2z_2} + 1}$$

where $z = 0.5 \log_e\{(1 + r_s)/(1 - r_s)\} = 0.9287$, $z_1 = z - 1.96/\sqrt{(n - 3)} = 0.2754$, and $z_2 = z + 1.96/\sqrt{(n - 3)} = 1.5820$.

Hence the confidence interval is from

$$\frac{0.7346}{2.7346} \text{ to } \frac{22.6651}{24.6651},$$

i.e. from 0.27 to 0.92. This is a very wide confidence interval, as we would expect from a small sample.

EXERCISES

The statements in questions 11.1–11.3 are either TRUE or FALSE.

11.1 Non-parametric tests are preferred to parametric tests when:

(a) The data are measured on an ordinal scale.
(b) The sample size is large.
(c) A more powerful test is required.
(d) It is difficult to establish the distribution of the data.
(e) The emphasis is on estimation rather than significance testing.

11.2 The Spearman rank correlation coefficient:
(a) Lies between −1 and +1.
(b) Measures the degree of association between two variables.
(c) Measures the degree of linear association between two variables.
(d) Requires that at least one of the variables be measured on a ranking scale.
(e) Is preferable to the Pearson correlation coefficient if the sample size is small.

11.3 In a preliminary investigation into the consequences of a treatment which altered growth hormone secretion, plasma insulin concentrations were measured in rabbits randomly assigned to treatment or control groups. There were five rabbits in each group. The rabbits' insulin levels (IU/dl) were measured before and after six weeks' treatment, and the difference in before and after concentration found for each rabbit. Which of the following tests is appropriate for comparing the treatment and control groups?
(a) The sign test.
(b) The Wilcoxon signed rank test.

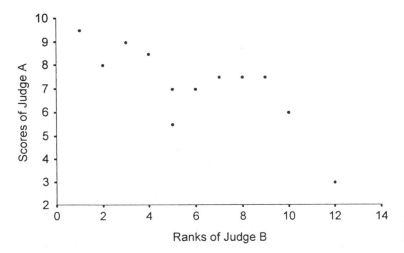

Fig. 11.4 Scatter diagram of two judges' assessments of 12 dogs.

(c) The Wilcoxon rank sum test.
(d) The paired *t*-test.
(e) The two-sample *t*-test.

11.4 Two methods were used to test the degree of fluorescence of spermatozoa treated with a fluorophore. The subjective method was an ordinal score (0 = no fluorescence, 1 = slight, 2 = clear, 3 = strong fluorescence) and the values are mean scores for 60 cells. The fluorimeter measurements are on a scale reflecting light intensity emitted by cells in suspension when irradiated by ultra-violet light and detected by a photo-multiplier cell. The results are shown in the Table 11.6.

(a) Examine the relationship between the two scores by plotting the data.
(b) Explain why it is more appropriate to calculate Spearman's rank correlation coefficient rather than Pearson's correlation coefficient as a measure of association.
(c) Estimate Spearman's rank correlation coefficient, and test the null hypothesis that its value in the population is zero. What do you conclude?

Table 11.6 Scores of fluorescence intensity of spermatozoa labelled with a fluorescent probe. The scores are made on an arbitrary scale by eye and by means of a fluorimeter.

Sample	Subjective score	Fluorimeter score
1	2.000	0.944
2	2.833	1.048
3	2.667	1.040
4	2.667	1.007
5	1.667	0.845
6	2.500	1.000
7	2.333	1.001
8	2.833	0.990
9	1.008	0.746
10	1.500	0.811
11	1.657	0.862
12	2.000	0.883

11.5 A dog breeder wanted to establish whether large litter size is inherited. He randomly selected a bitch pup from each of 9 large litters (litter size ≥5) and from 10 small litters (litter size

≤4). When each of these bitches reached adulthood, he counted the size of their second litters. The second litter sizes are shown below:

Bitches from large litters had litter sizes: 3, 7, 5, 6, 4, 6, 5, 7, 5
Bitches from small litters had litter sizes: 2, 3, 6, 4, 3, 4, 3, 5, 4, 5

Is there evidence to indicate that litter size is inherited?

11.6 Obesity is a problem in dogs kept as pets in the Western world. A novel weight control diet has been developed to address this problem. To test the diet, a veterinary surgeon investigates 18 successive obese dogs who present at her surgery, and she measures the dogs' weights (kg) at the time of presentation and after eight weeks on the weight control diet. The data are shown in Table 11.7. Use an appropriate hypothesis testing procedure to determine whether the novel diet is effective at promoting weight loss. Comment on the limitation of this design and the implication this has on your conclusion.

Table 11.7 Dogs' weights before and after a weight control diet.

Dog	Weight before (kg)	Weight after (kg)	Dog	Weight before (kg)	Weight after (kg)
1	26.5	24.3	10	12.1	11.7
2	16.5	16.1	11	17.4	17.7
3	36.1	31.8	12	21.1	20.4
4	28.0	27.0	13	19.2	19.0
5	23.5	21.4	14	13.1	13.4
6	8.3	9.7	15	16.0	15.4
7	17.7	18.9	16	29.1	27.3
8	15.8	15.1	17	13.1	12.6
9	14.3	14.3	18	19.0	18.8

11.7 This exercise follows on from exercise 11.6 which you should attempt first. In assessing the effect of a novel diet on weight in obese dogs, a veterinary surgeon randomly allocates 36 obese dogs who present at her surgery to two 'treatment' groups; either they receive the diet or they are prescibed a standard diet administered by the

Table 11.8 Dogs' weights before and after receiving the standard diet for eight weeks.

Dog	Weight before (kg)	Weight after (kg)	Dog	Weight before (kg)	Weight after (kg)
19	26.0	22.9	28	20.3	19.7
20	21.9	21.3	29	8.7	9.9
21	19.7	16.8	30	18.8	17.2
22	7.5	8.5	31	14.7	14.0
23	15.6	12.7	32	12.7	12.9
24	25.5	27.3	33	16.0	16.9
25	11.4	14.4	34	13.5	11.8
26	16.1	17.0	35	15.4	14.7
27	20.4	21.0	36	13.5	13.3

Table 11.9 Percentage of total aminopeptidase released into the culture medium by duodenal explants stimulated by gluten and phytohaemagglutinin. (Data adapted from O. Garden.)

Dog	Medium	Gluten (3 mg/ml)	PHA
Bonnie	11.8	8.4	13.0
Bertie	10.8	8.9	9.1
Billie	17.3	10.3	13.5
Bonker	21.9	9.4	17.5
Barton	12.0	8.1	8.4
Barker	17.0	3.5	8.1
Median (%)	14.50	8.65	11.05
Range (%)	10.8–21.9	3.5–10.3	8.1–17.5

owners in restricted quantities according to body weight and size. She measures the dogs' weights at the time of presentation and eight weeks after being put on the diet. The results for the novel diet group are shown in Table 11.7 in exercise 11.6. The results for the control group on the standard diet are shown in Table 11.8. What conclusions can you draw about the effectiveness of the novel diet in promoting weight loss?

11.8 In a study of gluten-sensitivity in Irish setter dogs, O. Garden (personal communication) has examined the activity of the enzyme, amino-petidase N, in cultured explants of the small intestine of affected dogs. We show in Table 11.9, some results of an experiment in which matched explants from six dogs were studied in medium alone (negative control), under stimulation by a gluten digest (3 mg/ml) and in the positive control, phytohaemagglutinin (PHA). The entries in the table are the percentages of total enzyme activity present in the medium after culture (a measure of cell damage).

(a) How would you analyse the data set, using a non-parametric approach, to determine whether the percentage enzyme activity released is affected by the treatments? State your null hypothesis clearly, and explain why you believe a non-parametric approach is suitable.

(b) If you have access to a computer, analyse the data. You should find that the appropriate non-parametric analysis, using all the data, gives $P = 0.006$. What are your conclusions?

Chapter 12

Further Aspects of Design and Analysis

12.1 LEARNING OBJECTIVES

By the end of this chapter you should be able to:

- Explain the purposes of data transformation, and choose an appropriate transformation and demonstrate its effect.
- Explain why sample size is an important design consideration.
- Use Altman's nomogram to determine optimal sample sizes for quantitative and qualitative data.
- Explain the terms sequential analysis, interim analysis and meta-analysis.
- Describe the conditions to be fulfilled for random sampling.
- Elaborate the different ways of selecting a sample.

12.2 TRANSFORMATIONS

By now you will be aware that not all data sets fulfil the inherent distributional assumptions of the required statistical procedure. Rather than turn immediately to a non-parametric analysis (see Chapter 11), we often consider transforming the data in order to be able to apply the statistical procedure. A **transformation** is a mathematical manipulation applied to each data point. The aim of the transformation is to produce a data set which satisfies the requirements of the procedure.

The most common reasons for transforming data are to attempt to Normalize data, to linearize a relationship and/or to stabilize variance. So, if the variable of interest is x, then we take a transformation of each individual x value to create a new variable, t_x, which is some func-

tion of x, e.g. its logarithm, reciprocal or square root. We give some examples of common transformations below.

12.2.1 Normalizing data

Many hypothesis tests and estimation procedures assume a Normal distribution of the variable of interest. There are various transformations that we can take in order to achieve a more nearly *Normal distribution* of t_x when the distribution of x is skewed. Two of the more common are:

1. **Log transformation** (Fig. 12.1(a),(b)). $t_x = \log x$ is a transformation which makes the distribution of x more nearly Normal if it is skewed to the right, in which case x is said to have a *Lognormal distribution* (see Section 3.5.3(f)). The logarithm may be taken either to base 10 (as is common in many branches of medical science) or to base e (the Napierian logarithm, written $\ln x$, which is often more convenient in mathematics). Always remember that logarithms can be taken only of positive numbers.
2. **Square transformation** (Fig. 12.1(c),(d)). $t_x = x^2$ makes a left skewed distribution of x closer to a Normal distribution.

12.2.2 Linearizing a relationship

It is much easier to analyse data and investigate a relationship between two variables when that relationship can be described by a straight line. The most common transformations which may help to **linearize** a relationship are:

(a)

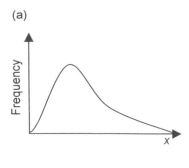

(b)

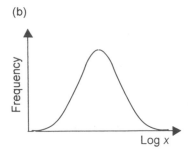

(c)

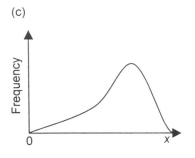

(d)

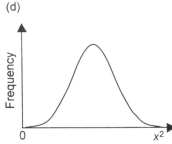

Fig. 12.1 Normalizing transformations.

1. **Log transformation** (Fig. 12.2(a),(b)). If there is an exponential relationship between y and another variable x, say, such that the slope of the curve (when y is plotted against x) increases for increasing values of x, then a logarithmic transformation of y, $t_y = \log y$, often produces a linear relationship between t_y and x.

2. **Square transformation** (Fig. 12.2(c),(d)). $t_x = x^2$ often linearizes a relationship with a consistently decreasing slope.

3. **Logit transformation** (Fig. 12.2(e),(f)). Proportions (or percentages) often have a tendency to be grouped towards the lower or upper ends of the scale. If p is a proportion which has a sigmoid relationship with another variable, x, the *logit* or *logistic* transformation, $t_p = \ln\{p/(1-p)\}$, produces a linear relationship between t_p and x.

4. **Arcsine transformation.** Another transformation of p which linearizes a sigmoid relationship is the *angular, inverse sine* or *arcsine* transformation, $t_p = \sin^{-1}\sqrt{p}$.

12.2.3 Stabilizing the variance

Equal variance is assumed in the two-sample *t*-test (see Section 7.4.2) and in the analysis of variance (see Section 8.6.1), and statistical analyses often assume that the residuals (see Section 10.4.3) have constant variance in different circumstances. The most common transformations which help to **stabilize variance** are:

1. **Log, reciprocal and square root transformations** (Fig. 12.3(a),(b)). If the variability of x tends to increase with increasing mean values of x (e.g. for groups defined by z), different transformations may be applied:
   (a) When the standard deviations of different samples are proportional to their means, then the logarithmic transformation, $t_x = \log x$, may stabilize the variance.
   (b) When the variability is particularly marked for increasing values of x, (e.g. if the standard deviation is proportional to the square of the mean) then the reciprocal transformation, $t_x = 1/x$, may stabilize the variance. The reciprocal transformation is often applied to survival times.
   (c) When the variances of different samples are proportional to their means, then the square root transformation, $t_x = \sqrt{x}$, is used; this transformation is appropriate when observations are in the form of counts which follow the Poisson distribution (see Section 3.4.3).

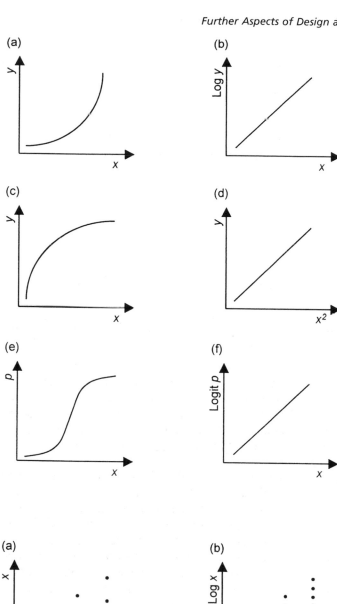

Fig. 12.2 Linearizing transformations.

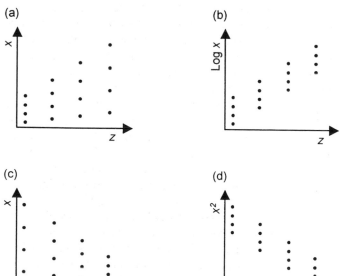

Fig. 12.3 Variance stabilizing transformations.

2. **Square transformation** (Fig. 12.3(c),(d)). $t_x = x^2$, is often used when the variability of the observations decreases with increasing values of x.
3. **Arcsine transformation**. The angular transformation of the proportion, $t_p = \sin^{-1}\sqrt{p}$, described under linearizing transformations, also has the important function of stabilizing variance.

12.3 SAMPLE SIZE

12.3.1 The importance of sample size

One of the most frequently asked questions of a statistician, and one of the hardest to answer, is 'How large a sample do I need if I am to conduct a particular experiment?' We usually design an experiment (see Section 5.4) to investigate the effect of a novel treatment (e.g. drug therapy or feeding regime) or, perhaps, an intervention (e.g. a surgical procedure or a changed management routine). Invariably, we wish to gauge whether it is superior to existing treatments, or the absence of treatment, and obtain some estimate of its effect.

Clearly, we should aim to have a sample size large enough to have a good chance of detecting any clinically important treatment differences, and yet not so large as to be wasteful of animals thereby creating ethical difficulties (see Section 5.9.7) and squandering resources. An inadequate sample size can lead to biologically or clinically meaningful treatment differences which are overlooked, and parameter estimates which lack precision.

Fortunately, statistical techniques exist for determining the optimal sample size in different circumstances for both experimental and observational studies. The downside, however, is that these calculations usually depend on our having some idea of the results we expect at the end of the experiment before we have conducted it! An added difficulty is that a statistical approach to the sample size problem may produce numbers which are not commensurate with the available resources, such as cost, time and the accessibility of animals. At the end of the day, it must be a combination of practical, ethical and statistical considerations which govern the final decision of the choice of sample size.

12.3.2 Methods for determining the optimal sample size

The standard statistical approach to determining the optimal sample size of an experiment relies on the direct relationship between its **power** and sample size. Power, you will remember (see Section 6.4), is the chance of detecting as statistically significant a true treatment difference of a given magnitude. The greater the sample size, the greater the power.

We can use statistical formulae, tables or a diagram (Altman's nomogram) to determine the numbers of animals we require in an experiment of a particular design if we are to have a prescribed power (typically exceeding 80%) of detecting a real treatment effect. All these procedures are based on the same theory and therefore require the same input (specification of the power, significance level, the difference of interest between the populations being compared, and the variability of the observations), details of which we provide in Section 12.3.3. It is a matter of personal preference as to which approach you use. Our favoured option is Altman's nomogram because of the ease with which we can determine the sample size of an experiment under slightly varying conditions (e.g. with different power specifications, at a different level of significance, etc.). Also, it is simple to reverse the procedure and determine the power of a study of a given sample size.

Alternatively, you may have access to the appropriate computer software (e.g. nQuery Advisor 2.0, Statistical Solutions Ltd, or SPSS Samplepower (1997)) which deals with both simple and complex designs including regression and survival analysis, and ANOVA. Computer programs speed up the process of sample size estimation, thus allowing us to produce, without any effort, power curves which show how the power varies as, for example, the sample size changes. However, bear in mind the fact that these computer programs require the same input as the other procedures, and it is acquiring this information which creates the real difficulties in sample size estimation.

You can find more on sample size estimation in Machin and Campbell (1987) and a full discussion in Cohen (1988). Altman (1982) introduces the nomogram, more details of which can be obtained in Altman (1991).

12.3.3 The nomogram

We can use **Altman's nomogram** to determine the optimal sample size for the comparison of two independent groups of animals (quantitative or qualitative data) or of paired observations (quantitative data). The calculations are for equally sized groups, but can be modified for unequal sample sizes.

The nomogram in Fig. 12.4 shows the relation between the total study size (N), the power, the level of significance (two-tailed) and what is termed the '**standardized difference**'. The formula for the standardized difference is specific to the particular comparison; essentially, it is the difference of interest divided by its standard deviation (details below). By drawing a straight line which joins a specified power and standardized difference, for a given level of significance, we can evaluate the required sample size. We can then easily appraise how variations in the power or the components of the standardized difference affect the sample size, or vice versa.

(a) Comparison of two independent groups – quantitative data

Suppose we wish to determine the sample size of our proposed trial if we are interested in comparing the means of a quantitative variable using two independent groups. This is achieved by the two-sample *t*-test (see Section 7.4) provided the variable is Normally distributed and each group has the same variance. In order to use the nomogram, we have to specify:

1. The power of the test (usually this should exceed 80%).

2. The two-sided significance level (usually 0.05 but sometimes 0.01).

3. The biologically or clinically relevant difference (δ); this treatment effect (see Section 6.3.1) is the difference in the means that is important to us and which we would not want to overlook. It is not necessarily the difference that we expect to find.

4. The standard deviation of the observations in each group (σ); here we are assuming constant variance, as in the two-sample *t*-test. This is where the real problem lies – we require an estimate of the standard deviation *before* we have collected the data. We can obtain this estimate either from a previous study that we may have performed which is similar to that which is proposed, from published papers or after we have conducted a pilot study (see Section 5.9.5).

Then the standardized difference = δ/σ, and N = the total number of observations.

Example

Suppose we want to compare the mean milk yields of Holstein-Friesian cows in Devon with those in Cheshire. The expected standard lactation (305 days) for cows in the UK from published figures is about 6500 kg. We want to know how many animals to sample from each of the two counties if we require an 85% chance of detecting a difference in mean milk yield of 250 kg (this is the minimum difference we would consider of importance to our investigation) at the 5% level of significance. Published information suggests that the standard deviation of milk yield is about 1425 kg.

Thus, $\delta = 250$, $\sigma = 1425$, and the standardized difference is 250/1425 = 0.175. If we mark 0.18 on the standardized difference axis, and 0.85 on the power axis of the nomogram, a line which joins these two points cuts the 0.05 significance level axis at $N = 1000$. Hence, each of the two random samples should comprise 500 cows.

(b) Comparison of two paired groups – quantitative data

Suppose we wish to determine the sample size of our proposed trial if we are interested in compar-

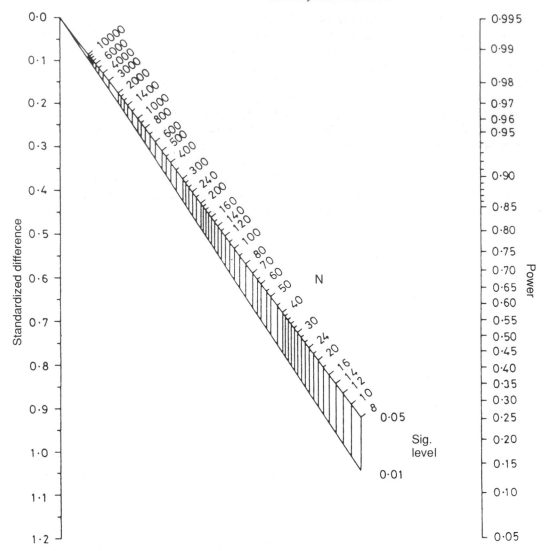

Fig. 12.4 The nomogram for sample size determination. (Reproduced from Altman, 1982, with permission.)

ing the measurements of a quantitative variable in two paired groups of observations. This is achieved by the paired *t*-test (see Section 7.5) provided the differences of the pairs are Normally distributed. In order to use the nomogram, we have to specify:

1. The power of the test (usually this should exceed 80%).
2. The two-sided significance level (usually 0.05 but sometimes 0.01).

3. The biologically or clinically relevant difference (δ).
4. The standard deviation of the *differences* (σ_d); this is likely to be very difficult to estimate and will probably have to be obtained from a pilot study.

Then the standardized difference = $2\delta/\sigma_d$.

Example

We want to measure the growth rate of weaner pigs under different growing conditions. We intend to choose matched pairs of weaners from pig litters and assign them to the two 'condition' groups. We want to know how many weaner pigs to select in order to have a 80% chance of detecting a difference in growth rates of 25 g per day (such a difference or a greater one would be considered biologically important) at the 5% level of significance. We believe, from a pilot study, that the standard deviation of the differences is about 45 g per day.

The standardized difference $= 2 \times 25/45 = 1.11$. If we mark 1.11 on the standardized difference axis of the nomogram, and 0.80 on the power axis, a line which joins these two points cuts the 0.05 significance level axis at approximately $N = 24$. Hence, we require about 24 pairs of weaners.

(c) Comparison of two independent groups – qualitative data

Suppose we wish to determine the sample size of our proposed trial if we are interested in comparing proportions in two independent groups of individuals; for example, those possessing a certain attribute, such as a disease, or having a particular outcome, such as death. This is achieved by the Chi-squared test (see Section 9.4). In order to use the nomogram, we have to specify:

1. The power of the test (usually this should exceed 80%).
2. The two-sided significance level (usually 0.05 but sometimes 0.01).
3. The clinically important difference in the two proportions, $p_1 - p_2$. So, if we know the proportion, p_1, that we expect in one group, we take the proportion, p_2, in the other group to be that which makes $p_1 - p_2$ represent a clinically relevant difference.

Then the standardized difference equals

$$\frac{p_1 - p_2}{\sqrt{\bar{p}(1 - \bar{p})}}$$

where

$$\bar{p} = \frac{p_1 + p_2}{2}$$

Example

Toxocara canis is a dog parasite which can cause blindness in children. We want to know whether the prevalence of *Toxocara canis* infestation is different in puppies under six months of age and dogs over one year of age in an urban setting. We expect the prevalence in puppies to be 30% and would be interested in detecting a difference of 25%, i.e. if we found that the prevalence in the dogs was 5%, we should regard this difference in prevalence to be biologically important. We need to know how many puppies and dogs to sample if we are to have a 90% chance of detecting this 25% difference at the 5% level of significance.

The mean prevalence

$$\bar{p} = \frac{0.30 + 0.05}{2} = 0.115$$

and the standardized difference equals

$$\frac{0.30 - 0.05}{\sqrt{0.115(1 - 0.115)}} = 0.78.$$

Connecting 0.78 on the standardized difference axis of the nomogram to a power of 0.90, we find that we will require about 70 animals in total if we are to achieve significance at the 5% level. Hence we need to take random samples of about 35 puppies and 35 dogs.

12.3.4 Sequential and interim analysis

The designs that we have considered so far have been **fixed sample size plans**; we make a decision about the approximate sample size in advance of performing the experiment. In certain circumstances, we can avoid choosing our sample size at the start of the investigation, and design the trial in such a way that the data are analysed as they are collected. We call this kind of trial, in which we have continuous monitoring of the treatment differences, a **sequential trial**. Generally, **sequential analysis** is performed on pairs of observations, one member of each pair being allocated at random to each of two treatments. We analyse the results from the pairs as they accumulate; we stop the trial when the evidence for one treatment is overwhelming or when we believe that it is unlikely that any difference will emerge. The stopping rules (determining when to 'stop') are defined by specifications of the null and the alternative hypotheses and of the significance level and power of the test. You may obtain full details in Armitage (1975).

Sequential trials tend, on average, to require smaller sample sizes than the equivalent fixed sample size plans. However, they are only amenable to the study of conditions in which the response to treatment can be evaluated soon after its administration. They are limited to trials in which there is only one response variable of predominant importance.

Sometimes we wish to design our trial as a fixed sample size study, but would like to have the option of terminating the trial before the end by performing a *predetermined* number of **interim analyses**. We must decide in advance when any intermediate analyses are to be carried out, and *not* be tempted to interrupt the investigation at whim. Then, if we find treatment differences which are convincingly large, we can stop the trial early, thereby ensuring:

- In the clinical setting, that the maximum number of animals receive the better treatment.
- In the experimental setting, that only a minimum number of animals are subjected to any adverse conditions.

Such a trial is also called a **group sequential design** (the data are analysed after the results of groups of animals become available, rather than after each pair as in the continuous sequential design) and is based on the idea of **repeated significance tests**. The significance test at each of the interim analyses uses the same form of test statistic as at the final stage, and not the stopping rules of sequential analysis. Multiple significance tests have the effect of increasing the chance of finding a significant difference when the treatments really are the same (see Section 8.6.3). In effect, we will increase the significance level at

the final stage after repeated significance tests unless we make appropriate adjustments. For example, if we have five repeated tests, each at the 5% level, the *overall* significance level becomes 14%, i.e. in effect we reject H_0 if $P < 0.14$. In order to keep this overall significance level at, say, 0.05, we must choose a more stringent *nominal* significance level for each of the repeated tests (an appropriate value <0.05). In particular, for our example of five repeated tests, the nominal level is 0.016. You can obtain further discussion of the method and the required nominal significance levels for varying numbers of interim analyses in Pocock (1983).

12.3.5 Meta-analysis

We may find that the results of a clinical trial are not statistically significant because its sample size is small and, hence, its power is low, even though there is a clinically important treatment difference. One way of improving the power of an investigation and increasing the precision of the estimates of treatment effects, without undertaking a much larger study, is to combine the results from similar trials in an appropriate manner. This is achieved by performing what is termed a **meta-analysis** or **overview** which provides a statistical summary of the numerical outcomes of the separate studies. A meta-analysis is a quantitative example of a **systematic review** which examines the literature in a rigorous and clearly defined manner; this contrasts with a traditional review which is often not very systematic and mixes together opinions and evidence.

Although meta-analyses are becoming increasingly popular in medicine, they are not without their critics. Several problems can arise: for example, the difficulty of deciding exactly which studies should be included (e.g. must they be randomized? Should poor quality trials be excluded?); the conclusions may be affected by **publication bias** (the tendency for journals to give substantially more space to papers in which the treatment effects are statistically significant) so that many trials with non-significant results are excluded from the meta-analysis, or the data summarized may not be homogeneous (e.g. because of methodological or clinical differences). However, if handled correctly, they will improve the reliability and accuracy of recommendations.

You can obtain a discussion of meta-analysis in three papers by Thompson (1995), Eysenck (1995), and Clarke and Stewart (1995) in Chalmers and Altman (1995).   ☐

12.4 SAMPLE SURVEYS

12.4.1 Introduction

When we are interested in certain features of a population, it is usually impractical to appraise the complete population, because of the constraints of time, finance or labour. Instead, we conduct a **sample survey** in which we study only a portion of the population. A sample survey is a particular type of observational study (see Section 5.2.1); it is usually concerned with providing estimates of the parameters in the population from which it is selected. The qualities that we require from a sample survey are that it should provide estimates of the population parameters which are **unbiased** (free from bias) and **precise**. If an estimate is free from bias, then the mean of its sampling distribution is equal to the value of the parameter in the population (see Section 4.4.3). The precision of an estimate is measured by its standard error, a more precise estimate having a smaller standard error.

We can ensure that the sample is free from selection bias if we take a **random sample** (see Section 1.8.2) comprising individuals with equal probabilities of selection chosen by a chance mechanism. Random sampling is sometimes called **probability sampling**. Then we build on the initial premise of random selection, using information about the structure of the population, and employ techniques which, for a given outlay of resources, improve the precision of the estimates of the parameters of interest. Alternatively, we can design the sample to attain a desired degree of precision for a minimum outlay of resources.

We only outline some of the basic ideas of sample surveys. You can obtain more detailed accounts in Moser and Kalton (1971), Cochran (1977) and Yates (1981).

12.4.2 Technical terms in sampling

An **element** is a single object or individual on which a measurement can be taken. The **population** from which we take our **sample** comprises an aggregate of **sampling units**. These are non-overlapping collections of elements, i.e. every element in the population belongs to only one unit. If each sampling unit contains only one element, then the sampling unit and the element are identical. The **frame** is a list of sampling units.

12.4.3 The more common sampling designs

You may find Fig. 12.5 helpful in conceptualizing the following descriptions of the more common sampling designs.

(a) **Simple random sampling** is the basic sampling design. The sampling units are chosen in such a way that:
  - The selection of one unit has no influence on the chance of any other being selected, i.e. they are *independent*.
  - Each possible sample of *n* units from the population of *N* units has an equal chance of being selected. This implies that every member of the population has an equal chance of being included in the sample.

  As an example, consider a trout farm in which scientists want to sample the trout from a pond for heavy metal contamination. A random sample is taken of sufficient size to be representative of the population. For example, for a stock of 8000 fish we might take a random sample of 2%, i.e. 160 fish.

(b) In **stratified sampling**, we divide the population into various sub-populations called strata. We select a simple random sample of units from each stratum, and compute parameter estimates from each stratum. We combine these estimates appropriately, using a weighted technique, to provide the required estimates of the parameters of interest. For example, in a wildlife population study in a particular location, the strata may be hedgerow, open field and woodland. These different habitats are likely to influence parameters such as population density, plumage and development rate. The sites would be identified and a simple random

(a) Random sampling

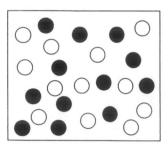

(b) Stratified sampling
(some units of all strata)

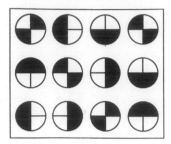

(c) Cluster sampling
(all units of selected clusters)

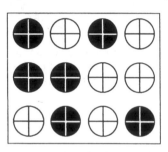

(d) Systematic sampling
(each unit in same relative
position)

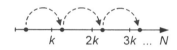

Fig. 12.5 Diagrammatic illustration of different sampling techniques.

sample taken from each. The estimates of each parameter of interest would be obtained from the three habitats and then combined to obtain an overall population estimate for this location.

Stratified sampling usually results in more precise estimates for a given cost than simple random sampling. For maximum precision, we construct the strata so that the strata means are as different as possible, and the units within each stratum are as alike as possible. Stratified sampling is the method most commonly employed in wildlife population surveys.

(c) In **cluster sampling**, we divide the population into clusters of units. We select a simple random sample of clusters from the population of clusters, and observe all the units in the selected clusters. As an example, suppose a veterinary practitioner wants to investigate the incidence of calving problems in his practice area. He could define the cattle farms on his books as the clusters, and note all the incidents of dystokia over the period of the study in a random selection of these farms.

Cluster sampling is less costly than simple or stratified random sampling if the clusters represent a geographically compact set of units, or if a frame which lists all population units is unavailable. However, the parameter estimates obtained from a cluster sample tend to be less precise than those of a simple random sample of the same number of units. We can maximize the precision of the estimates by choosing the clusters so that cluster means are as alike as possible, and the units within each cluster are as diverse as possible. Furthermore, we will obtain more precise estimates from a large number of small clusters than a small number of large clusters.

Although cluster sampling bears a superficial resemblance to stratified sampling in that a cluster, like a stratum, is a grouping of the units in the population, the two techniques are quite different. In stratified sampling, every stratum is represented in the final sample, and we select units at random from each sample; in cluster sampling, we select a random sample of clusters from a population of clusters in the same way as we select individual units from a population of units in simple random sampling. In cluster sampling we observe every unit in the selected clusters.

(d) We can extend cluster sampling by introducing one or more stages to the basic technique to obtain a **multi-stage sample**. For example, in two-stage sampling, we start by dividing the population into clusters. At the first stage, we select a random sample of clusters from the population of clusters. At the second stage, we select a random sample of units from the selected clusters rather than enumerating every unit in the selected clusters.

(e) In **systematic sampling**, we randomly select one unit from the first k units in the frame, and then every kth unit thereafter. In the strict sense, a systematic sample is not a true random sample because only the first unit is selected at random. Once the first unit has been selected, the remaining units are predetermined in that every one occupies the same relative position in each group of k units. A systematic sample is appealing because it is easy to draw and it ensures that the units in the sample are evenly distributed over the listed population. Hence systematic sampling is often more precise than simple random sampling. However, we cannot evaluate the precision of the estimates in a systematic sample, and we may obtain biased estimates if the population consists of a periodic trend and k coincides with the period or a multiple of it.

Multi-stage and systematic sampling have less use in veterinary and animal science than in human investigations. Systematic sampling depends on being able to list all the individuals. Unlike humans with their Voting Registers or National Insurance numbers, animals are usually more dispersed and less regimented. Moreover, the population density would rarely provide a

situation where multi-stage sampling would be appropriate.

You may be interested to note the relationship of systematic sampling to both stratified and cluster sampling. The systematic sample is almost equivalent to a stratified sample if we regard each stratum as a group of k consecutive units in the frame. Our sample comprises a single unit from each 'stratum', although only the first unit is selected at random. The systematic sample is equivalent to a cluster sample if we define the ith cluster ($i = 1, 2, 3, \ldots, k$) as that containing the ith unit in every group of k consecutive units in the frame. Then there exist k possible clusters to choose from, and in a systematic sample we are selecting a simple random sample of one cluster from this population of k clusters. □

12.4.4 Sampling from wildlife populations

It is important to be able to estimate the size of many wildlife populations for the study of growth, evolution and maintenance. There are a number of ways in which the estimate can be obtained.

(a) Capture–tag–recapture

The **capture–tag–recapture** method can be split into two types of sampling procedure: direct sampling and inverse sampling.

1. **Direct sampling**.
   (a) We take a random sample of size t from the wildlife population, tag each animal sampled, and return these animals to the population.
   (b) At some later date, we take a second random sample, this time of a predetermined size, n, from the population, and observe the number tagged, s.
   For example, suppose we want to estimate the pigeon population in Trafalgar Square. We take a random sample of $t = 500$ pigeons and ring (tag) them before release. A week later, we take another sample of $n = 200$ pigeons and note that $s = 29$ are ringed.

2. **Inverse sampling**.
   (a) We take a random sample of size t from the wildlife population, tag each animal sampled, and return these animals to the population.
   (b) At some later date, we select animals from the population, using random sampling, and observe whether or not the animals captured are tagged. We continue sampling until we observe exactly s (a predetermined number) tagged animals. Let us suppose that we need to select n animals in this second sample to obtain s tagged animals.
   Again we start by taking a random sample of $t = 500$ pigeons and ring them before release. We decide that we are going to capture $s = 25$ ringed pigeons one week later.

At that time we find that we have captured $n = 173$ pigeons of which $s = 25$ are ringed.

For both direct and inverse sampling

$$\text{Estimated population size} = \frac{t}{s/n}$$

where the denominator represents the proportion of tagged animals in the second sample, estimating the proportion of tagged animals in the population.

In our example, we estimate the pigeon population in Trafalgar Square to be

$$\text{Direct sampling, } \frac{t}{s/n} = \frac{500}{29/200} \approx 3448 \text{ pigeons}$$

$$\text{Inverse sampling, } \frac{t}{s/n} = \frac{500}{25/173} \approx 3460 \text{ pigeons}$$

However, the variance of the estimate is different in each case. The estimated variances of the estimated population size for direct and inverse sampling are, respectively

$$\frac{t^2 n(n-s)}{s^3} \text{ and } \frac{t^2 n(n-s)}{s^2(s+1)}$$

In our pigeon example, the standard errors of our estimates (i.e. the square roots of the variances) are approximately 592 and 628 for the direct and inverse methods, respectively. If the size of the second sample, n, is small compared to the overall population size, then inverse sampling provides a more precise estimate of the population size than direct sampling. However, if we know very little about the size of the population, then it is difficult to gauge the most appropriate t, which, if too great, could make n very large; in these circumstances, direct sampling is the preferred choice. Details of choosing sample sizes for direct and inverse sampling may be obtained from Mendenhall *et al.* (1971).

An explanation and further discussion of the methods of estimating wildlife population sizes is given by Greenwood (1996) and also by Southwood (1996). Greenwood, for example, explains how to estimate total population size by simultaneously tagging and recapturing animals by using traps of two different sorts in a closed population. The estimate is obtained by assessing, at the end point of the study, the relative numbers of animals caught in one type of trap from which they cannot escape, and from the other type in which the animals are tagged before they are allowed to escape.

Unfortunately, the methods which rely on tagging and recapturing the animals assume that all animals in the population have the same probability of recapture. This is often not the case, so that the population estimates may be inaccurate, and their calculated standard errors wildly off the mark. Sometimes, more reliable information can be obtained by estimating birth and survival rates having following the fortunes of a group of marked animals.

(b) Bootstrapping

Another approach to population studies is based on an iterative method, called **bootstrapping**, of estimating the parameters of interest. The underlying sampling process is often cluster sampling, the clusters being equivalent-sized areas derived from an appropriate map. The entire population in a random selection of areas is then counted within a short period, often by recruiting volunteer labour. For example, in a national survey of corn buntings (Donald and Evans, 1995), tetrads (2×2 km) were selected at random from areas which had previously been recorded as having the birds. Populations were calculated separately for 11 different regions representing Scotland, England and Wales to reduce geographical bias, and a national estimate of corn buntings obtained.

The estimate can be refined by using the bootstrap technique: the basic method uses computer simulation involving simple random resampling with replacement and recalculation of the population estimate. The procedure is repeated a large number of times (often 999 times as recommended by Manly, 1991), until the moving average of the estimates of the required parameter (e.g. the population size) becomes stable. The confidence interval for the parameter is then obtained from the percentiles of the simulated values. More details of territory mapping techniques are given in Bibby *et al.* (1992).

(c) Distance sampling

A variant sampling procedure is that of **distance sampling** from a transect line. A transect line is drawn and the number and frequency of species recorded by an observer along the transect. The method is based on the proposition that the detection of randomly distributed subjects declines with distance from the transect line; an increasing number of subjects will be undetected with increasing distance from the line. Distance sampling methods model the decline in detectability with distance for a given species, and arrive at an estimate of population based on the data. More details can be found in the volume by Bibby *et al.* (1992).

Childs *et al.* (1998) used both a capture–tag method and a distance sampling technique to make estimates of rural dog populations in the Philippines. They concluded that distance sampling was a simple and satisfactory method for estimating dog population density. ☐

12.5 MULTIVARIATE ANALYSIS

We have already introduced you to *multiple regression* (see Section 10.5) and *multiple logistic regression* (see Section 10.6), where we look at the effect of a number of explanatory variables on a single response variable. A similar model building approach, *log-linear analysis*, is used to investigate associations in multi-way contingency tables derived from a number of categorical variables (i.e. each individual is categorized with respect to several qualitative variables). Yet another model building approach to analysing data is the method of *multi-level modelling* which is a hierarchical (i.e. lower level observations are nested within higher level units) extension of regression analysis. It incorporates sophisticated techniques which are highly computational, allowing us to account for complex structures in the data by specifically modelling the effects of the different levels. In all these regression-type analyses, there is only a single dependent or response variable and so, strictly, these methods are termed *multivariable* or **univariate**.

The procedures gathered under the general heading '**multivariate analysis**' are traditionally directed at situations in which there are several response variables, and we wish to examine the variation in these variables simultaneously. Multivariate techniques are increasingly used, especially now that computer techniques can take the drudgery out of the calculations. As with all statistical procedures, you should aim to understand what the computer is doing, and how, before embarking on multivariate analyses.

Some of the more common analyses are:

- *Discriminant analysis* – given the existence of different groupings of the population, it uses the information from a sample of individuals, in which each individual is known to belong to a particular group, to devise a rule for allocating further individuals to the appropriate groups.
- *Cluster analysis* – determines whether there is a natural subdivision of the individuals into groups or clusters on the basis of the observations on several variables.
- *Factor analysis* – defines a model (with distributional and other assumptions) in which the k original variables are replaced by another set of $j < k$ variables (called factors), each of which

is a linear combination of the original variables together with a residual. In order to present the most economical model, j is chosen to be as small as possible.

- *Principal component analysis* – replaces the k original variables by another set of k variables (the principal components), each of which is a linear combination of the original variables. The first few principal components often account for most of the variability of the original data, so that the remaining principal components can be discarded and thereby reduce the dimensionality of the data.
- *Multidimensional scaling* – concerned with expressing the main content of the data in fewer dimensions with as little distortion as possible. It is based on the distances between the points, and is closely related to principal component analysis.
- *Canonical correlation* – concerned with investigating the interdependence between two sets of variables, $(y_1, y_2, y_3, \ldots, y_p)$ and $(x_1, x_2, x_3, \ldots, x_m)$.
- *Multivariate analysis of variance* (*MANOVA*) – an extension of the univariate ANOVA for multiple dependent variables. So, for example, in the one-way MANOVA, we test the null hypothesis that the population means are the same for all the dependent variables.

We suggest, if you require to utilize these multivariate analytical methods, you refer to books such as those by Marriott (1974), Chatfield and Collins (1980), Kendall (1980) or Manly (1986) before embarking on the analysis. The methods are sometimes difficult to understand, and need careful assessment to avoid misuse.

EXERCISES

The statements in questions 12.1–12.3 are either TRUE or FALSE.

12.1 The logarithmic transformation:
(a) Normalizes data which are skewed to the left.
(b) Linearizes an exponential relationship.

(c) Stabilizes variance when the variability of the data increases as the magnitude of the observations increases.

(d) Is particularly useful for transforming proportions.

(e) Is applied when the sample size is small.

12.2 You will need more animals to find a significant difference between two treatments in a clinical trial if (all other factors remaining constant):

(a) You increase the power of the test.

(b) You decrease the significance level from 0.05 to 0.01.

(c) You have been informed that the clinically important treatment difference is greater than you believed it to be.

(d) The response of interest is quantitative, and you have underestimated the standard deviation of the observations in each group.

(e) The standardized difference is increased.

12.3

(a) Sequential analysis is particulary appropriate when the response to treatment is prolonged.

(b) The nominal significance level in a group sequential design is always less than the overall significance level.

(c) Random allocation of animals to treatment groups is ensured by random sampling.

(d) A stratified sample is more precise than a simple random sample of the same size if it is designed so that the units within a stratum are as alike as possible, and the strata means are as different as possible.

(e) A cluster sample is more precise than a simple random sample of the same size if it is designed so that the units within a cluster are as alike as possible, and the cluster means are as different as possible.

12.4 The Indian water buffalo, like domestic cattle, suffers from gut parasite infestations, some of which cause severe anaemia. We want, therefore, to be able to detect a change in haemoglobin (Hb) content in buffalo blood. We know that the Hb content of buffalo blood has a mean value of 11.1 g/dl with an SD of

0.96 g/dl (Jain *et al.*, 1982). In an investigation comparing the effects of infestation with those in a control group, we want an 80% chance of detecting a change of, say, 1 g/dl. Will this be a one- or two-tailed test? How many animals would be needed to detect a change of this magnitude:

(a) At a significance level of 0.05 with a power of 80%?

(b) At a significance level of 0.05 with a power of 90%?

(c) At a significance level of 0.01 with a power of 80%?

(d) If the standard deviation was 1.3 g/dl, at a significance level of 0.05 with a power of 80%?

12.5 We want to compare two different exercise regimes for horses on a treadmill as judged by the plasma lactate concentration at the end of the exercise period. We will conduct a randomized cross-over trial (each horse undergoes both exercise regimes in a randomized order) on a group of randomly selected animals with two different cantering speeds for a period of 7 min. A difference in plasma lactate of 1 mmol/l is considered an important difference. From a previous pilot trial, we know that the SD of the differences in plasma lactate concentration under the two regimes is likely to be around 1.7 mmol/l.

(a) How many horses will we need to test in order to have a probability of 0.85 of detecting, at a 1% significance level, a difference in plasma lactate concentrations of 1.0 mmol/l between these exercise regimes?

(b) We actually have 20 horses available. What is the power of the test?

(c) Now what is the effect on power of changing the significance level to 5%?

12.6 A study is to be conducted on the effectiveness of attenuated canine parvovirus vaccine (A-CPV) to protect six-week-old puppies. It is anticipated that maternally-derived passive immunity would interfere with the establishment of an adequate immunity (titres greater than 1:80 in a haemaglutination-inhibition (HI) test) 1–2 weeks after vaccination. Puppies will be divided into seronegative (<1:10 HI titre) and seropositive (>1:20 HI titre) groups before vaccination. We anticipate that, in the seronegative group, a successful vaccination programme will produce a high percentage (i.e. >90%) of protected animals (>1:80 HI titre). If we find that vaccination in the seropositive group produces less than 50% protection, this will be considered a serious limitation. How many puppies will be required if we want a power of 90% of detecting this difference in protection rates at the 5% level of significance?

Chapter 13

Additional Topics

13.1 LEARNING OBJECTIVES

By the end of this chapter you should be able to:

- Define the terms 'sensitivity', 'specificity', 'predictive value' as used in diagnostic tests.
- Evaluate the performance of a diagnostic or screening test.
- Investigate both repeatability and method agreement in continuous data.
- Investigate agreement in categorical data using Cohen's kappa.
- Explain what is meant by a time series, and state the issues that are relevant for analysis.
- Identify the appropriate analysis for repeated measures.
- Recognize when a survival analysis should be performed.

13.2 DIAGNOSTIC TESTS

13.2.1 Introduction

We can often use the result of a test to diagnose a disease in a sick animal or as a screening device in a population of apparently healthy animals. Each animal either has the disease (is **positive**) or is disease-free (is **negative**). If the **diagnostic test** is based on a quantitative variable, then we may decide that the animal is likely to have the disease if the quantitative measurement for that animal exceeds or is below a certain value. Typically, this value will be the limit of a reference range (see Section 2.7). For example, we may use plasma thyroxin (T_4) measurements in the diagnosis of hypothyroidism in dogs. A dog could be diagnosed as having an underactive thyroid gland if its plasma thyroxin measurement was

less than 15 nmol/l, the lower limit of the reference range. Alternatively, our diagnostic test may be based on a qualitative response, such as the presence or absence of some symptom or sign. In either situation, we must be able to evaluate the performance of this diagnostic test. We want to know:

- How effective the test is at identifying animals with the disease (**sensitivity**).
- How effective the test is at identifying animals without the disease (**specificity**).
- How likely it is that the test will give a correct diagnosis, whether the animal is diseased or disease-free (**predictive value**).

The sensitivity and specificity of the test provide measures of the **validity** of the test whereas the predictive value gives an indication of the usefulness of the test.

13.2.2 Defining terms

The true or 'gold-standard' diagnosis may be made using a variety of information from sources such as clinical examination, laboratory or post-mortem results or an expert's opinion. Table 13.1 shows the observed frequencies in a general setting of such a test, and from this the terms can be defined.

- **Sensitivity** = $a/(a + c)$. The proportion of true (gold standard) positives identified by the test as positive. It gives an indication of the ability of the test to correctly identify those animals with the disease.
- **Specificity** = $d/(b + d)$. The proportion of true (gold standard) negatives identified by the test

Table 13.1 Table of observed frequencies.

		True diagnosis		
		Positive (diseased)	Negative (healthy)	Total
Test result	Positive	a	b	$a + b$
	Negative	c	d	$c + d$
	Total	$a + c$	$b + d$	$n = a + b + c + d$

as negative. It gives an indication of the ability of the test to correctly identify those animals without the disease.

- **Positive predictive value** (PPV) = $a/(a + b)$. The proportion of animals with a positive test result which really are positive.
- **Negative predictive value** (NPV) = $d/(c + d)$. The proportion of animals with a negative test result which really are negative.
- **Observed prevalence** = $(a + c)/n$. The proportion of animals in the study with the disease.

All these ratios are often multiplied by 100 and expressed as percentages.

Ideally, we should like a test which has both a high sensitivity and a high specificity. However, these two measures are usually not independent, so that as one increases, the other tends to decrease. The relative importance of the sensitivity and specificity of a test depends on the particular disease that is being tested and the implications of the animal either having or not having the disease.

- If we are concerned with identifying animals with the disease so that we can treat them, then we should use a test which has a high sensitivity, e.g. the glucose tolerance test in dogs to diagnose diabetes mellitus.
- If our concern is with excluding diseased animals and identifying those which are disease-free, then we require a test with a high specificity, e.g. tuberculin testing in cattle.

If our test is based on a quantitative variable, we can alter the sensitivity and the specificity of a diagnostic test by raising or lowering the cut-off

value for the variable, where this cut-off determines whether the test result is positive or negative. So, for example, in our hypothyroid example in dogs where a low T_4 level is taken as indicative of the existence of a pathological state, e.g. an inactive gland, we can increase the sensitivity and decrease the specificity if we raise the critical cut-off to a value above 15 nmol/l, the lower limit of 'normal'.

Sometimes a **receiver operating characteristic (ROC) curve** is plotted as a means of determining the best cut-off for comparing two or more tests. The ROC curve plots the sensitivity (the true positive rate) against one minus the specificity (the false positive rate) for different cut-off values. A 'good' test is one which has a high true positive rate and a low false positive rate and whose value, therefore, lies close to the top left-hand corner of the ROC curve. Further details may be found in Jekel *et al.* (1996) and similar texts.

The positive and negative predictive values of a test are affected by the prevalence of the disease. As the prevalence of the disease is raised, we have more animals with the disease in the population, and we have greater confidence that a positive test result is correct; the positive predictive value of the test is increased and the negative predictive value is decreased. The reverse is true as the prevalence of the disease is lowered. You should therefore not compare predictive values of tests which have been evaluated in populations in which the prevalence of the disease is different.

Generally, the sensitivity and specificity of the test are not affected by the prevalence of the disease. They provide measures of the validity of the test in relation to the 'gold-standard' diagnosis. However, if the gold-standard is not a true reflection of the real disease state of the animal, and the requirement is for measures of validity which relate to the true diagnosis, then sensitivity and specificity may be related to prevalence.

13.2.3 Example

Barber and Elliott (1998) investigated the aetiopathogenesis of renal secondary hyperpara-

Table 13.2 Results of the screening test for renal hyperparathyroidism (RHPTH) in cats diagnosed with chronic renal failure using plasma phosphate concentration. (Data from Barber and Elliott, 1998, with permission.)

| | 'True diagnosis' | | |
| | RHPTH (PTH > 25.5 pg/ml) | No RHPTH (PTH ≤ 25.5 pg/ml) | |
Screening test			Total
RHPTH (phosphate > 1.86 mmol/l)	43	1	44
No RHPTH (phosphate ≤ 1.86 mmol/l)	20	12	32
Total	63	13	76

Sensitivity = $\frac{43}{63}$ = 0.68   PPV = $\frac{43}{44}$ = 0.98   Observed prevalence = $\frac{63}{76}$ = 0.83

Specificity = $\frac{12}{13}$ = 0.92   NPV = $\frac{12}{32}$ = 0.38

thyroidism (RHPTH) in cats with chronic renal failure (CRF). We used this example in Section 11.6.2 to illustrate the Kruskal–Wallis test which compared the distributions of plasma parathyroid hormone (PTH) concentrations in the cats in three stages of CRF. We showed that the PTH concentrations were significantly higher in those groups of cats with a greater degree of renal dysfunction.

Assay of PTH is, at the moment, expensive and, as yet, not widely available. Barber and Elliott, therefore, investigated the use of more routine biochemical measurements to act as markers for the presence of RHPTH. In particular, they found that use of plasma phosphate concentrations was the most efficient screening test for RHPTH in feline CRF. As the 'gold standard', they used the upper limit of the reference range of PTH in an age-matched control group as the cut-off point for determining whether or not the cat suffered from RHPTH (a cat was thus defined as having RHPTH if its PTH > 25.5 pg/ml). Similarly, they used the upper limit of the reference range of phosphate (i.e. phosphate > 1.86 mmol/l) as the cut-off for the screening test. Table 13.2 shows the results they obtained in 76 cats with CRF.

Although the screening test based on plasma phosphate is well able to identify those CRF cats without RHPTH (specificity = 92%), its ability to detect RHPTH in CRF cats who have this complication is low (sensitivity = 68%). However, the PPV value of the test is very high (98%), indicating that if a CRF cat has a positive test result, it almost certainly does have RHPTH. Note that the prevalence of RHPTH is high (83%) in this group of CRF cats, so we would expect the PPV to be high as well.

Although this screening test has poor sensitivity, plasma phosphate concentrations proved to have superior efficiency compared to other variables that were investigated. It could certainly be used as a screen of CRF cats to institute dietary phosphate restriction. Monthly monitoring of phosphate would then be used to establish whether phosphate concentration can be stabilized within or above the normal range. The latter group, those with persistently high phosphate concentrations, are likely to have RHPTH which could then be confirmed by analysis of hormone levels.

13.3 MEASURING AGREEMENT

13.3.1 Repeatability and method agreement of quantitative measurements

Sometimes we are interested in assessing the similarity between two, three or more measurements of a quantitative variable.

- The **repeatability** of a method evaluates the extent to which the same observer obtains the same results in identical circumstances.
- A related problem is when we wish to investigate **method agreement**, often called

reproducibility. Do two methods of measurement agree with one another and can we obtain some quantity to describe this agreement? These methods may be, for example, different observers using the same technique or a single observer using different techniques.

In both cases, we shall assume that we are comparing *pairs* of measurements of a *quantitative* variable. For simplicity, we shall explain the approach comparing two successive measurements to assess repeatability; the approach is similar if we wish to compare single measurements from each of two methods or two observers. *Remember, it is necessary to establish that a method is repeatable before comparing two methods for reproducibility.* Bland and Altman (1986) give a detailed discussion of the problem; they explain how the approach can be modified when more than two measurements are to be compared, e.g. when each observer takes repeated measurements. We explain how to assess agreement between the values of a *categorical* variable in Section 13.3.2.

(a) Correct analysis of repeatability and method agreement

We calculate the difference between the pair of measurements for each individual. The mean of these differences ($\bar{d}$) is an estimate of the average **bias** of one method relative to the other. If this bias is zero (as established by the paired *t*-test – see Section 7.5), then the two measurements agree on average. However, this does not imply that they agree for each individual. In order to assess how well the measurements agree for the individual, we determine the limits within which most of the differences (typically, 95%) lie. These are called the **limits of agreement**. Provided the differences can be assumed to follow a Normal distribution, we calculate the limits as $\bar{d} \pm 2s_{diff}$, where $\bar{d}$ is the mean of the differences, and s_{diff} is the standard deviation of the differences. Based on clinical judgement of the particular problem at hand, we can decide whether the limits of agreement are acceptable, and therefore whether we are prepared to conclude

that the two measurements agree, and that the method is repeatable.

Clearly, we require these limits of agreement to be the same for all the measurements, whether they are large or small. In order to check that the relationship between the differences and the magnitude of the measurement is constant, we plot the difference in the two measurements in a pair against their average (Fig. 13.1). If the relationship is constant and there is no bias, we should see a random scatter of points around the line of zero difference, with no funnel effect as the mean of the two measurements increases. If the relationship is not constant, then we should take a transformation of the data (see Section 12.2) and repeat the process. Note that it is easier to spot outliers (see Section 5.9.2) in this plot than in the plot of the measurement of one method against the other. We should check the measurements for any outlier to determine if there is any obvious reason for its presence.

We can use the standard deviation of the differences, s_{diff}, as a **measure of agreement**. This is particularly relevant if we are concerned with assessing repeatability rather than method agreement, because we can use the measure to compare different methods to determine which is the more repeatable. The smaller the measure, the greater the repeatability. Alternatively, we can multiply it by 2 (an approximation to 1.96) and obtain the **British Standards Institution repeatability** (or, **reproducibility**, as relevant) **coefficient** which gives an indication of the maximum difference likely to occur between two measurements. We expect approximately 95% of the absolute differences to be less than the repeatability coefficient. Expressed another way, the repeatability coefficient is the value below which the difference between paired results may be expected to lie with 95% certainty. It is assumed that the results are obtained under the same conditions for repeatability, or on the same material using different methods for method agreement.

You may find that instead of the standard deviation of the differences, s_{diff}, being used as a measure of agreement or in the repeatability coefficient, the quantity $\sqrt{\sum d^2/n}$ is used instead.

This is derived from

$$s_{\text{diff}} = \sqrt{\left\{\sum (d - \bar{d})^2\right\}/(n-1)}$$

when $\bar{d} = 0$ and $(n-1)$ is replaced by n. Note that if there is no bias we would expect the mean of the differences to be zero, and if the sample size is reasonably large, $n-1$ is virtually the same as n.

Just to confuse the issue, Dahlberg's formula, $\sqrt{s_{\text{diff}}^2/2}$, is sometimes called the **standard error of measurement**. It is used in studies of repeatability to provide an estimate of the standard deviation of the *individual measurements*, s_{w}, rather than that of the *differences*. If there are many, rather than just two, repeated measurements on each individual, the standard error of measurement is equal to the square root of the residual variance, $\sqrt{s_{\text{w}}^2}$, in the one-way analysis of variance (see Section 8.5) in which the different individuals represent the groups.

It may be of interest to note that the British Standards Institution repeatability coefficient can also be calculated as 2.83 times the standard error of measurement (i.e. the coefficient is $2\sqrt{s_{\text{diff}}^2} = 2\sqrt{2s_{\text{w}}^2} = 2.83s_{\text{w}}$).

(b) Example of measuring agreement for a quantitative variable

We have two ways of evaluating sperm counts in the laboratory: we can count them directly using a haemocytometer (a time-consuming procedure) or we can count them indirectly using the calibration curve of optical density on a machine called a colorimeter. From time to time, however, we have to check that the colorimeter is giving the correct count. Table 13.3 shows the counts of sperm concentration in 22 samples of ram ejaculates using the two methods. Figure 13.1 is a scatter diagram of the difference in the counts plotted against their average. From Fig. 13.1, we can see that the scatter of the points is random, indicating that the size of the discrepancy between the two methods of counting is not related to the size of the count. Hence it is reasonable to calculate the limits of agreement for the two methods. These are the $\bar{d} \pm 2s_{\text{diff}}$, where the mean of the differences, $\bar{d} = 0.0136$ (10^9/ml), and the standard deviation of the differences, $s_{\text{diff}} = 0.1543$ (10^9/ml). Hence the limits are $0.0136 \pm 0.3086 = (-0.295, 0.322)$ 10^9/ml. These limits are shown as dotted lines in Fig. 13.1; we expect 95% of differences to lie within these limits. Expressed another way, we expect 95% of the absolute differences to be less than the reproducibility coefficient, $2s_{\text{diff}} = 0.31$ (i.e. 0.3086 corrected to two decimal places) 10^9/ml. This is satisfactory agreement, and we can use the colorimeter method with reasonable confidence.

(c) Erroneous analysis of repeatability and method agreement

You will find that a very common way of investigating repeatability and method agreement is by performing a paired *t*-test (see Section 7.5) on

Table 13.3 Sperm counts ($\times 10^9$/ml) of 22 sheep ejaculates using two methods of counting.

Colorimeter	Haemocytometer	Colorimeter	Haemocytometer
0.82	1.01	1.73	1.52
2.34	2.46	3.11	3.37
2.34	2.20	3.76	3.60
4.13	4.29	1.12	1.09
4.03	3.82	3.28	3.43
4.70	4.59	3.25	3.16
4.78	4.66	1.28	1.41
5.00	4.75	3.82	3.77
5.04	4.97	3.48	3.49
5.17	5.24	1.43	1.23
5.27	5.35	3.14	3.33

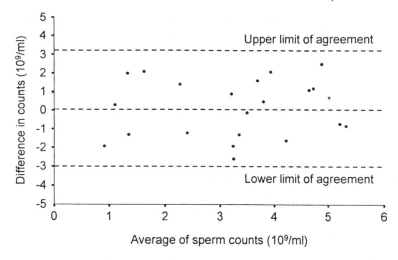

Fig. 13.1 The difference between the counts of sperm concentration using a colorimeter and a haemocytometer (C − H) plotted against their average (C + H)/2 in an investigation of method agreement.

the pairs of measurements to test the null hypothesis that there is agreement between them, and by calculating a correlation coefficient (see Section 10.3.1) to provide a measure of the agreement. This is *not* the way to proceed for the reasons which we outline below.

- The paired *t*-test tests the null hypothesis that the mean difference is zero. If the differences between the pairs are large (indicating that the two methods do not agree) but evenly scattered around zero, then we will obtain a non-significant result. We can conclude only that there is no *bias* (see Section 4.4.3), not that the methods agree.
- The correlation coefficient provides a measure of the linear association between the measurements obtained by the two methods. It gives us an indication of how close the observations in the scatter diagram (plotting the measurements of one method against the other) are to a straight line. To assess agreement, we need to know how close the points are to the line of equality, i.e. the 45° line.
- The value of the correlation coefficient depends on the range of values of the measurement. Thus, we could obtain a high value for the correlation coefficient simply because we have a wide range of measurements from each of the two methods.

13.3.2 The kappa measure of agreement for a categorical variable

We may be interested in comparing the values of a categorical variable when these values are obtained from two methods of measurement. This is similar to the problem of assessing the agreement between two different observers, raters or examiners after each observer has classified a number of animals into one of several groups; for example, the judging of dog and cat shows, or the judging of animals at agricultural shows. Let us suppose that we want to measure observer agreement.

(a) Cohen's kappa coefficient

The most usual measure of agreement is **Cohen's kappa coefficient**, written κ. It assesses overall observer agreement by relating the actual agreement obtained with that which would have been attained had the categorization been made at random, i.e. it compares the actual agreement with chance agreement, and may be interpreted as the chance corrected proportional agreement.

Unfortunately, there are a number of difficulties associated with using kappa.

(a) There are no objective criteria for judging kappa. Its maximum value of 1.00 represents perfect agreement. A value of zero indicates that the agreement is the same as chance agreement. A negative value, which rarely occurs, indicates that the agreement between the observers is less than chance agreement. Landis and Koch (1977) provide a reasonable approach to interpreting kappa. Very approximately, we might regard the agreement as:

- 'Poor' if $\kappa \leq 0.20$.
- 'Fair' if $0.21 \leq \kappa \leq 0.40$.
- 'Moderate' if $0.41 \leq \kappa \leq 0.60$.
- 'Substantial' if $0.61 \leq \kappa \leq 0.80$.
- 'Good' if it exceeds 0.80.

(b) The value of kappa depends on the proportion of individuals in each category. Thus different kappa values should not be compared in studies in which these proportions differ.

(c) Kappa depends on the number of categories that are used in its calculation, with its value being greater if there are less categories.

In order to calculate kappa, we arrange the data in a square two-way contingency table of frequencies (see Section 9.4.2 and Table 13.4). The rows represent the categories of response of one observer, and the columns represent the same categories of response of the second observer. Perfect agreement is obtained when both of the observers believe an animal belongs to the same category; the frequency with which this occurs is shown in the diagonal cells of the table. For each of the observed frequencies along this diagonal, we calculate the corresponding frequency we would expect if there were chance agreement. The calculations are similar to those for the Chi-squared statistic (see Section 9.5.3), i.e. each expected frequency is the product of the marginal totals divided by the overall total. The observed frequencies along the diagonal are added and their sum is divided by the total observed frequency to obtain a proportion which represents the 'observed agreement'. 'Chance agreement' is the sum of the expected frequencies along the diagonal, divided by the total observed frequency. Then

$$\kappa = \frac{\text{Observed agreement} - \text{Chance agreement}}{\text{Maximum agreement} - \text{Chance agreement}}$$

where maximum agreement = 1.

This unweighted kappa considers only perfect agreement of the observers, as demonstrated by the frequencies along the diagonal of the contingency table. It has the disadvantage that it takes no account of the *extent* to which the observers disagree. This is relevant if the categories are *ordered* so that observers differing by one category show less disagreement than if they differ by two categories, etc. Then the greater the discrepancy, the greater the distance of the cell from the diagonal in the contingency table. In these circumstances, we should calculate a **weighted kappa**; this is determined by assigning weightings to the animals about which the observers disagree according to the magnitude of the disagreement.

You can obtain full details of the calculations of kappa and the weighted kappa, together with formulae for standard errors from which confidence intervals can be derived, in Cohen (1960) and Cohen (1968).

(b) Example of the kappa measure of agreement

Scoring of body condition is routinely used in pig management. Generally, the score is on a subjective scale ranging from one to five (one is very poor condition, five implies a sow with excellent fat and muscle). To be consistent, the scoring system must be learned. Table 13.4 gives body condition scores of 160 pigs by two independent scorers. The first scorer is an experienced pigman, and the second is a trainee.

$$\text{Observed agreement} = \frac{4+7+15+36+3}{160}$$
$$= 0.406$$

Chance agreement
$$= \frac{0.400+1.463+7.813+29.656+4.400}{160}$$
$$= 0.273$$

Experienced pigman

Score	1	2	3	4	5	Total
1	**4** **(0.400)**	3	1	0	0	8
2	4	**7** **(1.463)**	5	2	0	18
3	0	2	**15** **(7.813)**	7	1	25
4	0	1	16	**36** **(29.656)**	12	65
5	0	0	13	28	**3** **(4.400)**	44
Total	8	13	50	73	16	160

Trainee

Table 13.4 Table of observed frequencies of body condition scores accorded to 160 pigs by a pigman and a trainee (expected frequencies are in brackets).

Hence, $\kappa = \dfrac{0.406 - 0.273}{1 - 0.273} = 0.183$

We can see that, with a kappa of only 0.18, the agreement between the assessors is poor; the trainee requires more experience and help!

13.4 MEASUREMENTS AT SUCCESSIVE POINTS IN TIME

13.4.1 Time series

A **time series** is a sequence of observations made at many successive time points. Generally these observations arc recorded on groups of animals or other phenomena of interest at each of the time points. Typical examples in agriculture are the average number of eggs per hen in a poultry farm in successive months, or the national herd or flock population in successive years. Sometimes, however, a time series is generated by recording observations on a single animal over many successive time points, e.g. the milk yield of a dairy cow throughout lactation. The *order* in which the observations are made is of particular relevance in a time series. Usually the successive observations are *dependent*, so that the expected value of an observation at one time point cannot

be regarded in isolation because it is likely to be related to the magnitude of the observation at the previous time point. This is known as an **autoregressive series**.

The aim of a statistical analysis of a time series is to describe it by constructing the appropriate mathematical model which explains both the systematic and the random, or unsystematic, variation. The systematic variation may comprise a trend or long-term movement, oscillations about the trend and/or a seasonal effect. From this model we may gain some insight into the causal mechanisms which generated the time series, and may be able to predict future observations.

Although it may seem appropriate to analyse a time series by regressing the variable of interest against time (see Section 10.4), this approach is rarely feasible. It is very unusual to find that a simple linear model is an adequate description of the time series. Furthermore, the fact that successive observations are dependent implies that these observations have deviations about any long-term trend which are associated. This so-called **serial correlation** violates the independence assumption underlying regression analysis. Therefore, special techniques have been devised to analyse time series. The details of this analysis are beyond the scope of this book, and we refer you to Chatfield (1989) or Diggle (1990) for further information.

13.4.2 The analysis of repeated measurements

(a) Correct analysis

Sometimes we are interested in analysing within-animal studies in which measurements of a quantitative variable are taken on each of a number of animals at pre-specified times. Typically, we may wish to compare such responses in two or more groups of animals. Although we could regard the serial measurements on any one animal as a time series, we do not use time series analysis (see Section 13.4.1) to evaluate the results because the series are generally too short, and because of the difficulty of combining the series from different animals.

There are a number of ways of analysing the data. We could perform a **repeated measures analysis of variance** (see Section 8.5.3) using the appropriate computer software, provided the design is completely balanced. The problem with this approach, and other suitable but elaborate analyses, is that the programs are relatively complex and the results are often not easy to interpret. The use of **summary measures** provides an alternative solution which is equally acceptable (Everitt, 1995). The approach based on summary measures is simpler to apply and to understand than the repeated measures ANOVA, and has much to recommend it.

The summary measures approach reduces the serial responses for each animal to a single statistic which describes some important aspect of that animal's response curve. For example, the summary measure might be:

- The maximum (or minimum) value.
- The time to maximum (or minimum) response.
- The time to reach a particular value.
- The difference between the initial and the final responses.
- The slope of the line.
- The area under the curve.
- The overall mean.

The summary measure should have some clear clinical or biological relevance and it should be chosen before the data are collected. The summary measure for each animal is then used in the analysis as if it is the raw data.

So, for example, suppose we wish to compare serial measurements over time in two groups of animals, with each group receiving a different treatment. We may decide that we are interested in determining whether the average time to reach the peak response is the same using both treatments. We find the time to reach the peak response in each animal, and perform a significance test (e.g. a two-sample *t*-test (see Section 7.4) or a Wilcoxon rank sum test (see Section 11.5)) on the times to peak response in the two groups to determine whether there is a treatment effect.

The statistical analysis is incomplete without a **graphical representation** of the data. However, it is often difficult to know how to provide this in an informative way. Avoid the temptation to draw the average curve for a group (i.e. by joining the mean responses for a group at successive time points) as it may not describe a typical curve for an animal. You should start by producing separate graphs of the responses against time for each animal. Then, perhaps, you could arrange them in some order or in a panel or grid with separate panels for each group. If the sample size is large, you could classify the curves in some meaningful way, and plot representative examples. Be sure that your examples are truly *representative* and not simply the best! It may also be helpful to plot the chosen summary measures; such as histograms for each measure or a scatter plot of any two summary measures, (e.g. the maximum value for each animal against the time that the maximum occurred).

(b) Incorrect analysis

Repeated measures data are frequently analysed inappropriately. The most usual approach when two groups are being compared is to apply separate two-sample tests (e.g. the two-sample *t*-test or the Wilcoxon rank sum test) at each time point. The main criticism of this approach is that:

- No account is taken of the fact that measurements at different time points are from the same animal, i.e. the within-animal changes are ignored.

- Successive observations on an animal are likely to be correlated, so that the results of significance tests at adjacent time points are not independent, which leads to difficulties in interpretation.
- A group may comprise different animals at various time points if there are different missing observations at these time points.

The most usual approach to the graphical display of the data is to draw the average curve for each group, often with error bars for each mean. As we point out in Section 13.4.2(a), this is generally inappropriate because the average curve may have quite a different shape from the individual curves, and individual variation will be obscured. One possibility is to represent all the individual curves in the background (e.g. in pastel colours) together with the average curve in bold.

(c) Example

In a study of the effect of thawing rate on the motility and survival of cryopreserved dog semen, the motility of the spermatozoa from individual dogs was recorded over a four-hour period. The semen from 6 of the dogs (chosen randomly from the 12) was thawed at 39°C, and the remaining semen samples were thawed at 70°C. The mean curves in Fig. 13.2(a) show the general trend but obscure the very real differences between dogs which are shown in Fig. 13.2(b) and Fig. 13.2(c). To address the problem of repeated measures data, the times for spermatozoa to reach a motility of 75% and 25% of the original values were measured from the plotted curves for each dog, and these summary measures were used for the statistical analysis to investigate differences in the two groups.

The times to reach a motility of 75% were 80.2, 53.5, 75.7, 57.8, 56.2, 55.8 min (median = 57.0 min) for the sperm of the six dogs thawed at

(a)

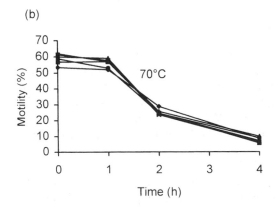

Fig. 13.2 Repeated measures data showing the effect of thawing rate on the motility of dog semen: (a) mean curves for thawing at 70°C and 39°C (mean ± SD at hourly intervals), (b) individual curves for thawing at 70°C, (c) individual curves for thawing at 39°C. (Data from England, 1992, with permission.)

(b)

(c)

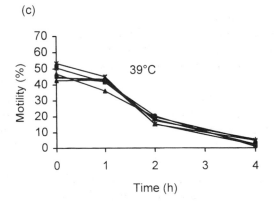

39°C, and 107.2, 63.0, 92.7, 97.0, 76.3, 80.5 min (median = 86.6 min) for the sperm of the six dogs thawed at 70°C. A Wilcoxon rank sum test (see Section 11.5) comparing the two distributions from which these samples were selected gives $P = 0.02$, indicating that the time to reach a motility of 75% is significantly greater in the sperm thawed at 70°C than in the sperm thawed at 39°C.

Furthermore, the times to reach a motility of 25% were 167.5, 124.3, 158.2, 170.2, 112.5, 140.3 min (median = 149.3 min) for the sperm of the six dogs thawed at 39°C, and 190.6, 160.0, 182.0, 195.0, 148.5, 186.0 min (median = 184.0 min) for the sperm of the six dogs thawed at 70°C. A Wilcoxon rank sum test comparing the two distributions from which these samples were selected gives $P = 0.04$, indicating that the time to reach a motility of 25% is also significantly greater in the sperm thawed at 70°C than in the sperm thawed at 39°C.

13.5 SURVIVAL ANALYSIS

Another form of statistical analysis which focuses on time is known as **survival analysis**. Here we are concerned with the time (the **survival time**) it takes for some critical event (the **failure**), such as death, to occur in an individual after a particular starting point, such as the initiation of treatment. The most common situation is when the failure can occur at most once in any individual. Examples of the 'individual' are a machine component in industrial reliability or a tooth filling; examples of the 'failure' are death, remission or recurrence. For purposes of discussion, we shall assume that the individual is an animal in a clinical trial, that the animal is being treated for a particular condition, and that the failure is death as a result of the condition. We may be interested in:

- Estimating the probability that an animal from a particular group survives for a given time period, say six months (the six-month survival rate).
- Estimating the median survival time for a given group of animals.

- Comparing the survival experience in two groups of animals receiving different treatments.

The analysis of survival times warrants special techniques because of **censored data**; these arise because some of the animals never experience the failure during the course of the clinical trial. Either they are alive at the end of the study period, or they are lost to follow-up (such animals are called **withdrawals**) or they die during the study period from some cause unrelated to the condition of interest. Furthermore, because the animals may be recruited into the trial at different times, and there is a single time point at which the study period ends, the animals are usually observed for varying lengths of time.

- One approach to the statistical analysis of survival data when survival times and censored times are grouped into intervals is to produce a **Berkson–Gage survival curve**, based on calculations of the actuarial life table.
- More often, we derive the **Kaplan–Meier survival curve** if the survival and censored times are known exactly. In both cases, the survival probability is plotted against the time from the starting point. Conventionally, the survival curve is drawn in steps, and the **median survival time**, corresponding to a survival probability of 0.5, may be read from it. This median survival time provides a reasonable summary of survival; the mean survival time should not be calculated when there are censored data.

Figure 13.3 is an illustration of a Kaplan–Meier survival curve depicting the survival of 31 uraemic cats in days following diagnosis; the data are discussed in Elliott and Barber (1998). The arrows indicate the censored data – these cats were still alive at the last follow-up at the times indicated (they were mostly lost to follow-up but one cat was alive at the end of the study period). The median survival time from diagnosis is 334 days (95% confidence interval is 176 to 492 days); this is the value on the horizontal axis which corresponds to a 50% survival on the vertical axis.

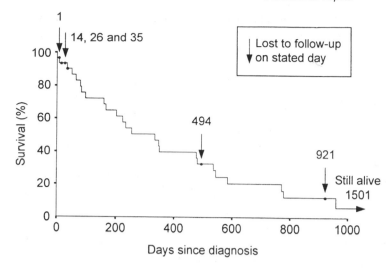

Fig. 13.3 Kaplan–Meier survival curve for uraemic cats. Numbers above arrows relate to individual cat identification codes. (Redrawn from Barber and Elliott, 1998, with permission.)

We often compare survival curves by using the non-parametric **logrank test**. It utilizes all the information in each curve but does not make assumptions about the shape of the curve. This approach is preferable to the much more restricted comparison of survival rates at a specific time (say, six months). If we wish to investigate the effect of several variables at the same time, we can use **Cox's proportional hazards model**. This is similar to multiple logistic regression (see Section 10.6) but allowances are made for the problems of censored data. Sometimes, we assume that we know the particular form of the survival curve, and fit the data to it so that we can estimate the parameters which define the model. We can then compare curves by comparing the estimated parameters.

The mathematical theory underlying survival analysis is relatively complex. We omit details of the calculations and refer you to Peto *et al.* (1976, 1977), Cox and Oakes (1984), and Chatfield (1989).

EXERCISES

The statements in questions 13.1–13.3 are either TRUE or FALSE.

13.1 The sensitivity of a screening test for a particular disease is 0.99. This means that:

(a) The proportion of animals correctly identified by the test as having the disease is 0.99.
(b) The proportion of animals with the disease, out of those which tested positive, is 0.99.
(c) The specificity of the test is 0.01.
(d) The test is particularly useful for identifying animals with a disease which is treatable.
(e) The prevalence of the disease in the population must be high.

13.2 The most appropriate way to investigate the agreement between two observers when each has measured a quantitative response on each of 20 animals is:
(a) To calculate Cohen's kappa.
(b) To perform a paired *t*-test.
(c) To calculate the correlation coefficient, and test its significance from zero.
(d) To calculate two times the standard deviation of the differences, and use this as a measure of agreement.
(e) To estimate the standard deviation of the individual measurements, s_w, and use this as a measure of agreement.

13.3 Suppose 16 animals are randomly allocated to one of two treatments, so that there are 8 animals in each treatment group. We take a single measurement of a quantitative variable at six successive time points on each animal. An appropriate analysis which investigates the treatment effect may be:

(a) A times series analysis.
(b) A repeated measures ANOVA.
(c) A two-sample *t*-test, comparing the observations in the two groups, at each time point.
(d) A two-sample *t*-test, comparing the changes from base-line in the two groups, at each time point.
(e) A two-sample *t*-test, comparing the differences between the initial and final responses in the two groups.

13.4 Quantitative determination of the corticosteroid-induced isoenzyme of alkaline phosphatase (CAP) was evaluated as a screening test for hyperadrenocorticism (HAC) in dogs (Solter *et al.*, 1993). A cut-off value of 90 U/l was selected for use for this assay as a screening test for HAC, with values of CAP greater than this cut-off value being indicative of HAC. This cut-off value was used in Harrogate on 46 dogs with a combination of historical and clinical signs of HAC and on 92 date-matched healthy control dogs (i.e. there were two controls for every HAC dog). The results are shown in Table 13.5.

(a) Determine the sensitivity and specificity of the test.
(b) Do you think that this cut-off is reasonable?
(c) What is the effect on sensitivity and specificity of raising the cut-off of CAP to >500 U/l (when, in this sample of dogs, 37 HAC dogs and 4 healthy dogs have CAP >500 U/l)?
(d) When the CAP cut-off value of 90 U/l was used on all canine serum samples submitted to the laboratory over a three-month period, the positive predictive value of the test was 21.4% and the negative predictive value was 100%. What do you infer from these results in terms of the usefulness of the CAP test as a diagnostic test rather than a screening test?
(e) Why do these predictive values not agree with what you would obtain if you were to calculate them using the information from Table 13.5?

13.5 A sheep farmer has a problem with foot rot. He decides to score the degree of foot rot in each

Table 13.5 Observed frequencies in two groups of dogs. Based on results of Solter *et al.*, 1993.

	HAC dogs	Healthy dogs	Total
CAP > 90 U/l	43	12	45
CAP ≤ 90 U/l	3	80	83
Total	46	92	138

sheep in his flock and then to treat them; later he scores them again to see if there has been any improvement. He scores them as follows: 1 = no lameness, perfect feet; 2 = no lameness, but at least one misshapen claw requiring trimming; 3 = mild lameness involving infection and damage to one foot only; 4 = severe lameness, foot rot and injury in more than one foot. Table 13.6 shows the frequency of occurrence of the scores before and after treatment. Conduct a suitable analysis

Table 13.6 Observed frequencies of scores of foot condition in sheep.

Score after treatment	Score before treatment				
	1	2	3	4	Total
1	34	78	27	4	143
2	1	16	36	13	66
3	0	6	14	49	69
4	0	0	2	3	5
Total	35	100	79	69	283

Table 13.7 Measurement of plasma glucose concentrations (mmol/l).

	First reading	Second reading
Sample 1	3.665	3.751
Sample 2	4.297	4.297
Sample 3	3.639	3.545
Sample 4	3.146	3.171
Sample 5	3.331	3.342
Sample 6	3.060	3.026
Sample 7	3.089	3.129
Sample 8	3.299	3.193
Sample 9	2.983	2.992
Sample 10	2.761	2.813
Sample 11	2.975	2.881

and present the result. Is it reasonable to presume that the treatment has helped to alleviate the problem of foot rot?

13.6 When conducting any sort of assay measurement, it is common to put duplicate samples through the assay. In an assay of plasma glucose concentration (mmol/l) in sheep blood, the duplicate results, shown in Table 13.7, were used to assess the repeatability of the method. Conduct an appropriate analysis to demonstrate repeatability and to assess its quality.

Solutions to Exercises

CHAPTER 1

1.1 (a) **F**: there are several sources of variation between animals, the most important being genetic variation. Biological variation describes it; it does not cause it (b) **T** (c) **F**: statistics deals with the problems of biological variation, but offers other benefits as well (d) **F**: since we can rarely sample whole populations, there will always be an element of uncertainty in the conclusions we draw about biological data. Statistics deals with the biological variation in such a way as to quantitate that uncertainty (e) **F**: no, this is known as technical error or fatigue!

1.2 (a) **F**: to achieve this, a sample would not have to be random (b) **F**: a sample cannot claim to represent the full range of the population (c) **F**: a sample does not claim to be made up of only 'normal' animals (d) **T**: yes, a random sample aims to be representative (e) **T**: a random sample excludes biases imposed by the process of selection.

1.3 (a) **T** (b) **F**: a nominal variable is a particular type of qualitative variable (c) **F**: a nominal scale relates to a qualitative variable which is not directly measurable (d) **F**: percentages are quantitative (e) **F**: ranked data are measured on an ordinal scale.

1.4 (a) **S**: enzyme activity is temperature dependent; if the temperature falls, the enzyme activity will be reduced. All samples will be similarly affected (b) **S**: the readings will be raised or lowered to the nearest 0.5 degree mark, which is not random (c) **S**: a zero offset will be present affecting every reading equally (d) **S**: the scales will have been calibrated by activation after the

load is placed. Should the scales be activated before the load is placed, this will probably induce a systematic error due to hysteresis (e) **R**: this is a random error caused by attempts to read beyond the sensitivity of the instrument.

1.5 (a) **H**: there is no existing population of treated cows (b) **R**: the population includes all horses at livery (c) **R**: all fleas on all dogs in Liverpool make up this population (d) **H**: there is no existing population of treated dogs (e) **R**: the population includes all blood glucose readings from diabetic dogs.

1.6 (a) **N**: nominal since the classes are descriptive (b) **C**: the percentage scale is continuous between 0 and 100, delimited only by the accuracy of the values (c) **C**: light absorbence is measured on a continuous but arbitrary scale (d) **O**: this arbitrary scale has only integer values, and a particular interval on the scale does not necessarily represent the same change in performance as we move up the scale. So, for example, the difference between 2 and 4 does not necessarily indicate the same change in performance as that between 5 and 7 (e) **C**: progesterone values are continuous, limited only by the sensitivity of the assay (f) **N**: two classes defined by appearance (g) **C**: optical density is another light intensity assay – a continuous scale (h) **D**: litter size is an integer scale $1 - n$ (i) **O**: body condition is a sliding scale with various classes given numerical values but without any expectation that the intervals between classes are identical (j) **D**: this is another integer scale which might be viewed as approximating a continuous scale if large numbers were involved (k) **D** or **C**: counts are considered to be on a continuous scale if the numbers of events in a sample are large and the integer intervals represent very small differences in the scale (l) **C**: time is a continuous scale, but since it is divided into days (integers), it could be considered to be D.

CHAPTER 2

2.1 (a) **T** (b) **F**: the pie chart is useful for categorical data (c) **T** (d) **F**: the bar chart is useful for categorical or discrete data (e) **T**.

2.2 (a) **F**: the mean will be unduly influenced by the extreme values and will overestimate the central tendency (b) **T** (c) **T**: this is the geometric mean (d) **T** (e) **T**: this is the median.

2.3 (a) **T** (b) **F** (c) **F**: for symmetrically distributed data, the range is approximately equal to four times the standard deviation (d) **T** (e) **F**: the SD is the square root of the variance.

2.4 (a) **F**: the reference range can be determined as the difference between the 2.5th and 97.5th percentiles if the data are skewed (b) **T** (c) **F**: the reference range is meant to be representative of the population of healthy animals. A small sample is inadequate (d) **F**: it is determined as mean ± 1.96SD, often approximated by mean ± 2SD (e) **F**: the difference between the largest and smallest observations is the range which may be unduly influenced by outliers.

2.5 (a) Class intervals of 1.0 l/min give eight classes and the data are shown to display a unimodal distribution (b) With a class interval of 0.2 l/min, there are 36 classes and only 25 data, too many class intervals to be useful (c) With a class interval of 5.0 l/m, nearly all the observations are in one class and only two classes are represented. We get no sense of the distribution of the data. Clearly (a) is the most appropriate.

2.6 (a) Both axes have inadequate labelling; the tick marks have no scales. (b) This is a histogram, but it is drawn as a bar chart. The vertical bars should be attributed to represent the continuous variable on the axis (c) Again, the *x*-axis is inad-

equately labelled; we are left to guess what are the units for the scale; they must be included (d) The slices of the pie chart neither give details of the numbers involved, nor the percentages represented by the slices. These figures should be added.

2.7 Arranged in ascending order, the rates are: 29.2, 34.2, 44.4, 64.2, 67.6, 75.0, 76.2, 80.0. There are nine observations, so the median is the $(9 + 1)/2 = 5$th observation in the ordered set, i.e. the median is 64.7%.

2.8 Mean = 761.2/16 = 47.58 g, median = 51.95 g (the arithmetic mean of 51.9 and 52.0). The mean and the median do not coincide, indicating that the data are skewed. The mean is less than the mean, indicating that the data are skewed to the left.

2.9 Range = 2.5 to 8.6 = 6.1 μmol/l, variance = 3.57 (μmol/l)^2, standard deviation = 1.89 μmol/l.

CHAPTER 3

3.1 (a) **F**: the Normal distribution is symmetrical (b) **T** (c) **F**: the limits which contain 95% of the distribution are mean ± 1.96SD (d) **F**: this is a particular Normal distribution, i.e. the Standard Normal distribution (e) **F**: the term 'Normal' in statistics describes the Gaussian distribution and not the 'normal' or healthy population.

3.2 (a) **F**: *z* is a continuous random variable because the Standard Normal distribution is a continuous distribution (b) **F**: the mean equals 0 and the standard deviation equals 1 (c) **T** (d) **F**: it is *x* which has a mean of μ and a standard deviation of σ if *z* has a Standard Normal distribution (e) **T**.

3.3 (a) **T** (b) **F**: it is the Normal distribution (c) **F**: a Normal distribution is a theoretical probability distribution and should not be confused with 'normal' or healthy individuals. In this case, the variable simply follows a Normal distribution (d) **F**: The Standard Normal distribution always has a mean of 0 and an SD of 1 (e) **F**: if data have a distribution which is skewed to the right, then a log transformation is likely to Normalize it. The data are then said to follow the Lognormal distribution.

3.4 (a) The probability of a six when she rolls one die = 1/6; the probability of a six in the second die = 1/6. The probability of a double six, using the multiplication rule, is $(1/6) \times (1/6) = 0.028$. Similarly, the probability of a double of any other number is also 0.028. Hence, using the addition rule, the probability of either a double six, or a double five or a . . . or a double one is $6 \times 0.028 = 0.17$. There is, therefore, a very small chance that they will purchase a bitch using this approach, and he is right to have second thoughts (b) The chance of a six in one roll of a single die is 1/6. The chance of not getting a six in one roll is 5/6. Using the multiplication rule, the chance of not getting a six in the five rolls of a single die is $(5/6)^5 = 0.69$. Hence, there is now a pretty good chance that they will get a bitch. These calculations are based on the model approach to probability.

3.5 (a) The data are approximately Normally distributed (b) The data are skewed to the right, but the log data are approximately Normally distributed.

3.6 The Poisson distribution; the mean and variance of the counts should be equal.

3.7 (a) SND = $(0.40 - 0.37)/0.066 = 0.45$. Reference to Table A.1 gives a two-tailed probability of 0.6527. Hence the required percentage is half this, i.e. 32.7% (b) SND = $(0.30 - 0.37)/0.066 = -1.061$. The two-tailed area in Table A.1 is 0.2891. Hence the required percentage is 14.5% (c) The percentage of values below 0.40 ml/ml is $100 - 32.7 = 67.3\%$, the percentage of values below 0.30 ml/ml is 14.5%; hence the required percentage = $67.3 - 14.5 = 52.8\%$ (d) The lower limit is the value below which 5% of the observations fall; it is derived from the equality $-1.64 = (x_1 - 0.37)/0.066$ which gives $x_1 = 0.26$ ml/ml. The upper limit is the value above which 5% of the observations fall; it is derived from the equality $1.64 = (x_2 - 0.37)/0.066$ which gives

$x_2 = 0.48$ ml/ml. The required range is therefore 0.26 to 0.48 ml/ml.

3.8 (a) (i) From Table A.1, $0.0455 \times 1/2 = 0.0228$ (ii) From Table A.1, $0.3173 \times 1/2 = 0.1587$ (b) (i) From Table A.2, 1.64 (ii) From Table A.2, −1.96.

CHAPTER 4

4.1 (a) **F**: the SEM relates to the precision of the sample mean, and not the individual observations (b) **F**: it is the standard deviation which measures the spread of the observations (c) **T** (d) **T** (e) **T**.

4.2 (a) **F**: it contains the population mean with 95% certainty (b) **T** (c) **F**: it is the reference range which contains, usually, 95% of the observations in the population (d) **F**: you should add and subtract two standard errors to the sample mean (e) **T**.

4.3 (a) **F**: it is the population mean plasma potassium which lies between these values (b) **T** (c) **T** (d) **F**: the confidence interval is for the population mean and does not relate to individual values (e) **F**: there is a 5% chance that the population mean lies outside the interval.

4.4
(a) 95% CI = $2.35 \pm 1.96 \times \sqrt{(0.16/100)} = 2.272$ to 2.428 mg/kg
     99% CI = $2.35 \pm 2.58 \times \sqrt{(0.16/100)} = 2.247$ to 2.453 mg/kg
(b) 95% CI = $34.8 \pm 2.064 \times 13.0/\sqrt{25} = 29.434$ to 40.166 ng/ml
     99% CI = $34.8 \pm 2.797 \times 13.0/\sqrt{25} = 27.528$ to 42.072 ng/ml

4.5 (a) The estimated proportion of joint lameness is 5/60 = 0.0833 (i.e. 8.33%) therefore 95% CI = $0.0833 \pm 1.96 \times \sqrt{(0.0833)(1-0.0833)/60}$ = 0.013 to 0.153 (b) Wider (c) Narrower.

CHAPTER 5

5.1 (a) **F**: randomization is used so that biases associated with the allocation of animals to the different treatments are avoided (b) **T** (c) **F**: a control group can be incorporated into the design whether or not randomization is used (d) **T** (e) **F**: blinding is another issue, unrelated to random allocation.

5.2 (a) **F**: treatment is given to each chicken so that this is an experimental study (b) **F**: the chickens are assessed both before and after they have received treatment, so the trial is longitudinal (c) **F**: the chickens are followed forward in time, so the study is prospective (d) **T** (e) **F**: a sample survey is a particular type of observational study and this is an experimental study.

5.3 (a) **F**: the wash-out period eliminates carry-over effect (b) **F**: the randomization ensures that there is no allocation bias. A wash-out period should eliminate carry-over effect (c) **F**: a parallel group design is one in which each animal receives only one treatment and the treatment comparison is made between animals (d) **T** (e) **F**: a between-animal comparison provides less precise treatment effects than a within-animal comparison.

5.4 (a) Longitudinal study – it follows the bitches forward in time (b) Experimental – there was an intervention in one of the groups (c) Neither – cohort and case-control studies are only observational studies (d) A case-control study in which incontinent bitches and matched controls are followed back in time to see whether they had been spayed.

5.5 The *laissez-faire* approach does not subject the cats to any stress comparable with the surgical intervention. Any differences, therefore, are not due solely to the surgical repair but to the stresses of anaesthesia, etc. The proper controls should be subjected to a sham operation although this would be ethically unacceptable with clinical cases.

5.6 (a) Dose levels in dogs should be investigated with stratified randomization allowing for the differences in body weight. Common strata are large, medium and toy dogs. It might be advisable to use restricted randomization within

each of the strata, particularly if the number of dogs available for study is not great (b) Grouped randomization (because it is a treatment for a worm infestation) with groups of, say four to eight animals penned in small subplots of the two plots. In addition it would be sensible to have restricted randomization of the groups to treatment or control to ensure balance (c) Each litter is a group. The litters are allocated at random to one of the two preparations (d) Despite the word 'group' in the description, this is not a group investigation. Animals are allocated using restricted randomization to each of the treatments at each location (which can be regarded as a stratagum); this should result in required balance.

CHAPTER 6

6.1 (a) **F**: the null hypothesis concerns the population means (b) **T** (c) **F**: it is only the result of the test which is or is not significant, not the null hypothesis (d) **F**: the null hypothesis is a statement of fact which may or may not be true (e) **F**: the null hypothesis is not expressed in terms of what is expected.

6.2 (a) **F**: it could also refer to the left-hand side, but not both sides (b) **F**: the tails of the test influence the *P*-value which is the probability of rejecting the null hypothesis when it is true, whereas the power is the probability of rejecting the null hypothesis when it is false (c) **F**: most tests are two-tailed because it is very unusual to be sure, in advance, that any treatment difference can be in only one direction (d) **T** (e) **F**: the decision to use a one-tailed test does not relate to the sample size but rather to the biological certainty that, if a treatment difference exists, it can only be in one direction.

6.3 (a) **F**: the *P*-value is the probability of obtaining a result as or more extreme than the one observed if the null hypothesis is true (b) **F**: the null hypothesis is a stated theory about the population parameter(s) which is either true or false (c) **F**: the *P*-value relates what is observed in the sample to what is hypothesized about the population; the null hypothesis is either true or false, and no probability can be attached to it (d) **T** (e) **T**.

6.4 (a) **F**: the null hypothesis is a statement about the population parameter(s) which is either true or false; there is no probability attached to it (b) **F**: the alternative hypothesis is also a statement about the population parameter(s) which is true or false (c) **T** (d) **F**: the *P*-value must relate what is observed in the sample to what is hypothesized in the population (e) **F**: see (a).

6.5 (a) **F**: the test statistic is a mathematical expression in which the sample values are substituted to determine a *P*-value. This is used to decide whether the null hypothesis about a population parameter (such as the mean) is likely to be true (b) **F**: see (a) (c) **T** (d) **F**: it is the *P*-value which has to be lower than a stated value (typically 0.05) in order for the result of the test to be significant (e) **F**: significance tests can be performed using small and large samples. The test is more powerful if the sample size is large.

6.6 The null hypothesis is that the mean muscle tension in the populations is the same when using the novel drug and when using the control. The alternative hypothesis is that the two population means are different. This is a two-sided alternative; there is no biological reason for presuming that any difference, should it exist, can be in only one direction. The null hypothesis is essentially the same when using an existing drug – it is that the mean muscle tension in the populations is the same on the novel drug as on the existing treatment. Again, the alternative hypothesis is that the two population means are different (direction unspecified).

6.7 The null hypothesis is that the proportions of ponies who fail the test are the same in the population of ponies who are trained by the new system and in the population of ponies who are trained in the traditional manner. The alternative hypothesis is that these two proportions are not equal (direction unspecified).

CHAPTER 7

7.1 (a) **F**: the sample sizes do not have to be equal but, if they are, the assumption of Normality is less important (b) **F**: it is used on independent groups of observations. Performing a two-sample *t*-test on paired or dependent data will lead to a loss of power (c) **F**: the null hypothesis assumes that the two population means are equal (d) **T** (e) **F**: the paired *t*-test should be used on dependent data rather than the two-sample *t*-test, irrespective of sample size.

7.2 (a) **T** (b) **T** (c) **F**: the paired *t*-test should be used on paired or related data, irrespective of sample size. However, if the sample size is very small, a non-parametric alternative may be preferred (d) **F**: the two-sample *t*-test should be used for comparing the means of independent groups of observations (e) **F**: the paired *t*-test makes the assumption that the differences between the pairs are Normally distributed.

7.3 (a) Paired comparison (b) H_0: the population mean difference in plasma lactate concentration when the horse is cantering and when it is on a treadmill is zero (c) The differences are approximately Normally distributed. Paired *t*-test test statistic = 2.51, $df = 9$, $P = 0.033$ (d) Reject the null hypothesis that the mean difference in the population is zero. We cannot consider the exercise exerted by the horses to be of similar metabolic demand in both situations. The 95% confidence interval for the mean difference is 0.077 to 1.503 mmol/l.

7.4 (a) Two independent groups (b) H_0: the population mean sperm numbers are the same using the two methods (c) The observations in each sample are approximately Normally distributed. The mean (SEM) sperm numbers using the AV and EE methods are 63.46 (6.72) and 43.90 (6.07), respectively. The two variances (587.63 and 368.76) are not significantly different (Levene's test gives $P = 0.471$). The two-sample *t*-test statistic is 2.09, $df = 21$, $P = 0.049$ (d) The 95% confidence interval for the difference in means is 0.12 to 39.00. The result of the test is just significant at the 5% level indicating that the

AV method is likely to be able to obtain more sperm, and the difference in means could be as great as 39 sperm.

7.5 This is a one-sample *t* test of the null hypothesis that there is no difference between the mean urea value from this laboratory in January and 9.5 mmol/l. The test statistic is $(9.5 - 9.7)/0.22 = 10.00$ on 139 degrees of freedom. Hence $P < 0.001$, and there is evidence to reject the null hypothesis. It would seem that the laboratory overestimated plasma urea in cats in January.

7.6 The design is inappropriate because there is no control group, i.e. horses who do not go through the breaking programme, but are followed for the same length of time in, otherwise, identical circumstances. In the given design, the increase in cardiopulmonary function could be a consequence of time alone, unrelated to the effect of the breaking programme. An appropriate design should include a control group; then the change in cardiopulmonary function after eight weeks should be evaluated for each horse, and the changes in the two groups compared using a two-sample test, such as the two-sample *t*-test.

CHAPTER 8

8.1 (a) **T** (b) **F** (c) **T** (d) **F**: the data should be analysed as a repeated measures ANOVA if the data are matched (e) **F**: the null hypothesis states that the population means are all the same.

8.2 (a) **F**: the test makes no assumptions about the means, only that the data are Normally distributed (b) **T** (c) **T** (d) **F**: the *F*-test compares variances and not means (e) **F**: the *F*-test compares variances. Equal variances is an assumption of the two-sample *t*-test, so the *F*-test may precede the *t*-test to validate this assumption, but will be followed by the *t*-test only if the intention is to compare two means.

8.3 The data are approximately Normally distributed in each sample. The estimated variances

of Group 1 and Group 2 are 0.671 and 2.313 kg^2, respectively. The sample sizes are 15 and 13, respectively. The ratio of these two variances, the larger over the smaller, is 3.345; this follows the *F*-distribution with 12 *df* in the numerator, and 14 *df* in the denominator. The percentage points in Table A.5(b) which correspond to two-sided *P*-values of 0.05 and 0.01 (i.e. we look at $P = 0.025$ and $P = 0.005$ in the table) are 3.05 and 4.43, respectively. Since the 3.345 lies between these two values, $0.01 < P < 0.05$; we reject the null hypothesis that the two variances are equal, and would have to perform a modified *t*-test or a non-parametric test to compare the average liver weights in the two groups.

8.4 The null hypothesis is that there is no difference between the true mean intensities in the three diluent solutions. The data are approximately Normally distributed in each group. Levene's test (performed on the computer, but you could do a series of *F*-tests by hand, adjusting the *P*-value using Bonferroni's correction) shows that the three variances are not significantly different (test statistic = 3.27, $P = 0.06$). A one-way ANOVA (see Display 8.2) gives an *F* ratio of 13.66, $df = 2, 18$, $P = 0.0002$ (the sig. = 0.000 in the output implies that $P < 0.001$). Hence there is a significant difference between at least two of the means, suggesting that egg yolk dilution affects the binding of the fluorophore to the sperm membrane. The sample means (SEM) of the 1%, 5% and 25% egg yolk solutions are 0.999 (0.017), 0.950 (0.078) and 0.846 (0.040), respectively. *Post hoc* Bonferroni's tests show that the 25% egg yolk solution has a mean intensity that is significantly less than either of the other two solutions ($P < 0.05$), but that no other two means are significantly different from each other ($P > 0.05$). The mean square of the within groups source of variation is 0.0029, and this is used as the combined estimate of variance in the calculation of confidence intervals (i.e. this is the s^2 in the formula for the CI given in Section 7.4.3). The 95% confidence intervals for the difference in means between the 25% and each of the 1% and 5% egg yolk solutions are (0.087, 0.219) and (0.085, 0.125), respectively.

CHAPTER 9

9.1 (a) **F**: the *t*-test is for comparing two means from quantitative data (b) **F**: the *F*-test is for comparing variances (c) **T**: (d) **F**: McNemar's test is for paired qualitative responses, and these data are not paired (e) **F**: the null hypothesis is not about a theoretical distribution.

9.2 (a) **F**: it is the expected frequencies that have to be greater than 5 (b) **F**: the degrees of freedom are $(2-1)(2-1) = 1$ (c) **T** (d) **F**: the null hypothesis is that there is no difference between these proportions (e) **F**: the data are binary qualitative, and cannot be Normally distributed.

9.3 This is a test of a single proportion; the null hypothesis is that the proportion of dairy cattle in the local area does not differ from the national proportion. The estimated proportion of dairy cows in the local area = $359/1375 = 0.261$. Thus

$$Test_6 = \frac{|0.261 - 0.29| - 1/2750}{\sqrt{0.261(1 - 0.261)/1375}} = 2.42.$$ Referring

this value to Table A.1, we find that $P = 0.0155$. Hence we reject the null hypothesis ($P = 0.02$) – it seems that the committee were right and this area has a lower percentage of dairy cows in the cattle population.

9.4 This is a test of two proportions; we can use the chi-squared test to test the null hypothesis that the true proportions of bitches which have mammary tumours are equal in those bitches which had MPA and in those without MPA. The table shows the observed frequencies; the expected frequencies are in brackets.

Hence $Test_7 = 6.21$ (with the continuity correction), and $P = 0.0127$. There is evidence to reject the null hypothesis ($P = 0.01$). From this retrospective study, we would conclude that MPA administration does appear to increase the chance of subsequent mammary tumours. Note that the estimated proportions which had tumours are $38/59 = 0.644$ and $60/137 = 0.438$ in the groups with and without MPA, respectively. The estimated difference in the two proportions is 0.206. The 95% CI for the difference in the true proportions is $(0.644 - 0.438) \pm 1.96 \times 0.075 = (0.058, 0.354)$.

Observed frequencies of tumours in bitches which have or have not previously been administered medroxy-progesterone acetate (MPA). Calculated expected frequencies are shown in parentheses.

	MPA +ve	MPA −ve	Total
With tumours	38 (29.5)	60 (68.5)	98
Without tumours	21 (29.5)	77 (68.5)	98
Total	59	137	196

9.5 We show the observed frequencies in the contingency table. We use McNemar's test: $Test_9 = (|16 - 14| - 1)^2/(16 + 14) = 1/30 = 0.03$. This has a chi-squared distribution on 1 degree of freedom. Referring to Table A.4, we find that $P > 0.05$. Hence we do not have evidence to reject the null hypothesis. The two sample proportions with positive results are $53/143 = 0.37$ by the egg-shedding approach, and $55/143 = 0.38$ by the ELISA test. The 95% confidence interval for the difference in the true proportions is

$$(0.38 - 0.37) \pm 1.96 \frac{1}{143} \sqrt{16 + 14 - \frac{(16 - 14)^2}{143}}$$
$$= 0.01 \pm 1.96 \times 0.038$$
$$= (-0.07, 0.09).$$

Numbers of sheep with (+ve) and without (−ve) liver fluke infestation and with a positive response to a diagnostic ELISA test.

	ELISA +ve	ELISA −ve	Total
Egg shedding +ve	39	14	53
Egg shedding −ve	16	74	90
Total	55	74	143

9.6 In order to calculate the Chi-squared goodness-of-fit statistic, we must combine some of the categories since there are expected values which are less than 5. Combining the frequencies for 0 to 3 pregnant ewes, and for 7 and 8 pregnant ewes, we find that $Test_8 = 3.9553 + 0.0127 + 0.0302 + 0.2582 + 0.9732 = 5.23$ with 4 *df*. Referring to Table A.4 we obtain $0.25 < P < 0.50$ (in fact, a computer analysis gives $P = 0.27$). Hence we can assume that the observed distribution of the number of pregnant ewes conforms with the binomial distribution with $\pi = 0.64$.

CHAPTER 10

10.1 (a) **F**: it lies between -1 and $+1$ (b) **F**: the assumption of Normality of at least one of the variables is important only for hypothesis testing; both variables should be Normally distributed if the confidence interval is to be calculated (c) **T** (d) **F**: it is zero if there is no linear relationship between the two variables; there could be a non-linear relationship (e) **F**: this is the interpretation of the regression coefficient, β.

10.2 (a) **F**: this is the function of the correlation coefficient (b) **T** (c) **T** (d) **F**: it assumes that the residuals are Normally distributed, and that y is Normally distributed for each value of x (e) **F**: the x variable is assumed capable of measurement without error and is used to predict the y variable. There is no distinction between the two variables in correlation analysis.

10.3 (a) **F**: the residuals should be Normally distributed (b) **T** (c) **T**: this is a particular application of multiple regression, the analysis of covariance, when the means can be compared whilst adjusting for other variables (d) **F**: the sample size should be about ten times greater than the number of independent variables (e) **F**: the reverse is true.

10.4 (a) **F**: the correlation coefficient lies between these limits (b) **F**: again, confusion with the correlation coefficient (c) **T** (d) **F**: this is R^2 (e) **F**: it is the correlation coefficient which is independent of the units of measurement.

10.5 (a) There appears to be an approximately linear relationship between CFT and ELISA (see Fig. 10.11(a)), with ELISA values increasing as the CFT values increase (b) The Model Summary table shows that the estimated correlation coefficient is 0.737 (c) From the Coefficients table, we find that the estimated regression line is ELISA = 1.21 + 0.020CFT (d) From the Model

Summary table, $R^2 = 0.54$; this is derived from $(137.467)/(253.269)$ obtained from the ANOVA table. Thus, 54% of the variation in ELISA values is explained by its relationship with CFT; 46% is unexplained. Since more that half the variation is explained, we might conclude that the model is a reasonable fit (e) From the boxplot (Fig. 10.11(b)) we see that, although there is a suggestion that the residuals are slightly skewed to the right, they may be regarded as being approximately Normally distributed. The residuals in the scatter diagram (Fig. 10.11(d)) appear to be randomly scattered around a mean of about zero, indicating that a linear relationship between CFT and ELISA is reasonable. The residuals in the scatter diagram (Fig. 10.11(c)) have constant variability for increasing predicted values of ELISA. There is only one pair of readings of ELISA and CFT for each donkey. Hence, we can conclude that all the assumptions underlying the linear regression are satisfied (f) The ANOVA table is testing the null hypothesis that the true slope of the line is zero. The P-value of 0.000 (i.e. $P < 0.001$) shows that there is evidence to reject this null hypothesis in favour of the alternative hypothesis that the true slope is not zero (g) The slope of the line (from the Coefficients table) is 0.0198 (i.e. 1.98E-02) with an estimated standard error of 0.002 and 95% CI = (0.017, 0.023). Thus, as we increase CFT by 1 unit, we increase the ELISA by 0.0198 units on average (although, we believe with 95% confidence, that this average increase could be as low as 0.017 or as great as 0.023) (h) The t-test in the Coefficients table (test statistic = 12.03) and the F-test in the ANOVA table (test statistic = 144.82) both give $P < 0.001$ (i.e. sig. = 0.000). Hence there is strong evidence to reject the null hypothesis that the true slope is equal to zero.

10.6 (a) The correlation coefficient measures the linear association between rugal fold thickness and body weight. A coefficient of 0 indicates there is no linear association. A coefficient of 1 indicates that there is perfect positive association. This coefficient is positive and, judged subjectively, quite large, suggesting that there is a strong positive linear association between the two variables (b) The P-value results from the hypothesis test that the true correlation coefficient is zero. Since $P < 0.001$ is very small, there is strong evidence to reject the null hypothesis (c) The slope of the line represents the average change in y per unit change in x; thus we estimate that as the dog's body weight increases by 1 kg, its rugal thickness increases, on average, by 0.069 mm (d) The fraction is the square of the correlation coefficient $= 0.71 \times 0.71 = 0.50$; thus 50% of the variance in y is explained by the regression, and 50% is unexplained (e) The regression line is a questionable fit as it explains only half the variance in y, in spite of the correlation coefficient being highly significant.

CHAPTER 11

11.1 (a) **T** (b) **F**: the reverse is true (c) **F**: nonparametric tests tend to be less powerful than their parametric counterparts if all the assumptions underlying the parametric test are satisfied (d) **T** (e) **F**: the tests do not generally incorporate parameter estimates in their calculation.

11.2 (a) **T** (b) **T** (c) **F** (d) **F**: the data on each variable are converted to ranks but they do not have to be initially measured on a ranking scale (e) **T**: then it is difficult to establish the distribution of the data.

11.3 The correct way to analyse these data is to consider the set of differences in each group. These differences are not related so that any test which relies on paired data is inappropriate (a) **F** (b) **F** (c) **T** (d) **F** (e) **F**: the sample size is probably too small to perform a two-sample t-test because it is difficult, if not impossible, to establish whether the data are Normally distributed in each group and whether there is constant variance.

11.4 (a) There is a strong positive relationship between the scores which appears to be approximately linear (b) The subjective method assigns arbitrary scores to measure the degree of fluorescence, i.e. they are on an ordinal scale (c) $r_s = 0.90$, $P < 0.002$ from Table A.7 since $0.90 > 0.8182$, the tabulated percentage point for signifi-

cance at the 0.2% level with a sample size of 12. Hence we reject the null hypothesis that the true correlation coefficient is zero, and conclude that there is a significant relationship between the two scoring systems. Note that the 95% confidence limits for the correlation coefficient are 0.67 to 0.97, which is quite wide (to be expected since the sample size is small). Although a significant association exists, the lower confidence limit indicates that it may be as low as 0.67.

11.5 A Wilcoxon rank sum test computer analysis gives $P = 0.035$ (although when corrected for ties, $P = 0.030$). If performing the test by hand, we rank the two groups together and find the sum of the ranks of the bitches from the larger litters $= 3.5 + 7.5 + 12 + 12 + 12 + 16 + 16 + 18 + 19 = 116$. (Note, the sum of the ranks of the bitches from the smaller litters $= 1 + 3.5 + 3.5 + 3.5 + 7.5 + 7.5 + 7.5 + 12 + 12 + 16 = 74$). Referring to Table A.9 with sample sizes of 9 and 10, we find that 116 exceeds the tabulated 5% significance level limits of 65–115 (or alternatively, with sample sizes of 10 and 9, 74 is less than the tabulated limits of 75–125). However, 116 lies within the 1% significance level limits of 58–122. Hence we reject the null hypothesis that the median litter sizes are the same in the populations, $0.01 < P < 0.05$. There is evidence to indicate that litter size is inherited. The median litter sizes for the bitches from the larger litters is 5 (range 3–7), and from the smaller litters is 4 (range 2–5).

11.6 We find the differences in weight (before − after). The differences are (kg): +2.2, +0.4, +4.3, +1.0, +2.1, −1.4, −1.2, +0.7, 0.0, +0.4, −0.3, +0.7, +0.2, −0.3, +0.6, +1.8, +0.5, +0.2. These differences are skewed to the right, so that a nonparametric test is advocated. The null hypothesis is that the true median of these differences is equal to zero which would indicate that the dogs' weight is unaffected by the diet. The alternative hypothesis is that this median is not zero. The ranks of the differences are 16, 5.5, 17, 11, 15, 13, 12, 9.5, (we ignore the zero difference) 5.5, 3.5, 9.5, 1.5, 3.5, 8, 14, 7, 1.5, respectively. There are only 4 negative differences, and there are 13 positive differences. The sum of the ranks of the negative differences $= 12 + 13 + 3.5 + 3.5 = 32$. We refer this sum to Table A.9, and find that $P < 0.05$ (since 32 lies outside 34–119) but $P > 0.02$ (since 32 lies within 28–125). Hence we reject the null hypothesis $0.02 < P < 0.05$. In fact, a computer analysis gives $P = 0.04$. The median weight loss (with 25th and 75th percentiles) is 0.45 (–0.08, 1.20) kg. On the basis of this analysis, we would conclude that the novel diet is effective in promoting weight loss. However, this is a poorly designed trial since there is no control group of dogs which do not receive the novel diet. Hence, we cannot be sure that the observed loss in weight can be attributed to the novel diet: perhaps the dogs would have lost weight without it. Question 11.7 shows the results in a control group of dogs without the diet.

11.7 We find the differences between the dogs' weights before and after (B − A) the standard diet. They are +3.1, +0.6, +2.9, −1.0, +2.9, −1.8, −3.0, −0.9, −0.6, +0.6, −1.2, +1.6, +0.7, −0.2, −0.9, +1.7, +0.7, +0.2 kg, respectively. They are not Normally distributed. The differences in weights for the dogs on the novel diet (exercise 11.6) are: +2.2, +0.4, +4.3, +1.0, +2.1, −1.4, −1.2, +0.7, 0.0, +0.4, −0.3, +0.7, +0.2, −0.3, +0.6, +1.8, +0.5, +0.2 kg. These differences are skewed to the right. The null hypothesis is that the distributions of the differences in weight loss between the dogs in the population on the novel diet and those on the standard diet are the same. This is a two-sample test of the differences; we can use the Wilcoxon rank sum test to test the null hypothesis. We rank the two groups together and find the sum of the ranks of one of the two groups, say the novel diet group. The sum of these ranks is $3 + 4.5 + 10 + 11 + 13 + 15 + 15 + 17 + 18 + 19 + 21 + 24.5 + 24.5 + 27 + 30 + 31 + 32 + 36 = 351.5$. We cannot refer this sum to Table A.10 because the sample sizes are too great. Instead, we find

$$Test_{14} = \frac{351.5 - 18(18 + 18 + 1)/2}{\sqrt{18(18)(18 + 18 + 1)/12}} = 0.59$$

which we refer to Table A.1 which gives $P = 0.56$. Hence we have insufficient evidence to reject the null hypothesis. Note, a computer analysis also

gives $P = 0.56$. Thus there is no evidence to indicate that the novel diet promotes weight loss in obese dogs. The median weight loss (25th, 75th percentiles) in the novel diet group of dogs is 0.45 (−0.08, 1.2) kg, and in the standard diet group it is 0.40 (−0.93, 1.63) kg.

11.8 (a) The Friedman two-way ANOVA is the appropriate analysis because the data are dependent – there is a response for each dog for each of the three conditions. The null hypothesis is that the percentage aminopeptidase responses in the three different conditions come from the same population or from populations with the same median. Because the data are not homoscedastic (i.e. the variances are not constant), and recognizing that both the numerator and the denominator of the variable of interest (the percentages) are random variables (leading to some theoretical difficulties), we would analyse the data using a non-parametric approach (b) The result of the Friedman ANOVA is significant ($P = 0.006$) so that we have evidence to reject the null hypothesis. We can infer that the aminopeptidase responses are not the same in the three conditions. We are particularly interested to know whether the response in the presence of gluten is different from that of either the negative or positive controls. Wilcoxon signed rank tests comparing the results of the gluten responses with the negative and the positive controls gives $P = 0.027$ for each comparison (if we employ the Bonferroni correction – see Section 8.6.3 – in each case (i.e. multiply the P-value by 2), we would only obtain borderline significance). It would seem that the aminopeptidase response in the presence of gluten is supressed, a surprising result and one which certainly deserves to be explored further.

CHAPTER 12

12.1 (a) **F**: it Normalizes data which are skewed to the right (b) **T** (c) **T**: in particular when the standard deviation is proportional to the mean (d) **F**: it is not used for proportions. The logistic transformation is appropriate (e) **F**: non-parametric tests are often applied when the sample size is small.

12.2 (a) **T**: if you increase the power, you have a greater chance of detecting a real difference (b) **T** (c) **F**: it is easier to detect, as significant, a large treatment difference than a small one, so that you will need less animals if the treatment effect is greater (d) **T**: if you have underestimated the standard deviation, then the treatment effect relative to the standard deviation will be smaller, and therefore harder to detect. Also, if there is more variability in the data, it will be harder to detect a treatment difference unless you increase the sample size (e) **F**: if the standardized difference is increased, this means that the treatment effect relative to the standard deviation is greater. As it is easier to detect a large difference, you can decrease the sample size.

12.3 (a) **F**: a long time-lag precludes an early decision and wastes information from further subjects (b) **T**: selection and allocation are two different processes, and one does not imply the other (c) **F**: (d) **T** (e) **F**: a cluster sample is less precise than a simple random sample. The greatest precision is achieved if it is designed so that the units within a cluster are as different as possible, and the cluster means are as alike as possible.

12.4 This is a two-tailed test. Even though we are interested in the decline in Hb content, we cannot exclude the possibility that the Hb content of the blood might rise in the course of the investigation (a) The standardized difference = $1/(0.96) = 1.04$; hence we need about 30 animals (15 per group) (b) About 40 animals would be required to raise the power to 90%, i.e. 20 per group (c) About 44 animals would be required, i.e. 22 per group (d) The standardized difference is now $1/(1.3) = 0.77$; hence about 55 animals would be required, i.e. 28 per group.

12.5 (a) The standardized difference = $2 \times (1.0)/(1.7) = 1.18$, so we require about 26 horses for this trial (b) Only 55%, i.e. too low to be of any real use (c) For a sample size of 20, the power of the test increases to just over 75%.

12.6 The standardized difference is $(90 - 50)/\sqrt{70(100 - 70)} = 0.87$. This trial will require about 55 animals in total, with 28 in each group.

CHAPTER 13

13.1 (a) **T** (b) **F**: this is the positive predictive value (c) **F**: although the sensitivity and the specificity of a test are related, so that as one is increased, the other will tend to decrease, there is no simple relationship between them (d) **T** (e) **F**: the sensitivity and specificity of a test are not affected by the prevalence of the disease.

13.2 (a) **F**: this is for a categorical variable (b) **F**: this only determines whether bias is present (c) **F**: the correlation coefficient does not assess how close the points are to the line of equality (d) **T**: this measure gives an indication of the maximum likely difference between two measurements. We can use this measure to determine the limits of agreement (e) **F**: we are interested in the differences if we are investigating agreement, so s_w should not be used as the actual measure of agreement. Note that it is possible to calculate the appropriate measure of agreement from this quantity.

13.3 (a) **F**: there are too few points in the series (b) **T** (c) **F**: the information on the changes that a given animal undergoes is lost. Multiple comparisons may lead to spurious P-values (d) **F**: multiple comparisons may lead to spurious P-values. The results of successive tests are not independent (e) **T**: the use of summary measures is the correct approach. The difference between the initial and final response in an animal may be the correct summary measure in a particular circumstance.

13.4 (a) For a cut-off value of >90 U/l, sensitivity $= 100 \times (43/46) = 93.5\%$, specificity $= 100 \times (80/92) = 87.0\%$ (b) This cut-off value produces a test with both a high sensitivity and a high specificity, and is a worthwhile screening test (c) With a cut-off value of >500 U/l, sensitivity $= 100 \times (37/46) = 80.4\%$, specificity $= 100 \times (88/92) = 95.7\%$. Hence, when the cut-off value is raised, the sensitivity is compromised so that the test has a lesser ability to detect HAC, although the specificity of the test is substantially the same (d) The PPV is very low, indicating that it is unlikely that a dog with a positive test result actually has HAC. Thus, the test is unreliable for establishing whether the dog has HAC. However, because the NPV = 100%, then we would expect all dogs with CAP ≤ 90 U/l not to have HAC. It would seem that the CAP test should not be used as a diagnostic tool but is a useful screening device (after which more specific tests could be used for diagnosis) (e) Using the data in the table, we find that PPV = $100 \times (43/45) = 95.6\%$ and NPV = $100 \times (80/83) = 96.4\%$. The PPV is very different from what was obtained from the serum samples submitted to the laboratory in the three-month period because the prevalence of HAC is very different in the two data sets. In the original investigations, the results of which are shown in the table, the observed prevalence is $100 \times (46/138) = 33.3\%$. In the wider population, the prevalence is very much lower, so that the PPV is also lower.

13.5 The frequencies that we would expect if there were chance agreement along the diagonal (starting from the top) are 17.69 (i.e. this is $35 \times 143/283$), 23.32, 19.26, 1.22. Observed agreement along the diagonal = $(34 + 16 + 14 + 3)/283 = 67/283 = 0.267$; chance agreement = $(17.69 + 23.32 + 19.26 + 1.22)/283 = 61.49/283 = 0.217$; so kappa = $(0.267 - 0.217)/(1 - 0.217) = 0.025$. This repre-

sents poor agreement. Poor agreement implies that the scores before and after treatment are dissimilar. We can see from the table of results that the scores tend to improve after treatment. Hence we can presume that the treatment has improved the condition of foot rot in this flock.

13.6 We find the differences between the duplicate readings (these are, corrected to two decimal places, −0.09, 0.00, 0.09, −0.02, −0.01, 0.03, −0.04, 0.11, −0.01, −0.05, 0.09 mmol/l, respectively). We also find the average of the duplicate readings (these are, corrected to two decimal places, 3.71, 4.30, 3.59, 3.16, 3.34, 3.04, 3.11, 3.25, 2.99, 2.79, 2.93 mmol/l, respectively). When we plot the differences against their averages, we obtain a random scatter of points approximately evenly scattered around the zero difference line. In fact, the mean of these differences is 0.0095 mmol/l and the estimated standard deviation of the differences is 0.0645 mmol/l. A paired *t*-test investigating the differences between the readings gives a test statistic of 0.49 and $P = 0.623$, indicating that there is no bias. The limits of agreement are $0.0095 \pm 2 \times 0.0645 = -0.120$ mmol/l to 0.139 mmol/l. We expect 95% of the differences to lie between these limits; the maximum likely difference between two readings is $2 \times 0.0645 = 0.129$ mmol/l. Thus, we can see that this assay is highly repeatable. Although the repeatability is confirmed, we have no evidence of accuracy.

References

Altman, D.G. (1982) How large a sample? In: *Statistics in Practice*, (eds S.M. Gore & D.G. Altman). British Medical Association, London.

Altman, D.G. (1991) *Practical Statistics for Medical Research*. Chapman and Hall, London.

Altman, D.G. & Bland, J.M. (1997) Units of analysis. *British Medical Journal*, **314**, 1874.

Armitage, P. (1975) *Sequential Medical Trials*, 2nd edn. Blackwell Scientific Publications, Oxford.

Armitage, P. & Berry, G. (1994) *Statistical Methods in Medical Research*, 3rd edn. Blackwell Scientific Publications, Oxford.

Barber, P.J. & Elliott, J. (1998) Feline chronic renal failure: calcium homeostasis in 80 cases diagnosed between 1992 and 1995. *Journal of Small Animal Practice*, **39**, 108–16.

Bibby, C.J., Burgess, N.D. & Hill, D.A. (1992) *Bird Census Techniques*. Academic Press, London.

Bland, D.G. & Altman, D.G. (1994) Matching. *British Medical Journal*, **309**, 1128.

Bland, D.G. & Kerry, S.M. (1997) Sample size in cluster randomisation. *British Medical Journal*, **315**, 600.

Bland, J.M. & Altman, D.G. (1986) Statistical methods for assessing agreement between two methods of clinical measurement. *Lancet*, (**1986**) **i**, 307–10.

Burton, S.A., Lemke, K.A., Ihle, S.L. & MacKenzie, A.L. (1997) Effects of medetomidine on serum insulin and plasma glucose concentrations in clinically normal dogs. *American Journal of Veterinary Research*, **58**, 1440–2.

Chalmers, I. & Altman, D.G. (eds) (1995) *Systematic reviews*. British Medical Journal, London.

Chatfield, C. (1989) *The Analysis of Time Series: An Introduction*, 4th edn. Chapman and Hall, London.

Chatfield, C. & Collins, A.J. (1980) *Introduction to Multivariate Analysis*. Chapman and Hall, London.

Childs, J.E., Robinson, L.E., Sadek, R., Madden, A., Miranda, M.E. & Miranda, N.L. (1998) Density estimates of rural dog populations and an assessment of marking methods during a rabies vaccination campaign in the Phillipines. *Preventative Veterinary Medicine*, **33**, 207–18.

Ciba-Geigy, Ltd. (1990) *Geigy Scientific Tables*, Vol. 2, 8th edn. Ciba-Geigy Ltd, Basle.

Clarke, M.J. & Stewart, L.A. (1995) Obtaining data from randomised controlled trials: how much do we need for reliable and informative meta-analysis? In: *Systematic Reviews*, (eds I. Chalmers & D.G. Altman). British Medical Journal, London.

Cochran, W.G. (1977) *Sampling Techniques*, 3rd edn. Wiley, New York.

Cochran, W.G. & Cox, G.M. (1957) *Experimental Designs*, 2nd edn. Wiley, New York.

Cohen, J. (1960) A coefficient of agreement for nominal scales. *Educational and Psychological Measurement*, **20**, 37–46.

Cohen, J. (1968) Weighted kappa: nominal scale ageement with provision for scale disagreement or partial credit. *Pyschological Bulletin*, **70**, 213–20.

Cohen, J. (1988) *Statistical Power Analysis for the Behavioral Sciences*, 2nd edn. Laurence Erlbaum Associates, Hillsdale, New Jersey.

Corveleyn, S., Deprez, P., van der Weken, G., Baeyens, W. & Remon, J.P. (1996) Bioavailability of ketoprofen in horses after rectal administration. *The Journal of Veterinary Pharmacology and Therapeutics*, **19**, 359–63.

Coyne, R., Hiney, M. & Smith, P. (1996) Transient presence of oxytetracycline in blue mussels (*Mytilus edulis*) following its therapeutic use at a marine Atlantic salmon farm. *Aquaculture*, **149**, 175–81.

Cox, D.R. (1958) *Planning of Experiments*. Wiley, New York.

Cox, D.R. & Oakes, D. (1984) *Analysis of Survival Data*. Chapman and Hall, London.

Diggle, P.J. (1990) *Time Series – A Biostatistical Introduction*. Clarendon Press, Oxford.

Donald, P.F. & Evans, A.D. (1995) Habitat selection and population size of Corn Buntings *Milaria calandra* breeding in Britain in 1993. *Bird Study*, **42**, 190–204.

Donner, A. (1987) Statistical methodology for paired cluster designs. *American Journal of Epidemiology*, **126**, 972–9.

Donner, A., Birkett, N. & Buck, C. (1981) Randomisation by cluster: samples size requirements and analysis. *American Journal of Epidemiology*, **114**, 906–14.

Draper, N.R. & Smith, H. (1981) *Applied Regression Analysis*, 2nd edn. Wiley, New York.

Elliott, J. & Barber, P.J. (1998) Feline chronic renal failure: clinical findings in 80 cases diagnosed between 1992 and 1995. *Journal of Small Animal Practice*, **39**, 78–85.

England, G.C.W. (1992) *The cryopreservation of dog semen*. Fellowship thesis, Royal College of Veterinary Surgeons, London.

Everitt, B.S. (1995) The analysis of repeated measures: a practical review with examples. *The Statistician*, **44**, 113–35.

Eysenck, H.J. (1995) Problems with meta-analysis. In: *Systematic Reviews*, (eds I. Chalmers & D.G. Altman). British Medical Journal, London.

Gardiner, W.P. & Gettinby, G. (1998) *Experimental Design Techniques in Statistical Practice*. Horwood Publishing, Chichester.

Gardner, M.J. & Altman, D.G. (eds) (1989) *Statistics with Confidence: Confidence intervals and statistical guidelines*. British Medical Journal, London.

Greenwood, J.J.D. (1996) Basic techniques. In: *Ecological Census Techniques. A Handbook*, (ed. W.J. Sutherland). Cambridge University Press, Cambridge.

Gunning, R.F. & Walters, R.J.W. (1994) 'Flying scapulas', a post turnout myopathy in cattle. *Veterinary Record*, **135**, 433–4.

Haber, M., Logini, I.M. & Halloran, M.E. (1991) *International Journal of Epidemiology*, **20**, 300–10.

Halloran, M.E. & Struchiner, C.J. (1991) Study designs for dependent happenings. *Epidemiology*, **2**, 331–38.

Hawkins, T., Gala, R.R. & Dunbar, J.C. (1993) The effect of neonatal sex hormone manipulation on the incidence of diabetes in non-obese diabetic mice. *The Proceedings of the Society for Experimental Biology and Medicine*, **202**, 201–5.

Hiraga, A., Kai, A., Kubo, K. & Sugano, S. (1997) Effects of low intensity exercise during the breaking period on cardiopulmonary function in Thoroughbred yearlings. *Journal of Equine Science*, **8**, 21–4.

Hoeben, D., Mitjen, P. & de Kruif, A. (1997) Factors influencing complications during Caesarean section on the standing cow. *Veterinary Quarterly*, **19**, 88–92.

Hseih, F.Y. (1988) Sample size formulae for intervention studies with the cluster as unit of randomisation. *Statistics in Medicine*, **8**, 1195–201.

Jackson, B., Eastell, R., Russell, R.G.G., Lanyon, L.E. & Price, J.S. (1996) Measurement of bone specific alkaline phosphatase in the horse: a comparison of two techniques. *Research in Veterinary Science*, **61**, 160–4.

Jain, N.C., Vegad, J.L., Jain, N.K. & Shrivastava, A.B. (1982) Haematological studies on normal lactating Indian buffaloes. *Research in Veterinary Science*, **32**, 52–6.

Jakovljevic, S. & Gibbs, C. (1993) Radiographic assessment of gastric mucosal fold thickness in dogs. *American Journal of Veterinary Research*, **54**, 1827–30.

Jekel, J.F., Elmore, J.G. & Katz, D.L. (1996) *Epidemiology, Biostatistics and Preventive Medicine*. Saunders, Philadelphia.

Kendall, M.G. (1980) *Multivariate Analysis*, 2nd edn. Griffin, London.

Kerry, S.M. & Bland, D.G. (1998) Sample size in cluster randomisation. *British Medical Journal*, **316**, 549.

Kleinbaum, D.G., Kupper, L.L. & Muller, K.E. (1988) *Applied Regression Analysis and Other Multivariate Methods*, 2nd edn. PWS-Kent, Boston.

Knuth, U.A., Yeung, C.-H., Nieschlag, E. (1987) Computerized semen analysis: objective measurement of semen characteristics is biassed by subjective parameter setting. *Fertility and Sterility*, **48**, 118–24.

Ko, J.C., Nicklin, C.F., Heaton-Jones, T.G. & Kuo, W.C. (1998) Comparison of sedative and cardiorespiratory effects of diazepam, acepromazine, and xylazine in ferrets. *Journal of the American Animal Hospital Association*, **34**, 234–41.

Kulkarni, D.D., Bhikane, A.U., Shaila, M.S., Varalakshmi, P., Apte, M.P. & Nailadkar, B.W. (1996) Peste des petits ruminants in goats in India. *Veterinary Record*, **138**, 187–8.

Landis, J.R. & Koch, G.C. (1977) The measurement of observer agreement for categorical data. *Biometrics*, **33**, 159–74.

Ley, S.J., Waterman, A.E. & Livingston, A. (1995) A field study of the effect of lameness on mechanical nociceptive thresholds in sheep. *Veterinary Record*, **137**, 85–7.

Little, T.W.A., Richards, M.S., Hussaini, S.N. & Jones, T.D. (1980) The significance of Leptospiral antibodies in calving and aborting cattle in south west England. *Veterinary Record*, **106**, 221–4.

Lukacs, N.W., McCorkle, F.M. & Taylor, R.L. (1987) Monoamines suppress the phytohemagglutinin wattle response in chickens. *Dev. Comp. Immunol.*, **11**, 759–68.

Machin, D. & Campbell, M.J. (1987) *Statistical Tables for the Design of Clinical Trials*. Blackwell Scientific Publications, Oxford.

Manly, B.F.J. (1986) *Multivariate Statistical Methods, A Primer*. Chapman and Hall, London.

Manly, B.F.J. (1991) *Randomisation and Monte Carlo Methods in Biology*. Chapman and Hall, London.

Marriott, F.H.C. (1974) *The Interpretation of Multiple Observations*. Academic Press, London.

Martin, G.S., Strand, E. & Kearney, M.T. (1996) Use of statistical models to evaluate racing performance in Thoroughbreds. *Journal of the American Veterinary Medical Association*, **209**, 1900–6.

McCoy, M.A., Goodall, E.A. & Kennedy, D.G. (1996) Incidence of bovine hypomagnesaemia in Northern Ireland and methods of magnesium supplementation. *Veterinary Record*, **138**, 41–3.

Menard, S. (1995) Applied logistic regression analysis. *Sage University Paper series on Quantitative Applications in the Social Sciences*, series No. 07-106. Sage University Press, Thousand Oaks, California.

Mendenhall, W., Ott, L. & Scheaffer, R.L. (1971) *Elementary Survey Sampling*. Wadsworth, Belmont.

Merrell, B. (1998) Improving lamb survival on hill and upland farms. *SVS Congress Veterinary Times*, Peterborough, pp. 6–7.

Moser, C.A. & Kalton, G. (1971) *Survey Methods in Social Investigation*, 2nd edn. Heinemann, London.

Nanda, A.S., Dodson, H. & Ward, W.R. (1990) Relationship between an increase in plasma cortisol during transport-induced stress and failure of oestradiol to induce a luteinising hormone surge in dairy cows. *Res. Vet. Sci.*, **49**, 25–8.

Nelson, R.W., Duesberg, C.A., Ford, S.L., Feldman, E.C., Davenport, D.J., Kiernan, C. & Neal, L. (1998) Effect of dietary insoluble fibre on control of glycemia in dogs with naturally acquired diabetes mellitus. *Journal of the American Veterinary Medical Association*, **212**, 380–6.

Nicholas, F.W. (1987) *Veterinary Genetics*. Oxford University Press, Oxford.

Parker, B.N.J., Foulkes, J.A., Jones, P.C., Dexter, I. & Stephens, H. (1988) Prediction of calving times from plasma progesterone concentration. *Veterinary Record*, **122**, 88–9.

Pearson, E.S. & Hartley, H.O. (1966) *Biometrika Tables for Statisticians*, 3rd edn. Cambridge University Press, Cambridge.

Pearson, R.A. & Ouassat, M. (1996) Estimation of the liveweight and body condition of working donkeys in Morocco. *Veterinary Record*, **138**, 229–33.

Peto, R., Pike, M.C., Armitage, P., Breslow, N.E., Cox, D.R., Howard, S.V., Mantl, N., McPherson, K., Peto, J. & Smith, P.G. (1976) Design and analysis of randomised clinical trials requiring prolonged observation of each patient: I. Introduction and design. *British Journal of Cancer*, **34**, 585–612.

Peto, R., Pike, M.C., Armitage, P., Breslow, N.E., Cox, D.R., Howard, S.V., Mantl, N., McPherson, K., Peto, J. & Smith, P.G. (1977) Design and analysis of randomised clinical trials requiring prolonged observation of each patient: II. Analysis and examples. *British Journal of Cancer*, **35**, 1–39.

Pocock, S.J. (1983) *Clinical Trials: A Practical Approach*. Wiley, Chichester.

Scavelli, T.D., Patnaik, A.K., Mehlhaff, C.J. & Hayes, A.A. (1985) Hemangiosarcoma in the cat: retrospective evaluation of 31 surgical cases. *Journal of the American Veterinary Medical Association*, **187**, 817–19.

Schönmann, N.J., BonDurant, R.H., Gardner, I.A., Van Hoosear, K., Baltzer, W. & Kachulis, C. (1994) Comparison of sampling and culture methods for the diagnosis of *Tritrichomonas foetus* infection in bulls. *Veterinary Record*, **134**, 620–2.

Schroeder, L.D., Sjoquist, D.L. & Stephan, P.E. (1986) Understanding regression analysis: An introductory guide. *Sage University Paper series on Quantitative Applications in the Social Sciences*, series No. 07-057. Sage University Press, Beverly Hills, California.

Schwartz, D., Flamant, R. & Lellouch, J. (1980) *Clinical Trials*. Academic Press, London.

Senn, S. (1993) *Cross-over Trials in Clinical Research*. Wiley, Chichester.

Siegel, S. & Castellan, N.J. (1988) *Nonparametric Statistics for the Behavioral Sciences*, 2nd edn. McGraw-Hill, New York.

Sloet van Oldruitenborgh-Oosterbaan, M.M. & Barneveld, A. (1995) Comparison of the workload of Dutch warmblood horses ridden normally and on a treadmill. *Veterinary Record*, **137**, 136–9.

Solter, P.F., Hoffman, W.E., Hungerford, L.L., Peterson, M.E. & Dorner, J.L. (1993) Assessment of corticosteroid-induced alkaline phosphatase isoenzyme as a screening test for hyperadrenocorticism in dogs. *Journal of the American Veterinary Medical Association*, **203**, 534–8.

Southwood, T.R.E. (1966) *Ecological Methods*. Methuen, London.

Stookey, G.K., Warrick, J.M. & Miller, L.L. (1995) Effects of sodium hexametaphosphate on dental calculus formation in dogs. *American Journal of Veterinary Research*, **56**, 913–18.

Stroving, M., Moe, L., Gattre, E. (1997) A population-based case-control study of canine mammary tumours and clinical use of medroxyprogesterone acetate. *APMIS*, **105**, 590–6.

Tamuli, M.K. & Watson, P.F. (1994) Cold resistance in the live acrosome-intact subpopulation of boar spermatozoa acquired during incubation after ejaculation. *Veterinary Record*, **135**, 160–2.

Thompson, S.G. (1995) Why sources of heterogeneity in meta-analysis should be investigated. In: *Systematic Reviews*, (eds I. Chalmers & D.G. Altman). British Medical Journal, London.

Thrusfield, M. (1995) *Veterinary Epidemiology*, 2nd edn. Blackwell Scientific Publications, Oxford.

Warriss, P.D. & Edwards, J.E. (1995) Estimating the live weight of sheep from chest girth measurements. *Veterinary Record*, **137**, 123–4.

Watson, P.F. (1979) An objective method for measuring fluorescence of individual sperm cells labelled with 1-anilinonaphthalene-8-sulphonate (ANS) by means of photomicrography and densitometry. *Journal of Microscopy*, **117**, 425–9.

Welch, R.D., Smith, P.H., Malone, J.B., Holmes, R.A. & Geaghan, J.P. (1987) Herd evaluation of *Fasciola hepatica* infection levels in Louisiana cattle by an enzyme-linked immunosorbent assay. *American Journal of Veterinary Research*, **48**, 345–7.

Wilesmith, J.W., Wells, G.A.H., Ryan, J.B.M., Gavier-Widen, D. & Simmons, M.M. (1997) A cohort study to examine maternally associated risk factors for bovine spongiform encephalopathy. *Veterinary Record*, **141**, 239–43.

Yates, F. (1981) *Sampling Methods for Censuses and Surveys*, 4th edn. Griffin, London.

COMPUTER PACKAGES MENTIONED

Borenstein, M., Rothstein, H. & Cohen, J. (1997) *Samplepower 1.0*. SPSS Inc., Chicago.

nQuery Advisor 2.0. Statistical Solutions Ltd.

SPSS, version 8. SPSS Inc. Chicago.

Appendices

ACKNOWLEDGEMENTS

Table A.1 Modified from Altman (1991) *Practical Statistics for Medical Research.* Chapman and Hall, London, with permission.

Table A.3 Modified from *Geigy Scientific Tables*, Vol. 2 (1990) 8th edn, Ciba-Geigy Ltd, Basle, with permission.

Table A.4 Condensed from Table 8 of Pearson, E.S. and Hartley, H.O. (1966*) Biometrika Tables for Statisticians*, 3rd edn, Cambridge University Press, Cambridge, by permission of Oxford University Press on behalf of Biometrika Trustees.

Table A.5 Condensed from Geigy Scientific Tables, Vol. 2 (1990) 8th edn, Ciba-Geigy Ltd, Basle, with permission.

Table A.6 Modified from *Geigy Scientific Tables*, Vol. 2 (1990) 8th edn, Ciba-Geigy Ltd, Basle, with permission.

Table A.7 Modified from Altman, D.G. (1991) *Practical Statistics for Medical Research.* Chapman and Hall, London, with permission

Table A.8 Condensed from Siegel, S. and Castellan, N.J. (1988) *Nonparametric Statistics for the Behavioral Sciences*, 2nd edn, McGraw-Hill, New York, and used with permission of the McGraw-Hill Companies.

Table A.9 Reproduced from Altman, D.G. (1991) *Practical Statistics for Medical Research.* Chapman and Hall, London, with permission.

Table A.10 Extracted from *Geigy Scientific Tables*, Vol. 2 (1990) 8th edn, Ciba-Geigy Ltd, Basle, with permission.

Appendix A

Statistical Tables

TABLE A.1 THE STANDARD NORMAL DISTRIBUTION (TWO-TAILED *P*-VALUES FROM VALUES OF *z*, THE SND)

The tabulated value is the *P*-value in the two tails of the Standard Normal distribution corresponding to a specified value (critical value or percentage point) of the Standardized Normal Deviate

$$z = \frac{x - \mu}{\sigma}$$

where *x* is a Normally distributed variable with mean = μ and standard deviation = σ (see Section 3.5.3(c)).

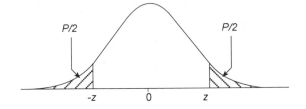

Example: If $z = 1.96$, then the two-tailed *P*-value = 0.05 ($P = 0.025$ in each tail).

Table A.1 The Standard Normal distribution (two-tailed *P*-values from values of *z*, the SND).

z	P	z	P	z	P	z	P	z	P	z	P
0.00	1.0000	0.53	0.5961	1.04	0.2983	1.56	0.1188	2.08	0.0375	2.59	0.0096
0.01	0.9920	0.54	0.5892	1.05	0.2937	1.57	0.1164	2.09	0.0366	2.60	0.0093
0.02	0.9840	0.55	0.5823	1.06	0.2891	1.58	0.1141	2.10	0.0357	2.61	0.0091
0.03	0.9761	0.56	0.5755	1.07	0.2846	1.59	0.1118	2.11	0.0349	2.62	0.0088
0.04	0.9681	0.57	0.5687	1.08	0.2801	1.60	0.1096	2.12	0.0340	2.63	0.0085
0.05	0.9601	0.58	0.5619	1.09	0.2757	1.61	0.1074	2.13	0.0332	2.64	0.0083
0.06	0.9522	0.59	0.5552	1.10	0.2713	1.62	0.1052	2.14	0.0324	2.65	0.0080
0.07	0.9442	0.60	0.5485	1.11	0.2670	1.63	0.1031	2.15	0.0316	2.66	0.0078
0.08	0.9362	0.61	0.5419	1.12	0.2627	1.64	0.1010	2.16	0.0308	2.67	0.0076
0.09	0.9283	0.62	0.5353	1.13	0.2585	1.65	0.0989	2.17	0.0300	2.68	0.0074
0.10	0.9203	0.63	0.5287	1.14	0.2543	1.66	0.0969	2.18	0.0293	2.69	0.0071
0.11	0.9124	0.64	0.5222	1.15	0.2501	1.67	0.0949	2.19	0.0285	2.70	0.0069
0.12	0.9045	0.65	0.5157	1.16	0.2460	1.68	0.0930	2.20	0.0278	2.71	0.0067
0.13	0.8966	0.66	0.5093	1.17	0.2420	1.69	0.0910	2.21	0.0271	2.72	0.0065
0.14	0.8887	0.67	0.5029	1.18	0.2380	1.70	0.0891	2.22	0.0264	2.73	0.0063
0.15	0.8808	0.68	0.4965	1.19	0.2340	1.71	0.0873	2.23	0.0257	2.74	0.0061
0.16	0.8729	0.69	0.4902	1.20	0.2301	1.72	0.0854	2.24	0.0251	2.75	0.0060
0.17	0.8650	0.70	0.4839	1.21	0.2263	1.73	0.0836	2.25	0.0244	2.76	0.0058
0.18	0.8572	0.71	0.4777	1.22	0.2225	1.74	0.0819	2.26	0.0238	2.77	0.0056
0.19	0.8493	0.72	0.4715	1.23	0.2187	1.75	0.0801	2.27	0.0232	2.78	0.0054
0.20	0.8415	0.73	0.4654	1.24	0.2150	1.76	0.0784	2.28	0.0226	2.79	0.0053
0.21	0.8337	0.74	0.4593	1.25	0.2113	1.77	0.0767	2.29	0.0220	2.80	0.0051
0.22	0.8259	0.75	0.4533	1.26	0.2077	1.78	0.0751	2.30	0.0214	2.81	0.0050
0.23	0.8181	0.76	0.4473	1.27	0.2041	1.79	0.0735	2.31	0.0209	2.82	0.0048
0.24	0.8103	0.77	0.4413	1.28	0.2005	1.80	0.0719	2.32	0.0203	2.83	0.0047
0.25	0.8026	0.78	0.4354	1.29	0.1971	1.81	0.0703	2.33	0.0198	2.84	0.0045
0.26	0.7949	0.79	0.4295	1.30	0.1936	1.82	0.0688	2.34	0.0193	2.85	0.0044
0.27	0.7872	0.80	0.4237	1.31	0.1902	1.83	0.0672	2.35	0.0188	2.86	0.0042
0.28	0.7795	0.81	0.4179	1.32	0.1868	1.84	0.0658	2.36	0.0183	2.87	0.0041
0.29	0.7718	0.82	0.4122	1.33	0.1835	1.85	0.0643	2.37	0.0178	2.88	0.0040
0.30	0.7642	0.83	0.4065	1.34	0.1802	1.86	0.0629	2.38	0.0173	2.89	0.0039
0.31	0.7566	0.84	0.4009	1.35	0.1770	1.87	0.0615	2.39	0.0168	2.90	0.0037
0.32	0.7490	0.85	0.3953	1.36	0.1738	1.88	0.0601	2.40	0.0164	2.91	0.0036
0.33	0.7414	0.86	0.3898	1.37	0.1707	1.89	0.0588	2.41	0.0160	2.92	0.0035
0.34	0.7339	0.87	0.3843	1.38	0.1676	1.90	0.0574	2.42	0.0155	2.93	0.0034
0.35	0.7263	0.88	0.3789	1.39	0.1645	1.91	0.0561	2.43	0.0151	2.94	0.0033
0.36	0.7188	0.89	0.3735	1.40	0.1615	1.92	0.0549	2.44	0.0147	2.95	0.0032
0.37	0.7114	0.90	0.3681	1.41	0.1585	1.93	0.0536	2.45	0.0143	2.96	0.0031
0.38	0.7039	0.91	0.3628	1.42	0.1556	1.94	0.0524	2.46	0.0139	2.97	0.0030
0.39	0.6965	0.92	0.3576	1.43	0.1527	1.95	0.0512	2.47	0.0135	2.98	0.0029
0.40	0.6892	0.93	0.3524	1.44	0.1499	1.96	0.0500	2.48	0.0131	2.99	0.0028
0.41	0.6818	0.94	0.3472	1.45	0.1471	1.97	0.0488	2.49	0.0128	3.00	0.0027
0.42	0.6745	0.95	0.3421	1.46	0.1443	1.98	0.0477	2.50	0.0124	3.10	0.00194
0.43	0.6672	0.96	0.3371	1.47	0.1416	1.99	0.0466	2.51	0.0121	3.20	0.00137
0.44	0.6599	0.97	0.3320	1.48	0.1389	2.00	0.0455	2.52	0.0117	3.30	0.00097
0.45	0.6527	0.98	0.3271	1.49	0.1362	2.01	0.0444	2.53	0.0114	3.40	0.00067
0.46	0.6455	0.99	0.3222	1.50	0.1336	2.02	0.0434	2.54	0.0111	3.50	0.00047
0.47	0.6384	1.00	0.3173	1.51	0.1310	2.03	0.0424	2.55	0.0108	3.60	0.00032
0.48	0.6312	1.01	0.3125	1.52	0.1285	2.04	0.0414	2.56	0.0105	3.70	0.00022
0.49	0.6241	1.02	0.3077	1.53	0.1260	2.05	0.0404	2.57	0.0102	3.80	0.00014
0.50	0.6171	1.03	0.3030	1.54	0.1236	2.06	0.0394	2.58	0.0099	3.90	0.00010
0.51	0.6101			1.55	0.1211	2.07	0.0385			4.00	0.00006
0.52	0.6031										

TABLE A.2 THE STANDARD NORMAL DISTRIBUTION (VALUES OF *z*, THE SND, FROM *P*-VALUES)

The one-tailed *P*-value is that in which the total probability is contained in the tail area to the right of the Standardized Normal Deviate

$$z = \frac{x - \mu}{\sigma}$$

where *x* is a Normally distributed variable with mean = μ and standard deviation = σ. The two-tailed *P*-value is that in which half of the total probablity is contained in the tail area to the right of *z*, the SND, and the other half is contained in the tail area to the left of $-z$ (see Section 3.5.3(d)).

Table A.2 Tail area probabilites and corresponding values of the SND, *z*.

Two-tailed probability	SND, *z*	One-tailed probability
1.00	0.00	0.50
0.90	0.13	0.45
0.50	0.67	0.25
0.25	1.15	0.125
0.20	1.28	0.10
0.15	1.44	0.075
0.10	1.64	0.05
0.05	1.96	0.025
0.02	2.33	0.01
0.01	2.58	0.005
0.005	2.81	0.0025
0.001	3.29	0.0005

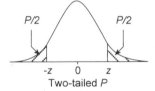

Two-tailed *P*

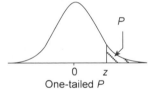

One-tailed *P*

TABLE A.3 THE *t*-DISTRIBUTION

This table contains the critical value (percentage point), t_p, of the *t*-distribution which corresponds to a particular two-tailed *P*-value for specified degrees of freedom. If the test statistic follows the *t*-distribution with known degrees of freedom, then the *P*-value for the two tailed hypothesis test is calculated by determining where the observed test statistic lies in relation to the critical values in the table. If the observed test statistic is greater than the critical value, then the *P*-value for the test is less than the relevant tabulated P-value. If the observed test statistic lies between two adjacent critical values, then the *P*-value for the test lies between the corresponding tabulated *P*-values.

Example: If the observed test statistic = 2.72 on 15 degrees of freedom, then since 2.72 > 2.602, $P < 0.02$. Furthermore, since 2.72 lies between 2.602 and 2.947, $0.01 < P < 0.02$.

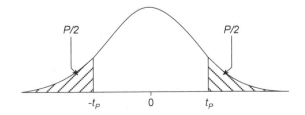

Table A.3 Percentage points of the t-distribution.

df	Two-tailed P-values												
	0.9	0.8	0.7	0.6	0.5	0.4	0.3	0.2	0.1	0.05	0.02	0.01	0.001
1	0.158	0.325	0.510	0.727	1.000	1.376	1.963	3.078	6.314	12.706	31.821	63.657	636.619
2	0.142	0.289	0.445	0.617	0.816	1.061	1.386	1.886	2.920	4.303	6.965	9.925	31.598
3	0.137	0.277	0.424	0.584	0.765	0.978	1.250	1.638	2.353	3.182	4.541	5.841	12.924
4	0.134	0.271	0.414	0.569	0.741	0.941	1.190	1.533	2.132	2.776	3.747	4.604	8.610
5	0.132	0.267	0.408	0.559	0.727	0.920	1.156	1.476	2.015	2.571	3.365	4.032	6.869
6	0.131	0.265	0.404	0.553	0.718	0.906	1.134	1.440	1.943	2.447	3.143	3.707	5.959
7	0.130	0.263	0.402	0.549	0.711	0.896	1.119	1.415	1.895	2.365	2.998	3.499	5.408
8	0.130	0.262	0.399	0.546	0.706	0.889	1.108	1.397	1.86	2.306	2.896	3.355	5.041
9	0.129	0.261	0.398	0.543	0.703	0.883	1.100	1.383	1.833	2.262	2.821	3.250	4.781
10	0.129	0.260	0.397	0.542	0.700	0.879	1.093	1.372	1.812	2.228	2.764	3.169	4.587
11	0.129	0.260	0.396	0.540	0.697	0.876	1.088	1.363	1.796	2.201	2.718	3.106	4.437
12	0.128	0.259	0.395	0.539	0.695	0.873	1.083	1.356	1.782	2.179	2.681	3.055	4.318
13	0.128	0.259	0.394	0.538	0.694	0.870	1.079	1.350	1.771	2.160	2.650	3.012	4.221
14	0.128	0.258	0.393	0.537	0.692	0.868	1.076	1.345	1.761	2.145	2.624	2.977	4.140
15	0.128	0.258	0.393	0.536	0.691	0.866	1.074	1.341	1.753	2.131	2.602	2.947	4.073
16	0.128	0.258	0.392	0.535	0.690	0.865	1.071	1.337	1.746	2.120	2.583	2.921	4.015
17	0.128	0.257	0.392	0.534	0.689	0.863	1.069	1.333	1.741	2.110	2.567	2.898	3.965
18	0.127	0.257	0.392	0.534	0.688	0.862	1.067	1.330	1.734	2.101	2.552	2.878	3.922
19	0.127	0.257	0.391	0.533	0.688	0.861	1.066	1.328	1.729	2.093	2.539	2.861	3.883
20	0.127	0.257	0.391	0.533	0.687	0.860	1.064	1.325	1.725	2.086	2.528	2.845	3.850
21	0.127	0.257	0.391	0.532	0.686	0.859	1.063	1.323	1.721	2.080	2.518	2.831	3.819
22	0.127	0.256	0.390	0.532	0.686	0.858	1.061	1.321	1.717	2.074	2.508	2.819	3.792
23	0.127	0.256	0.390	0.532	0.685	0.858	1.060	1.319	1.714	2.069	2.500	2.807	3.767
24	0.127	0.256	0.390	0.531	0.685	0.857	1.059	1.318	1.711	2.064	2.492	2.797	3.745
25	0.127	0.256	0.390	0.531	0.684	0.856	1.058	1.316	1.708	2.060	2.485	2.787	3.725
26	0.127	0.256	0.390	0.531	0.684	0.856	1.058	1.315	1.706	2.056	2.479	2.773	3.707
27	0.127	0.256	0.389	0.531	0.684	0.855	1.057	1.314	1.703	2.052	2.473	2.771	3.690
28	0.127	0.256	0.389	0.530	0.683	0.855	1.056	1.313	1.701	2.048	2.467	2.763	3.674
29	0.127	0.256	0.389	0.530	0.683	0.854	1.055	1.311	1.699	2.045	2.462	2.756	3.659
30	0.127	0.256	0.389	0.530	0.683	0.854	1.055	1.310	1.697	2.042	2.457	2.750	3.646
40	0.126	0.255	0.388	0.529	0.681	0.851	1.050	1.303	1.684	2.021	2.423	2.704	3.551
50	0.126	0.255	0.388	0.528	0.679	0.849	1.047	1.299	1.676	2.009	2.403	2.678	3.497
100	0.126	0.254	0.386	0.526	0.677	0.845	1.042	1.291	1.661	1.984	2.364	2.626	3.391
200	0.126	0.254	0.385	0.525	0.676	0.843	1.039	1.286	1.653	1.972	2.345	2.601	3.340
∞	0.126	0.253	0.385	0.524	0.674	0.842	1.036	1.282	1.645	1.960	2.326	2.576	3.291

TABLE A.4 THE CHI-SQUARED (χ^2)-DISTRIBUTION

This table contains the critical value (percentage point), χ^2_P, of the χ^2-distribution which corresponds to a particular *P*-value for specified degrees of freedom. Note that the *P*-value relates to the upper tail of the χ^2-distribution. If the test statistic follows the χ^2-distribution with known degrees of freedom, then the *P*-value for the hypothesis test is calculated by determining where the observed test statistic lies in relation to the critical values in the table. If the observed test statistic is greater than the critical value, then the *P*-value for the test is less than the tabulated *P*-value. If the observed test statistic lies between two adjacent critical values, then the *P*-value for the test lies between the corresponding tabulated *P*-values.

Example: If the observed test statistic = 20.3 on 10 degrees of freedom, then since 20.3 > 18.307, $P < 0.05$. Furthermore, since 20.3 lies between 18.307 and 21.161, $0.02 < P < 0.05$.

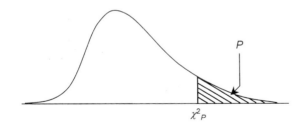

Table A.4 The Chi-squared (χ^2)-distribution.

df	\multicolumn{7}{c}{Two-tailed *P*-value}
	0.500	0.250	0.100	0.050	0.025	0.010	0.001
1	0.45	1.32	2.71	3.84	5.02	6.63	10.83
2	1.39	2.77	4.61	5.99	7.38	9.21	13.82
3	2.37	4.11	6.25	7.81	9.35	11.34	16.27
4	3.36	5.39	7.78	9.49	11.14	13.28	18.47
5	4.35	6.63	9.24	11.07	12.83	15.09	20.52
6	5.35	7.84	10.64	12.59	14.45	16.81	22.46
7	6.35	9.04	12.02	14.07	16.01	18.48	24.32
8	7.34	10.22	13.36	15.51	17.53	20.09	26.12
9	8.34	11.39	14.68	16.92	19.02	21.67	27.88
10	9.34	12.55	15.99	18.31	20.48	23.21	29.59
11	10.34	13.70	17.28	19.68	21.92	24.72	31.26
12	11.34	14.85	18.55	21.03	23.34	26.22	32.91
13	12.34	15.98	19.81	22.36	24.74	27.69	34.53
14	13.34	17.12	21.06	23.68	26.12	29.14	36.12
15	14.34	18.25	22.31	25.00	27.49	30.58	37.70
16	15.34	19.37	23.54	26.30	28.85	32.00	39.25
17	16.34	20.49	24.77	27.59	30.19	33.41	40.79
18	17.34	21.60	25.99	28.87	31.53	34.81	42.31
19	18.34	22.72	27.20	30.14	32.85	36.19	43.82
20	19.34	23.83	28.41	31.41	34.17	37.57	45.32
21	20.34	24.93	29.62	32.67	35.48	38.93	46.80
22	21.34	26.04	30.81	33.92	36.78	40.29	48.27
23	22.34	27.14	32.01	35.17	38.08	41.64	49.73
24	23.34	28.24	33.20	36.42	39.36	42.98	51.18
25	24.34	29.34	34.38	37.65	40.65	44.31	32.62
26	25.34	30.43	35.56	38.89	41.92	45.64	54.05
27	26.34	31.53	36.74	40.11	43.19	46.96	55.48
28	27.34	32.62	37.92	41.34	44.46	48.28	56.89
29	28.34	33.71	39.09	42.56	45.72	49.59	58.30
30	29.34	34.80	40.26	43.77	46.98	50.89	59.70
40	39.34	45.62	51.80	55.76	59.34	63.69	73.40
50	49.33	56.33	63.17	67.50	71.42	76.15	86.66
60	59.33	66.98	74.40	79.08	83.30	88.38	99.61
70	69.33	77.58	85.53	90.53	95.02	100.42	112.32
80	79.33	88.13	96.58	101.88	106.63	112.33	124.84
90	89.33	98.64	107.56	113.14	118.14	124.12	137.21
100	99.33	109.14	118.50	124.34	129.56	135.81	149.45

TABLE A.5 THE *F*-DISTRIBUTION

Tables A.5(a) and A.5(b) contain the critical values (percentage points) of the *F*-distribution, F_p, which correspond to a specified *P*-value for v_1 degrees of freedom in the numerator and v_2 degrees of freedom in the denominator. If the test statistic follows the *F*-distribution with known degrees of freedom, then we can calculate the *P*-value by determining where the observed test statistic lies in relation to the critical values in the table. Note that the tabulated *P*-value relates to the *upper* tail of the *F*-distribution.

For a *one-sided* hypothesis test (as in the ANOVA), if the observed test statistic is greater than the critical value, then the *P*-value for the one-sided test is less than the tabulated *P*-value. If the observed test statistic lies between two adjacent critical values, then the *P*-value lies between the corresponding tabulated *P*-values. We are more likely to use Table A.5(a) if the test is one-sided.

Example: For a *one-sided* test, if the observed test statistic = 4.41 on 5 (numerator) and 6 (denominator) degrees of freedom, then since 4.41 > 4.39, $P < 0.05$. Furthermore, since 4.41 lies between 4.39 and 8.75, $0.01 < P < 0.05$.

Occasionally, we have a *two-sided* hypothesis test (e.g. when comparing two variances from independent groups). To determine significance at a given *P* level, we have to compare our observed test statistic with the critical value in the table that corresponds to the tabulated *P*/2. Thus, a two-sided *P*-value of 0.05 corresponds to the tabulated $P = 0.025$; a two-sided *P*-value of 0.01 corresponds to the tabulated $P = 0.005$. We are more likely in this situation to use Table A.5(b).

Example: For a *two-sided* test, if the observed test statistic = 6.0 on 2 (numerator) and 9 (denominator) degrees of freedom, then since 6.0 lies between 5.71 (the critical value for $P = 0.025$) and 10.11 (the critical value for $P = 0.005$), then $0.01 < P < 0.05$.

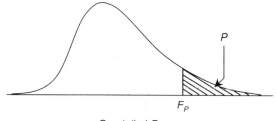

One-tailed *P*

Table A.5(a)   Percentage points of the F-distribution ($P = 0.05$ and $P = 0.01$).

df denominator, v_2	P	\multicolumn{11}{c}{df numerator, v_1}

df denominator, v_2	P	1	2	3	4	5	6	7	8	12	24	∞
1	0.05	161.4	199.5	215.7	224.6	230.2	234.0	236.8	238.9	243.9	249.1	254.3
	0.01	**4052**	**5000**	**5403**	**5625**	**5764**	**5859**	**5928**	**5981**	**6106**	**6235**	**6366**
2	0.05	18.51	19.00	19.16	19.25	19.30	19.33	19.35	19.37	19.41	19.45	19.50
	0.01	**98.50**	**99.00**	**99.17**	**99.25**	**99.30**	**99.33**	**99.36**	**99.37**	**99.42**	**99.46**	**99.50**
3	0.05	10.13	9.55	9.28	9.12	9.01	8.94	8.89	8.85	8.74	8.64	8.53
	0.01	**34.12**	**30.82**	**29.46**	**28.71**	**28.24**	**27.91**	**27.67**	**27.49**	**27.05**	**26.60**	**26.13**
4	0.05	7.71	6.94	6.59	6.39	6.26	6.16	6.09	6.04	5.91	5.77	5.63
	0.01	**21.20**	**18.00**	**16.69**	**15.98**	**15.52**	**15.21**	**14.98**	**14.80**	**14.37**	**13.93**	**3.46**
5	0.05	6.61	5.79	5.41	5.19	5.05	4.95	4.88	4.82	4.68	4.53	4.36
	0.01	**16.26**	**13.27**	**12.06**	**11.39**	**10.97**	**10.67**	**10.46**	**10.29**	**9.89**	**9.47**	**9.02**
6	0.05	5.99	5.14	4.76	4.53	4.39	4.28	4.21	4.15	4.00	3.84	3.67
	0.01	**13.75**	**10.92**	**9.78**	**9.15**	**8.75**	**8.47**	**8.26**	**8.10**	**7.72**	**7.31**	**6.88**
7	0.05	5.59	4.74	4.35	4.12	3.97	3.87	3.79	3.73	3.57	3.41	3.23
	0.01	**12.25**	**9.55**	**8.45**	**7.85**	**7.46**	**7.19**	**6.99**	**6.84**	**6.47**	**6.07**	**5.65**
8	0.05	5.32	4.46	4.07	3.84	3.69	3.58	3.50	3.44	3.28	3.12	2.93
	0.01	**11.26**	**8.65**	**7.59**	**7.01**	**6.63**	**6.37**	**6.18**	**6.03**	**5.67**	**5.28**	**4.86**
9	0.05	5.12	4.26	3.86	3.63	3.48	3.37	3.29	3.23	3.07	2.90	2.71
	0.01	**10.56**	**8.02**	**6.99**	**6.42**	**6.06**	**5.80**	**5.61**	**5.47**	**5.11**	**4.73**	**4.31**
10	0.05	4.96	4.10	3.71	3.48	3.33	3.22	3.14	3.07	2.91	2.74	2.54
	0.01	**10.04**	**7.56**	**6.55**	**5.99**	**5.64**	**5.39**	**5.20**	**5.06**	**4.71**	**4.33**	**3.91**
12	0.05	4.75	3.89	3.49	3.26	3.11	3.00	2.91	2.85	2.69	2.51	2.30
	0.01	**9.33**	**6.93**	**5.95**	**5.41**	**5.06**	**4.82**	**4.64**	**4.50**	**4.16**	**3.78**	**3.36**
14	0.05	4.60	3.74	3.34	3.11	2.96	2.85	2.76	2.70	2.53	2.35	2.13
	0.01	**8.86**	**6.51**	**5.56**	**5.04**	**4.69**	**4.46**	**4.28**	**4.14**	**3.80**	**3.43**	**3.00**
16	0.05	4.49	3.63	3.24	3.01	2.85	2.74	2.66	2.59	2.42	2.24	2.01
	0.01	**8.53**	**6.23**	**5.29**	**4.77**	**4.44**	**4.20**	**4.03**	**3.89**	**3.55**	**3.18**	**2.75**
18	0.05	4.41	3.55	3.16	2.93	2.77	2.66	2.58	2.51	2.34	2.15	1.92
	0.01	**8.29**	**6.01**	**5.09**	**4.58**	**4.25**	**4.01**	**3.84**	**3.71**	**3.37**	**3.00**	**2.57**
20	0.05	4.35	3.49	3.10	2.87	2.71	2.60	2.51	2.45	2.28	2.08	1.84
	0.01	**8.10**	**5.85**	**4.94**	**4.43**	**4.10**	**3.87**	**3.70**	**3.56**	**3.23**	**2.86**	**2.42**
30	0.05	4.17	3.32	2.92	2.69	2.53	2.42	2.33	2.27	2.09	1.89	1.62
	0.01	**7.56**	**5.39**	**4.51**	**4.02**	**3.70**	**3.47**	**3.30**	**3.17**	**2.84**	**2.47**	**2.01**
40	0.05	4.08	3.23	2.84	2.61	2.45	2.34	2.25	2.18	2.00	1.79	1.51
	0.01	**7.31**	**5.18**	**4.31**	**3.83**	**3.51**	**3.29**	**3.12**	**2.99**	**2.66**	**2.29**	**1.80**
60	0.05	4.00	3.15	2.76	2.53	2.37	2.25	2.17	2.10	1.92	1.70	1.39
	0.01	**7.08**	**4.98**	**4.13**	**3.65**	**3.34**	**3.12**	**2.95**	**2.82**	**2.50**	**2.12**	**1.60**
120	0.05	3.92	3.07	2.68	2.45	2.29	2.17	2.09	2.02	1.83	1.61	1.25
	0.01	**6.85**	**4.79**	**3.95**	**3.48**	**3.17**	**2.96**	**2.79**	**2.66**	**2.34**	**1.95**	**1.38**
∞	0.05	3.84	3.00	2.60	2.37	2.21	2.10	2.01	1.94	1.75	1.52	1.00
	0.01	**6.63**	**4.61**	**3.78**	**3.32**	**3.02**	**2.80**	**2.64**	**2.51**	**2.18**	**1.79**	**1.00**

Table A.5(b) Percentage points of the *F*-distribution ($P = 0.05$ and $P = 0.01$).

df denominator, v_2	P	df numerator, v_1										
		1	2	3	4	5	6	7	8	12	24	∞
1	0.025	647.8	799.5	864.2	899.6	921.8	937.1	948.2	956.7	976.7	997.2	1018
	0.005	**16211**	**20000**	**21615**	**22500**	**23056**	**23437**	**23715**	**23925**	**24426**	**24940**	**25465**
2	0.025	38.51	39.00	39.17	39.25	39.30	39.33	39.36	39.37	39.41	39.46	39.50
	0.005	**198.5**	**199.0**	**199.2**	**199.2**	**199.3**	**199.3**	**199.4**	**199.4**	**199.4**	**199.5**	**199.5**
3	0.025	17.44	16.04	15.44	15.10	14.88	14.73	14.62	14.54	14.34	14.12	13.90
	0.005	**55.55**	**49.80**	**47.47**	**46.19**	**45.39**	**44.84**	**44.43**	**44.13**	**43.39**	**42.62**	**41.83**
4	0.025	12.22	10.65	9.98	9.60	9.36	9.20	9.07	8.98	8.75	8.51	8.26
	0.005	**31.33**	**26.28**	**24.26**	**23.15**	**22.46**	**21.97**	**21.62**	**21.35**	**20.70**	**20.03**	**19.32**
5	0.025	10.01	8.43	7.76	7.39	7.15	6.98	6.85	6.76	6.52	6.28	6.02
	0.005	**22.78**	**18.31**	**16.53**	**15.56**	**14.94**	**14.51**	**14.20**	**13.96**	**13.38**	**12.78**	**12.14**
6	0.025	8.81	7.26	6.60	6.23	5.99	5.82	5.70	5.60	5.37	5.12	4.85
	0.005	**18.63**	**14.54**	**12.92**	**12.03**	**11.46**	**11.07**	**10.79**	**10.57**	**10.03**	**9.47**	**8.88**
7	0.025	8.07	6.54	5.89	5.52	5.29	5.12	4.99	4.90	4.67	4.42	4.14
	0.005	**16.24**	**12.40**	**10.88**	**10.05**	**9.52**	**9.16**	**8.89**	**8.68**	**8.18**	**7.65**	**7.08**
8	0.025	7.57	6.06	5.42	5.05	4.82	4.65	4.53	4.43	4.20	3.95	3.67
	0.005	**14.69**	**11.04**	**9.60**	**8.81**	**8.30**	**7.95**	**7.69**	**7.50**	**7.01**	**6.50**	**5.95**
9	0.025	7.21	5.71	5.08	4.72	4.48	4.32	4.20	4.10	3.87	3.61	3.33
	0.005	**13.61**	**10.11**	**8.72**	**7.96**	**7.47**	**7.13**	**6.88**	**6.69**	**6.23**	**5.73**	**5.19**
10	0.025	6.94	5.46	4.83	4.47	4.24	4.07	3.95	3.85	3.62	3.37	3.08
	0.005	**12.83**	**9.43**	**8.08**	**7.34**	**6.87**	**6.54**	**6.30**	**6.12**	**5.66**	**5.17**	**4.64**
12	0.025	6.55	5.10	4.47	4.12	3.89	3.73	3.61	3.51	3.28	3.02	2.72
	0.005	**11.75**	**8.51**	**7.23**	**6.52**	**6.07**	**5.76**	**5.52**	**5.35**	**4.91**	**4.43**	**3.90**
14	0.025	6.30	4.86	4.24	3.89	3.66	3.50	3.38	3.29	3.05	2.79	2.49
	0.005	**11.06**	**7.92**	**6.68**	**6.00**	**5.56**	**5.26**	**5.03**	**4.86**	**4.43**	**3.96**	**3.44**
16	0.025	6.12	4.69	4.08	3.73	3.50	3.34	3.22	3.12	2.89	2.63	2.32
	0.005	**10.58**	**7.51**	**6.30**	**5.64**	**5.21**	**4.91**	**4.69**	**4.52**	**4.10**	**3.64**	**3.11**
18	0.025	5.98	4.56	3.95	3.61	3.38	3.22	3.10	3.01	2.77	2.50	2.19
	0.005	**10.22**	**7.21**	**6.03**	**5.37**	**4.96**	**4.66**	**4.44**	**4.28**	**3.86**	**3.40**	**2.87**
20	0.025	5.87	4.46	3.86	3.51	3.29	3.13	3.01	2.91	2.68	2.41	2.09
	0.005	**9.94**	**6.99**	**5.82**	**5.17**	**4.76**	**4.47**	**4.26**	**4.09**	**3.68**	**3.22**	**2.69**
30	0.025	5.57	4.18	3.59	3.25	3.03	2.87	2.75	2.65	2.41	2.14	1.79
	0.005	**9.18**	**6.35**	**5.24**	**4.62**	**4.23**	**3.95**	**3.74**	**3.58**	**3.18**	**2.73**	**2.18**
40	0.025	5.42	4.05	3.46	3.13	2.90	2.74	2.62	2.53	2.29	2.01	1.64
	0.005	**8.83**	**6.07**	**4.98**	**4.37**	**3.99**	**3.71**	**3.51**	**3.35**	**2.95**	**2.50**	**1.93**
60	0.025	5.29	3.93	3.34	3.01	2.79	2.63	2.51	2.41	2.17	1.88	1.48
	0.005	**8.49**	**5.79**	**4.73**	**4.14**	**3.76**	**3.49**	**3.29**	**3.13**	**2.74**	**2.29**	**1.69**
120	0.025	5.15	3.80	3.23	2.89	2.67	2.52	2.39	2.30	2.05	1.76	1.31
	0.005	**8.18**	**5.54**	**4.50**	**3.92**	**3.55**	**3.28**	**3.09**	**2.93**	**2.54**	**2.09**	**1.43**
∞	0.025	5.02	3.69	3.12	2.79	2.57	2.41	2.29	2.19	1.94	1.64	1.00
	0.005	**7.88**	**5.30**	**4.28**	**3.72**	**3.35**	**3.09**	**2.90**	**2.74**	**2.36**	**1.90**	**1.00**

TABLE A.6 PEARSON'S CORRELATION COEFFICIENT (*r*)

This table contains critical values of the sample correlation coefficient, r; it is used to test the null hypothesis that the true correlation coefficient (ρ) is equal to zero. For a given sample size (number of pairs), if the absolute value (i.e. ignoring its sign) of the sample correlation coefficient, r, is greater than the critical value, then the two-tailed P-value of the test is less than the tabulated P-value. If the sample correlation coefficient lies between two adjacent critical values, then the P-value for the test lies between the corresponding tabulated P-values. See Sec-

tion 10.3.2(b) if the sample size is greater than 150.

Note: This table can also be used to test the significance of Spearman's rank correlation coefficient (see Section 11.7.4), provided the sample size is greater than ten pairs. If the sample size is ten or less, refer to Table A.7.

Example: If the sample size is 14 and $r = 0.70$, then since $0.70 > 0.6614$, $P < 0.01$. Furthermore, since 0.70 lies between 0.6614 and 0.7800, $0.001 < P < 0.01$.

Table A.6   Critical values of Pearson's correlation coefficient (r).

Sample size	Two-tailed *P*-value			Sample size	Two-tailed *P*-value		
	0.05	0.01	0.001		0.05	0.01	0.001
3	0.9969	0.9999	1.0000	23	0.4132	0.5256	0.6402
4	0.9500	0.9900	0.9990	24	0.4044	0.5151	0.6287
5	0.8783	0.9587	0.9911	25	0.3961	0.5052	0.6177
6	0.8114	0.9172	0.9741	26	0.3882	0.4958	0.6073
7	0.7545	0.8745	0.9509	27	0.3809	0.4869	0.5974
8	0.7067	0.8343	0.9249	28	0.3739	0.4785	0.5880
9	0.6664	0.7977	0.8983	29	0.3673	0.4705	0.5790
10	0.6319	0.7646	0.8721	30	0.3610	0.4629	0.5703
11	0.6021	0.7348	0.8471	35	0.3338	0.4296	0.5322
12	0.5760	0.7079	0.8233	40	0.3120	0.4026	0.5007
13	0.5529	0.6835	0.8010	45	0.2940	0.3801	0.4742
14	0.5324	0.6614	0.7800	50	0.2787	0.3610	0.4514
15	0.5139	0.6411	0.7604	55	0.2656	0.3445	0.4317
16	0.4973	0.6226	0.7419	60	0.2542	0.3301	0.4143
17	0.4821	0.6055	0.7247	70	0.2352	0.3060	0.3850
18	0.4683	0.5897	0.7084	80	0.2199	0.2864	0.3611
19	0.4555	0.5751	0.6932	90	0.2072	0.2702	0.3412
20	0.4438	0.5614	0.6788	100	0.2172	0.2830	0.3569
21	0.4329	0.5487	0.6652	150	0.1603	0.2097	0.2660
22	0.4227	0.5368	0.6524				

TABLE A.7 SPEARMAN'S RANK CORRELATION COEFFICIENT (r_s)

This table contains critical values for Spearman's rank correlation coefficient, r_s, for small samples; it is used to test the null hypothesis that the true correlation coefficient (ρ_s) is equal to zero. If the sample size (number of pairs) is greater than ten, refer to Table A.6, which provides a good approximation. For a given sample size, if the absolute value (i.e. ignoring its sign) of the sample rank correlation coefficient, r_s, is greater than the critical value, then the two-tailed P-value of the test is less than the tabulated P-value. If the sample rank correlation coefficient lies between two adjacent critical values, then the two-tailed P-value for the test lies between the corresponding tabulated P-values.

Example: If the sample size is 6 and $r_s = 0.85$, since $0.85 > 0.83$, $P < 0.05$. Furthermore, since $0.8286 < 0.85 < 0.8857$, $0.02 < P < 0.05$.

Table A.7 Critical values of Spearman's rank correlation coefficient.

Sample size	\multicolumn{5}{c}{Two tailed P-value}				
	0.1	0.05	0.02	0.01	0.002
4	0.8000	–	–	–	–
5	0.8000	0.9000	0.9000	–	–
6	0.7714	0.8286	0.8857	0.9429	–
7	0.6786	0.7450	0.8571	0.8929	0.9643
8	0.6190	0.7143	0.8095	0.8571	0.9286
9	0.5833	0.6833	0.7667	0.8167	0.9000
10	0.5515	0.6364	0.7333	0.7818	0.8667
11	0.5273	0.6091	0.7000	0.7455	0.8364
12	0.4965	0.5804	0.6713	0.7273	0.8182
13	0.4780	0.5549	0.6429	0.6978	0.7912
14	0.4593	0.5341	0.6220	0.6747	0.7670
15	0.4429	0.5179	0.6000	0.6536	0.7464

TABLE A.8 THE SIGN TEST

This table contains two-tailed P-values for the sign test of the null hypothesis that the proportion of positive (or negative, whichever is the smaller) differences is equal to one half. k is the number of positive differences; n is the number of non-zero differences. Note that probabilities less than 0.001 are omitted.

Example: if $k = 3$ and $n = 10$, $P = 0.344$.

Table A.8 Two-tailed P-values for the sign test.

n	\multicolumn{10}{c}{k}
	0	1	2	3	4	5	6	7	8	9
4	0.125	0.624	1.00	–	–	–	–	–	–	–
5	0.062	0.376	1.00	–	–	–	–	–	–	–
6	0.032	0.218	0.688	1.00	–	–	–	–	–	–
7	0.016	0.124	0.454	1.00	–	–	–	–	–	–
8	0.008	0.070	0.290	0.726	1.00	–	–	–	–	–
9	0.004	0.040	0.180	0.508	1.00	–	–	–	–	–
10	0.002	0.022	0.110	0.344	0.754	1.00	–	–	–	–
11	0.001	0.012	0.066	0.226	0.548	1.00	–	–	–	–
12	–	0.006	0.038	0.146	0.388	0.774	1.00	–	–	–
13	–	0.004	0.022	0.092	0.266	0.582	1.00	–	–	–
14	–	0.002	0.012	0.058	0.180	0.424	0.790	1.00	–	–
15	–	–	0.008	0.036	0.118	0.302	0.608	1.00	–	–
16	–	–	0.004	0.022	0.076	0.210	0.554	0.804	1.00	–
17	–	–	0.002	0.012	0.050	0.144	0.332	0.630	1.00	–
18	–	–	0.002	0.004	0.030	0.096	0.238	0.480	0.814	1.00
19	–	–	–	0.004	0.020	0.064	0.168	0.360	0.648	1.00
20	–	–	–	0.002	0.012	0.042	0.116	0.264	0.504	0.824

TABLE A.9 THE WILCOXON SIGNED RANK TEST

This table contains the critical values for a two-tailed Wilcoxon signed rank test of n non-zero differences (see Section 11.4). It uses the sum of the positive ranks, T_+, or the negative ranks, T_-, of the differences. Then if T_+ (or T_-) is equal to or lies outside the tabulated critical values, the P-value for the two-sided test is less than tabulated P-value.

Example: If the number of non-zero differences is 10, and $T_+ = 5$, then since $5 < 8$, $P < 0.05$. However, since $5 > 3$, $P > 0.01$.

	Two-tailed P-value				
n	0.1	0.05	0.02	0.01	0.001
4	–	–	–	–	–
5	0–15	–	–	–	–
6	2–19	0–21	–	–	–
7	3–25	2–26	0–28	–	–
8	5–31	3–33	1–35	0–36	–
9	8–37	5–40	3–42	1–44	–
10	10–45	8–47	5–50	3–52	–
11	13–53	10–56	7–59	5–61	0–66
12	17–61	13–65	9–69	7–71	1–77
13	21–70	17–74	12–79	9–82	2–89
14	25–80	21–84	15–90	12–93	4–101
15	30–90	25–95	19–101	15–105	6–114
16	35–101	29–107	23–113	19–117	9–127
17	41–112	34–119	28–125	23–130	11–142
18	47–124	40–131	32–139	27–144	14–157
19	53–137	46–144	37–153	32–158	18–172
20	60–150	52–158	43–167	37–173	21–189
21	67–164	58–173	49–182	42–189	26–205
22	75–178	66–187	55–198	48–205	30–223
23	83–193	73–203	62–214	54–222	35–241
24	91–209	81–219	69–231	61–239	40–260
25	100–225	89–236	76–249	68–257	45–280

Table A.9 Critical values for the Wilcoxon signed rank test.

TABLE A.10 THE WILCOXON RANK SUM TEST

This table contains the critical values for a two-tailed Wilcoxon rank sum test comparing two samples of size n_1 and n_2, with $n_1 < n_2$ (see Section 11.5). Suppose T_1 is the sum of the ranks of the smaller sample. If $T_1 \leq$ the lower critical value, or if $T_1 \geq$ the upper critical value, then the two-tailed P-value of the test is less than the relevant tabulated P-value.

Example: If $n_1 = 10$, $n_2 = 14$ and $T_1 = 83$, then since 83 lies outside the limits 91–159, then $P < 0.05$; since 83 lies within the limits 81–169, then $P > 0.01$. Hence $0.01 < P < 0.05$.

Table A.10(a)   Critical values for the Wilcoxon rank sum test. Two-tailed $P = 0.05$.

n_1	4	5	6	7	8	9	10	11	12	13	14	15
n_2												
4	10–26	16–34	23–43	31–53	40–64	49–77	60–90	72–104	85–119	99–135	114–152	130–170
5	11–29	17–38	24–48	33–58	42–70	52–83	63–97	75–112	89–127	103–144	118–162	134–181
6	12–32	18–42	26–52	34–64	44–76	55–89	66–104	79–119	92–136	107–153	122–172	139–191
7	13–35	20–45	27–57	36–69	46–82	57–96	69–111	82–127	96–144	111–162	127–181	144–201
8	14–38	21–49	29–61	38–74	49–87	60–102	72–118	85–135	100–152	115–171	131–191	149–211
9	14–42	22–53	31–65	40–79	51–93	62–109	75–125	89–142	104–160	119–180	136–200	154–221
10	15–45	23–57	32–70	42–84	53–99	65–115	78–132	92–150	107–169	124–188	141–209	159–231
11	16–48	24–61	34–74	44–89	55–105	68–121	81–139	96–157	111–177	128–197	145–219	164–241
12	17–51	26–64	35–79	46–94	58–110	71–127	84–146	99–165	115–185	132–206	150–228	169–251
13	18–54	27–68	37–83	48–99	60–116	73–134	88–152	103–172	119–193	136–215	155–237	174–261
14	19–57	28–72	38–88	50–104	62–122	76–140	91–159	106–180	123–201	141–223	160–246	179–271
15	20–60	29–76	40–92	52–109	65–127	79–146	94–166	110–187	127–209	145–232	164–256	184–281
16	21–63	30–80	42–96	54–114	67–133	82–152	97–173	113–195	131–217	150–240	169–265	190–290
17	21–67	32–83	43–101	56–119	70–138	84–159	100–180	117–202	135–225	154–249	174–274	195–300
18	22–70	33–87	45–105	58–124	72–144	87–165	103–187	121–209	139–233	159–257	179–283	200–310
19	23–73	34–91	46–110	60–129	74–150	90–171	107–193	124–217	143–241	163–266	184–292	205–320
20	24–76	35–95	48–114	62–134	77–155	93–177	110 200	128–224	147–249	167–275	188–302	211–329

Table A.10(b) Critical values for the Wilcoxon rank sum test. Two-tailed $P = 0.01$.

n_1	4	5	6	7	8	9	10	11	12	13	14	15
n_2												
4	–	–	21–45	28–56	37–67	46–80	57–93	68–108	81–123	94–140	109–157	125–175
5	–	15–40	22–50	29–62	38–74	48–87	59–101	71–116	84–132	98–149	112–168	128–187
6	10–34	16–44	23–55	31–67	40–80	50–94	61–109	73–125	87–141	101–159	116–178	132–198
7	10–38	16–49	24–60	32–73	42–86	52–101	64–116	76–133	90–150	104–169	120–188	136–209
8	11–41	17–53	25–65	34–78	43 93	54–108	66–124	79–141	93–159	108–178	123–199	140–220
9	11–45	18–57	26–70	35–84	45–99	56–115	68–132	82–149	96–168	111–188	127–209	144–231
10	12–48	19–61	27–75	37–89	47–105	58–122	71–139	84–158	99–177	115–197	131–219	149–241
11	12–52	20–65	28–80	38–95	49–111	61–128	73–147	87–166	102–186	118–207	135–229	153–252
12	13–55	21–69	30–84	40–100	51–117	63–135	76–154	90–174	105–195	122–216	139–239	157–263
13	13–59	22–73	31–89	41–106	53–123	65–142	79–161	93–182	109–203	125–226	143–249	162–273
14	14–62	22–78	32–94	43–111	54–130	67–149	81–169	96–190	112–212	129–235	147–259	166–284
15	15–65	23–82	33–99	44–117	56–136	69–156	84–176	99–198	115–221	133–244	151–269	171–294
16	15–69	24–86	34–104	46–122	58–142	72–162	86–184	102–206	119–229	136–254	155–279	175–305
17	16–72	25–90	36–108	47–128	60–148	74–169	89–191	105–214	122–238	140–263	160–288	180–315
18	16–76	26–94	37–113	49–133	62–154	76–176	92–198	108–222	125–247	144–272	164–298	184–326
19	17–79	27–98	38–118	50–139	64–160	78–183	94–206	111–230	129–255	148–281	168 308	189–336
20	18–82	28–102	39–123	52–144	66–166	81–189	97–213	114–238	132–264	152–290	172–318	193–347

Table A.11   Table of random numbers.

77267	67258	38499	94709	46989	44360	46788	62666	67551	79212
72309	70484	25843	72251	82013	70561	14058	38073	53571	91594
54395	89438	92622	45780	29108	53340	85537	50232	28477	93512
98270	62867	44084	98370	59635	25367	30528	58516	78666	83753
66032	31218	29309	26890	34700	43168	09914	47240	51526	51115
57277	70054	60345	84988	24257	19358	39083	63075	67491	55733
85981	87059	50122	80180	98114	64749	75696	59666	43806	52538
75254	50278	61364	84524	18067	94064	42011	21085	79258	44419
71820	17948	38074	48411	63605	34244	96320	36384	80985	79176
55759	77728	41765	61731	27045	81464	44584	11390	85593	69342
92725	91260	25468	94632	44972	96413	93134	29630	70497	71787
18169	44658	95643	71214	61018	90640	59106	76377	90625	15455
55710	88227	84684	33948	29576	57306	96961	90832	52720	38631
49556	24412	93967	63006	69252	52089	29551	62555	54033	39961
87891	87778	61646	24558	16210	81147	16734	24214	45062	64957
18699	87766	21808	40788	77612	97617	34199	86693	51631	17475
96353	24916	71714	97492	42680	14894	87091	51667	10183	28272
58932	54779	81765	17127	76773	52970	52430	56064	62116	48515
60376	97508	91787	84684	39870	12608	11299	30277	87317	61131
71521	34632	82603	56428	71537	10548	10765	51679	45875	12404
17760	37556	52225	68445	18626	67414	62242	51329	80427	11747
36901	23375	21348	32148	47612	60511	24558	91901	50626	65405
17488	34113	69144	24953	13842	90301	38518	59852	96747	96478
16435	63514	78929	62326	89294	48853	35503	43729	89186	36601
79145	37322	17054	61899	74394	58695	77454	81735	98688	91397
96388	61117	31714	58107	85666	47675	33123	08943	75625	06598
38147	23339	32981	80989	96940	44860	39707	84883	26243	59861
95893	06491	95520	91538	35285	17192	80784	32664	49226	25919
53544	31391	23798	36857	16786	19639	93659	66776	34108	74268
03513	34015	78337	46158	92198	99481	70804	73939	39152	44116
92737	89927	81721	33548	78029	62464	53482	54191	95898	66099
10688	61502	73817	63841	87058	23377	24045	99470	17509	26636
51658	59565	61280	48120	38438	57832	25639	84632	38523	89459
53916	57066	46906	18657	79932	93039	62470	22405	78427	92145
40912	63211	63856	61644	18635	02946	30842	24031	36992	37917
75159	14888	59932	74222	39075	33201	33747	53800	79883	26609
25224	72513	58746	52366	73436	74699	80799	56699	16557	58671
82703	53196	34797	28093	97105	56797	39992	67944	00310	49311
51627	41127	86363	48078	27726	37269	21629	21785	25822	95264
02574	68647	82762	80442	70966	95743	56140	58213	78202	60038

Appendix B

Tables of Confidence Intervals

Table B.1 95%* Confidence intervals from a single sample: summary of results (see relevant sections for assumptions and explanation of notation).

Parameter	95% confidence interval	Section
Mean (μ)	$\bar{x} \pm t_{0.05}\text{SEM} = \bar{x} \pm t_{0.05}\dfrac{s}{\sqrt{n}}$ where degrees of freedom $= n - 1$	4.5
Proportion (π)	$p \pm 1.96\sqrt{\dfrac{p(1-p)}{n}}$ where $\quad p = \dfrac{r}{n}$	4.7
Correlation coefficient (ρ)	$\dfrac{e^{2z_1}-1}{e^{2z_1}+1} \quad \text{to} \quad \dfrac{e^{2z_2}-1}{e^{2z_2}+1}$ where $\quad z = \dfrac{1}{2}\log_e\dfrac{1+r}{1-r}$ $z_1 = z - \dfrac{1.96}{\sqrt{(n-3)}}, \quad z_2 = z + \dfrac{1.96}{\sqrt{(n-3)}}$	10.3.2(b)
Regression coefficient (β)	$b \pm t_{0.05}\text{SE}(b)$ where degrees of freedom $= n - 2$ $\text{SE}(b) = \dfrac{s_{\text{res}}}{\sqrt{\sum(x-\bar{x})^2}}$ $s_{\text{res}} = \sqrt{\dfrac{\sum(y-Y)^2}{n-2}}$	10.4.6

* Replace 1.96 by appropriate percentage point of the Standard Normal distribution (Table A.2) if a different CI is required, e.g. replace 1.96 by 2.58 for a 99% CI. Similarly, replace $t_{0.05}$ by $t_{0.10}$ for a 99% confidence interval.

Table B.2 95%* Confidence intervals from two samples: summary of results (see relevant sections for assumptions and explanation of notation).

Parameter	95% confidence interval	Section
Difference in means ($\mu_1 - \mu_2$):		
(a) Independent samples (equal variances)	$(\bar{x}_1 - \bar{x}_2) \pm t_{0.05} SE(\bar{x}_1 - \bar{x}_2)$ where degrees of freedom $= n_1 + n_2 - 2$ $$SE(\bar{x}_1 - \bar{x}_2) = \sqrt{s^2\left(\frac{1}{n_1} + \frac{1}{n_2}\right)}$$ $$s^2 = \frac{(n_1 - 1)s_1^2 + (n_2 - 1)s_2^2}{n_1 + n_2 - 2}$$	7.4.3
(b) Paired samples	$\bar{d} \pm t_{0.05} \dfrac{s_d}{\sqrt{n}}$ where degrees of freedom $= n - 1$ and s_d is the SD of the differences	7.5.3
Difference in proportions ($\pi_1 - \pi_2$):		
(a) Independent samples	$(p_1 - p_2) \pm 1.96\sqrt{\dfrac{p_1(1 - p_1)}{n_1} + \dfrac{p_2(1 - p_2)}{n_2}}$	9.4.3(c)
(b) Paired samples	$(p_1 - p_2) \pm 1.96\dfrac{1}{m}\sqrt{(f + g) - \dfrac{(f - g)^2}{m}}$ where e, f, g and h are defined in Table 9.4 and $p_1 = \dfrac{e + f}{m}$ and $p_2 = \dfrac{e + g}{m}$ so $p_1 - p_2 = \dfrac{f - g}{m}$	9.6.3

*The above are 95% CIs. For a different CI, replace the 1.96 in the formula by the appropriate percentage point in the table of the Standard Normal distribution (Table A.2), e.g. for a 90% CI, replace 1.96 by 1.64. Similarly, replace $t_{0.05}$ by $t_{0.10}$ for a 90% CI.

Appendix C

Flow Charts for Selection of Appropriate Tests

Fig. C.1 Flow chart for choosing appropriate statistical analysis (section number in brackets).

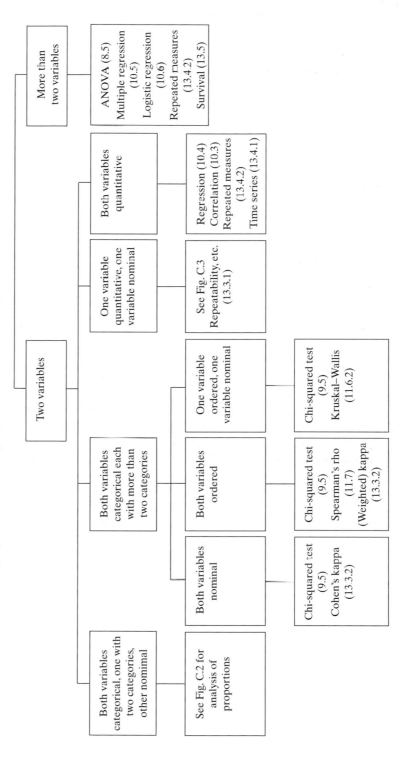

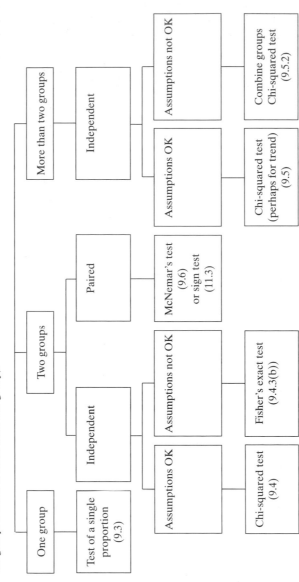

Fig. C.2 Flow chart for choosing appropriate tests for proportions derived from a binary variable (a nominal variable defines the groups if there is more than one group).

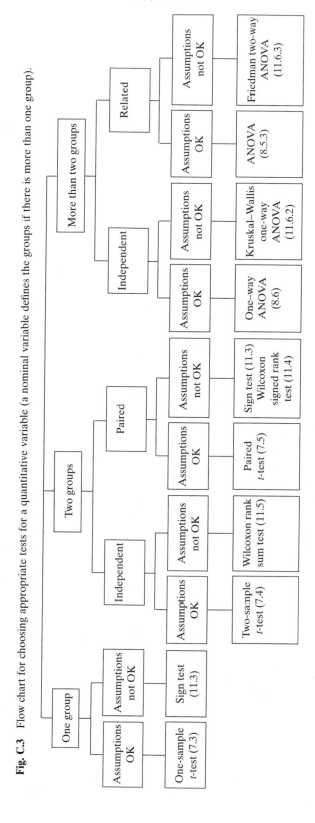

Fig. C.3 Flow chart for choosing appropriate tests for a quantitative variable (a nominal variable defines the groups if there is more than one group).

Appendix D

Glossary of Notation

We have used algebraic and mathematical notation throughout this book. The following glossary may help you understand some of that notation.

∞	Infinity.
$\pm$	This means that, in turn, we add and subtract the quantity following the sign to the quantity preceding it, to obtain two separate quantities. Hence, $x \pm y$ gives $(x + y)$ and $(x - y)$.
$\geq$	The value preceeding the sign is greater than or equal to the value after it.
$\leq$	The value preceeding the sign is less than or equal to the value after it.
$\log x$	This is the logarithm (log) of the number x. Sometimes we put brackets around the x if it aids clarification. See Section 12.2 for the uses of the logarithmic transformation. Logarithms can take different bases, the most usual ones being 10 and e (see below). In general terms, if $\log_y(x) = z$, then $x = y^z$, where the base of the logarithm is the number y. As long as we are consistent in using a particular base of a logarithm, and specify which base we are using, we can use the logarithm to any base. *Remember that the log of zero is infinity, and that we can only take logs of positive numbers.* We can obtain the values of logarithms from special tables or more usually from hand calculators. If we have two numbers a and b, say, then

(a) the log of their product is equal to the sum of the logs,

$$\log(ab) = \log(a) + \log(b)$$

(b) the log of their quotient is equal to the difference of their logs,

$$\log(a/b) = \log(a) - \log(b).$$

$\log_e x$	This is the Napierian or natural logarithm of x to base e, often written as $\ln x$, where e is the constant 2.71828. The logarithm to base e of a quantity x is the value z such that $x = e^z$. These logs are used most often in statistics and are generally used in computer packages.
$\log_{10} x$	This is the common logarithm to base 10 of x. If $\log_{10}(x) = z$, then $x = 10^z$. So, for example, $\log_{10}(10) = 1$ and $\log_{10}(100) = 2$. Logs to base 10 were used to simplify multiplication and division, relying on addition and subtraction instead, but are rarely used for this purpose now because of the advent of hand-held calculators.
e^x	This is the exponential function, sometimes written exp (x). If $x = \log_e(y)$, then $y = e^x$ is the antilogarithm of x. Thus, if we have taken a logarithmic transformation of a variable, we can transform back to the original scale by taking the antilog, using the exponential function of a calculator. Note that if we have taken logs to base 10 as a transformation, we can transform back to the original scale by using the antilog function 10^x.
$\|x\|$	The vertical lines to the left and right of the x indicate that we should ignore the sign of x, i.e. we should consider its 'absolute value'. So, for example, $\|-15.5\| = \|15.5\| = 15.5$.
x_i	If x denotes the value of a variable, such as age or systolic blood pressure, then the subscript, i, indicates that we are referring to the value of that variable for the ith individual in the sample or the population. If there are n individuals in the sample, then the sample values for that variable are $(x_1, x_2, x_3, \ldots, x_n)$.
$\displaystyle\sum_{i=1}^{n} x_i$	Commonly abbreviated to Σx. The Greek letter 'sigma', Σ, indicates that we are summing the values of the variable, x, for all the n individuals in the sample, i.e. from $i = 1$ to $i = n$. The abbreviation which omits the values of i both above and below the summation sign, and as the subscript of x, is used when no confusion can result. Clearly,

$$\sum_{i=1}^{n} x_i = x_1 + x_2 + x_3 + \ldots + x_n$$

$\bar{x}$	The sample mean of the variable, x. It is pronounced 'x bar', and is equal to the sum of all the values of x in the sample divided by the number of observations, n, in the sample (see Section 2.6.1). Hence

$$\overline{x} = \frac{x_1 + x_2 + x_3 + \ldots + x_n}{n} = \frac{1}{n}\sum_{i=1}^{n} x_i, \text{ often written as } \frac{1}{n}\sum x$$

μ The lower case Greek letter 'mu'. It represents the population mean. If there are N observations on the variable, x, in the population, then

$$\mu = \frac{1}{N}\sum_{i=1}^{N} x_i$$

$\sum_{i=1}^{n}(x_i - \overline{x})^2$ Commonly abbreviated to $\Sigma(x - \overline{x})^2$. It is called the sum of squared deviations, the corrected sum of squares or simply the sum of squares. We take the sample mean, $\overline{x}$, from each value of x in the sample, and then square this difference; repeating this procedure for all n values of x in the sample, we obtain a set of n squared differences which we then add up.

s The estimated population standard deviation obtained from a sample of n observations, thus

$$s = \sqrt{\frac{\sum_{i=1}^{n}(x_i - \overline{x})^2}{n-1}}$$

Its square, s^2, is the estimated population variance.

σ The population standard deviation. If there are N observations on the variable, x, in the population, then

$$\sigma = \sqrt{\frac{\sum_{i=1}^{N}(x_i - \mu)^2}{N}}$$

Its square, σ^2, is the population variance.

SD   The standard deviation of a set of observations.

SEM   The standard error of the sample mean.

SE(b)   The standard error of a statistic, b.

CI   Confidence interval; it contains the parameter of interest with a prescribed probability.

SND   A Standardized Normal Deviate given by

$$z = \frac{x - \mu}{\sigma}$$

where the variable, x, is Normally distributed with mean $= \mu$ and SD $= \sigma$. The SND has a Normal distribution with mean $= 0$ and SD $= 1$.

RCT   A randomized controlled trial.

R^2 The coefficient of determination. It is the proportion of the variance of the response variable, y, explained by it relationship with the explanatory variables in a multiple regression analysis

r The sample estimate of Pearson's product moment correlation coefficient, expressed as

$$r = \frac{\sum(x - \overline{x})(y - \overline{y})}{\sqrt{\sum(x - \overline{x})^2 \sum(y - \overline{y})^2}}$$

ρ The Greek letter 'rho'. The population value of the Pearson's product moment correlation coefficient.

r_s The sample estimate of Spearman's rank correlation coefficient. It is equal to the Pearson product moment correlation coefficient between the ranks of the observations in the sample.

ρ_s The population value of Spearman's rank correlation coefficient.

p The proportion of 'successes' in a sample, i.e. the proportion of individuals in the sample possessing some characteristic.

π The Greek letter 'pi'. The proportion of individuals in the population possessing some characteristic.

b Often used to refer to an estimated regression coefficient.

β The Greek letter 'beta'. It usually refers to the true value of a regression coefficient representing the gradient of the line.

α The Greek letter 'alpha'. It may refer to the constant term in a regression equation; alternatively, it sometimes refers to the significance level of a hypothesis test (the cut-off value for the P-value leading to rejection of the null hypothesis).

κ The Greek letter 'kappa'. A measure of agreement for categorical variables.

δ The Greek letter 'delta'. Sometimes used to refer to a difference of interest in the population.

PPV   The positive predictive value of a diagnostic or screening test – the proportion of those testing positive who actually have the disease.

NPV   The negative predictive value of a diagnostic or screening test – the proportion of those testing negative who really are disease free.

P The P-value; the probability of obtaining the observed results (or more extreme results) if the null hypothesis is true.

H_0 The null hypothesis (H nought).

$Test_i$ The test statistic used to test a particular null hypothesis ($i = 1, 2, \ldots, 14$).

df The degrees of freedom of a statistic, i.e. the number of independent observations contributing to the value of the statistic.

χ^2 Chi-squared; a particular continuous probability distribution

F A particular continuous probability distribution

t A particular continuous probability distribution

$t_{0.05}$ This is the percentage point or critical value of the t-distribution (see Table A. 3) which gives a total tail area probability of 0.05, i.e. 2.5% of the total area under the curve is contained in the tail to the left of $-t_{0.05}$, and 2.5% is contained in the tail to the right of $t_{0.05}$.

Appendix E

Glossary of Terms

***a priori* probability** a way of evaluating the probability of an outcome solely on the basis of a theoretical model. Hence it may be called the model definition of probability.

accuracy refers to how well the observed value of a quantity agrees with the true value.

addition rule the probability of either of two mutually exclusive events occurring is the sum of the probability of each event.

adjusted R^2 a corrected value of R^2 (see coefficient of determination) which allows multiple regression models with differing numbers of explanatory variables to be compared when assessing goodness-of-fit.

all subsets selection the process of determining an optimal regression model which examines all the possible models for the various combinations of the explanatory variables of interest.

alternative hypothesis the proposition (statement) which disagrees with the hypothesis under test (the null hypothesis).

Altman's nomogram a graphic representation showing the relationship between sample size, power and standardized difference; it can be used to determine any one with knowledge of the other two. The standardized difference is a reflection of the variability of the observations and the minimum magnitude of the treatment effect considered important.

analysis of covariance (ANCOVA) an extension to the analysis of variance which takes account of the values of one or more subsidiary variables (the covariates).

analysis of variance (ANOVA) a powerful collection of parametric statistical procedures for the analysis of data, essentially comparing the means of various groups of data. It relies on separating the total variation of a variable into

its component parts which are associated with defined sources of variation.

ANCOVA *see* analysis of covariance.

angular transformation *see* arcsin transformation.

ANOVA *see* analysis of variance.

arcsine transformation a transformation for a proportion, p, to $\sin^{-1}\sqrt{p}$. It linearizes a sigmoid curve and stabilizes variance. Also called the angular transformation or inverse sine transformation.

arithmetic mean (usually abbreviated to the **mean**) a measure of location; it is the sum of the observations divided by the number of observations in the set.

artificial pairing two different animals which have been matched with respect to any variables that may be thought to influence response.

attributable risk the proportion of the total risk of the disease that is attributable to a factor.

autoregressive series a time series in which the value of an observation is dependent on the preceding observation(s).

average a measure of location of a set of observations which describes central tendency, e.g. mean, median, mode.

backward step-down selection the process of selecting an optimal regression model in which, starting with all the explanatory variables in the model, we remove them sequentially (beginning with the variable which contributes the least) until the deletion of a variable significantly increases the residual variance.

bar chart a diagram in which every category of a variable is represented by the length of a bar depicting the number or percentage of individuals belonging to that category.

Berkson–Gage survival curve   a survival curve based on actuarial life tables; its calculations require knowledge of the time intervals within which the critical events (e.g. death) occur.

bias   systematic distortion of the data.

bimodal   a distribution which has two modes or modal groups.

binary variable   a discrete random variable with only two possible values. Also called a dichotomous variable.

Binomial distribution   a discrete probability distribution of a variable representing the number of successes in trials in which there are only two outcomes – success (with a fixed probability) and failure.

biological (clinical) importance   the considered judgement of what is relevant in the particular circumstances of the investigation; it should be contrasted with statistical significance.

biological variation   an inherent variability in biological material such that measurements taken from different individuals will rarely be identical.

biometry   a broad numerical approach to biology including study design, data collection, analysis, display and the drawing of appropriate conclusions (*see* statistics).

blind   either the carer of the animals in a clinical trial or the investigator, or both, have no knowledge of the specific treatments the animals receive.

block   a group of individuals in an experimental design which are observed in particular circumstances (e.g. after individuals are allocated a treatment). Blocks are usually created to isolate sources of variability, so that the individuals within a block exhibit less variability than in the general population.

blocked randomization   a method of randomly allocating individuals to treatments with the aim of achieving approximately equal numbers of individuals in each treatment group. Also called restricted randomization.

Bonferroni's correction   a method of reducing the risk of a Type I error when using multiple comparisons; it involves multiplying the *P*-value obtained from any one test by the number of multiple comparisons.

bootstrapping   an iterative method of estimating parameters of interest based on resampling.

box-and-whisker plot   a diagram which shows the distribution of data. It usually comprises a box whose horizontal limits are defined by the upper and lower quartiles enclosing the central 50% of the observations, with the median marked by a horizontal line within the box. The whiskers are vertical lines extending from the box as low as the 2.5th percentile and as high as the 97.5th percentile.

British Standards Institution repeatability coefficient   a measure of the repeatability of a method; it gives an indication of the maximum difference likely to occur between two measurements.

capture–tag–recapture method   a method of estimating the size of a wildlife population.

case-control study   a form of observational study. At the start of the investigation, we identify animals as being either diseased (cases) or healthy (controls). Then we assess whether the animals in the two groups have differences in past exposure to various risk factors.

censored data   animals in survival analysis who are alive at the end of the study or who are lost to follow up.

central tendency   indicates a position which represents the middle of a group of observations.

Chi-squared (χ^2) distribution   a continuous probability distribution which is often used in hypothesis testing of proportions.

Chi-squared (χ^2) test   a non-parametric test, based on the Chi-squared distribution, which is often used to compare proportions.

Chi-squared (χ^2) test for trend   a specific chi-squared test used to determine whether there is a linear trend in proportions classified by an ordinal variable.

clinical field trial   a comparative study involving new treatments or preventive measures applied under natural, field or semi-field conditions.

clinical trial   a form of experimental study in controlled conditions which is designed to assess the effectiveness of one or more treatments or preventive measures when these are applied to humans or animals.

cluster sampling a form of random sampling in which subdivisions or clusters of the population are identified; a simple random sample of clusters is selected and all the units within the selected clusters studied.

coefficient of determination (R^2) the proportion of the total variance of the dependent variable, y, in a regression model which is explained by the regression.

coefficient of variation (CV) the standard deviation expressed as a percentage of the mean.

Cohen's kappa coefficient a measure of the agreement between two categorical assessments.

cohort study a form of observational study. We start by defining groups (cohorts) of animals by the exposure of the animals in the groups to the factors of interest; we usually follow these animals forward in time and observe the outcome (e.g. disease).

collinearity (multicollinearity) when two or more of the explanatory variables in a multiple regression model exhibit a linear relationship and are very highly correlated.

complete randomized block design each block in the experimental design contains a complete set of treatments.

confidence band, region or interval for the line the region around a linear regression line within which we believe the true line lies with a prescribed degree of certainty.

confidence interval the range of values which contains a population parameter (e.g. the mean) with a given probability.

confidence limits the upper and lower values of the confidence interval.

confounder an explanatory variable which is related both to the response of interest and to another (or more than one) explanatory variable so that it is impossible to separate the effects of the two explanatory variables on the response.

contemporary control animals are assigned to control or test treatment at the same time.

contingency table a table of frequencies which shows how individuals are classified into the different categories of two or more factors.

continuity correction a correction applied to a test statistic to facilitate the approximation of a discrete distribution (of the test statistic) to a continuous distribution (such as the Chi-squared distribution).

continuous scale all values are theoretically possible (perhaps limited by an upper and/or lower boundary), e.g. height, weight.

continuous variable one which can take an infinite set of possible values in a range.

control group a group of individuals in an experimental study who receive either the standard treatment or no active treatment; it is used as a basis for comparison with the group of individuals receiving the active treatment(s).

controlled clinical trial a clinical trial which includes a control group.

correlation coefficient Pearson's correlation coefficient measures of the degree of linear association between two variables. *See also* Spearman's correlation coefficient.

covariate a factor that may influence the response. Also called an explanatory or independent variable.

Cox's proportional hazards model an advanced regression approach to survival analysis, used when we desire to investigate the effect of several variables on survival and also to take censored data into account.

critical value (or percentage point) the value of a test statistic, determined from a theoretical probability distribution, which corresponds to a given tail area probability (say, 0.05).

cross-over trial two or more treatments are applied in random order to each individual animal. The aim is to examine the effects of the treatments within the animals, rather than between animals, thereby enhancing the precision of the estimate of the differences between treatments.

cross-sectional study one in which we take all our measurements on the individuals included in the study at a given point in time.

cumulative relative frequency distribution shows the accumulated proportions of individuals which are contained in a category (class) and in all lower categories.

cumulative relative frequency polygon a

diagram showing a cumulative relative frequency distribution. It is formed by joining cumulative relative frequencies which correspond to the class midpoints.

degrees of freedom (*df*)　the number of independent observations contributing to the value of a statistic, i.e. the number of observations available to evaluate that statistic minus the number of restrictions on those observations.

dependent variable　the variable in a regression model which can be predicted by the explanatory (independent) variable(s). Also called the response or outcome variable.

descriptive statistics　that branch of statistics concerned with describing and characterizing the data distribution and summarizing and displaying the findings.

design　the plan of the study or experiment which should take into account any factors which may affect the response of interest.

diagnostic service　analyses animal samples for the benefit of health monitoring and diagnosis of disease.

diagnostic test　a procedure that is able to distinguish between diseased and healthy animals.

diagram　a means of displaying data pictorially.

digit preference　when there is an element of judgement involved in making readings from instruments, certain digits between 0 and 9 are more commonly chosen than others; it varies from individual to individual.

discrete (discontinuous) scale　data can take only integer values, typically counts, e.g. litter size, clutch size, parity.

discrete variable　taking only a finite set of possible values.

distance sampling　a method of estimating parameters of interest using a sampling procedure which obtains estimates by recording the number and frequency of species from a transect line. The method is based on the proposition that the detection of randomly distributed subjects declines with distance from the transect line.

distribution　*see* empirical frequency distribution and probability distribution.

distribution-free tests　*see* non-parametric methods.

dot diagram/plot　used to show the distribution of a data set. Each observation is marked as a dot on a line calibrated in the units of measurement of the variable.

double-blind　neither the carer(s) of the animals in a clinical trial nor the assessor of response to treatment (test or control) is aware of which treatment each animal is receiving.

dummy　*see* placebo.

Duncan's multiple range test　a multiple comparisons test of the means in three or more independent groups.

effect　a measure of the compaison of interest. *See also* treatment effect.

element　a single object or individual or unit of investigation.

empirical frequency distribution　shows the frequency of occurrence of the observations in a data set.

epidemiological study　a particular form of an analytical sample survey; it is concerned with investigating the aetiology of a disease by determining whether various factors (termed risk factors) are associated with the occurrence and distribution of the disease in the population.

estimation　the process of generating an approximation of a population parameter using sample data.

experimental study　we intervene in the study; we then observe the effect of our intervention on the response of interest, usually with a view to establishing whether a change in response may be directly attributable to our action.

experimental unit　the basic subject for experimentation; it is usually the individual, but may be a group. The entire assembly of the experimental units is the population from which a sample may be taken.

explanatory variable　*see* independent variable.

***F*-test**　*see* variance ratio test.

***F*-distribution**　a continuous probability distribution; it is used to compare variances.

factor　a variable with one or more categories

(levels) into which individuals can be classified.

Fisher's exact test a test for which the exact *P*-value is calculated in a hypothesis test of data presented in a contingency table; this approach is preferable to using the Chi-squared approximation to the Chi-squared test statistic when the expected frequencies in the table are very small.

fixed sample size plans study designs in which the sample size is predetermined before the data are collected.

forward step-up selection the process of selecting an optimal regression model; we start with the explanatory variable which contributes the most to the explained variation in *y*, and include more variables in the equation, progressively, until the addition of an extra variable does not significantly improve the situation.

frame a complete list of sampling units.

frequency the number of times a particular value (or range of values) of a variable occurs.

frequency definition of probability relies on counting the frequency of occurrence of the event in a large number of repetitions of similar trials.

frequency distribution *see* distribution.

Friedman two-way ANOVA a non-parametric equivalent to the two-way ANOVA.

Gaussian distribution *see* Normal distribution.

geometric mean a measure of location. It is the antilog of the arithmetic mean of the log transformed values of a variable.

goodness-of-fit examines the agreement between an observed set of values and another set of values which are derived under some theory or hypothesis.

group a collection of animals or experimental units.

group randomization the randomization process is applied to the whole group of units rather than to the individual units within a group.

group sequential design involves interim analyses of the data.

herd immunity if the experimental unit is the animal rather than the group, the protection afforded the vaccinated animals leads to a reduced prevalence of disease in the group environment, resulting in a reduced incidence of disease in the control animals.

heteroscedasticity the variances of the observations in different groups are not equal.

histogram a two-dimensional diagram illustrating a frequency distribution of a continuous variable. Usually, the horizontal axis represents the units of measurement of the variable; rectangles above each class interval (of constant width) indicate the frequency for that class by their height.

historical control animals are not assigned to control or test treatment(s) contemporaneously; information from historical controls is obtained from past records.

homoscedasticity the variances of the observations in different groups are equal.

human error variability in the measurements due to human mistakes.

hypothesis testing the process of formulating and testing a proposition about the population using the sample data.

hypothetical (or infinite) population the population does not exist but can be conceptualized (e.g. the population of animals who might receive a novel treatment).

hysteresis the phenomenon whereby a series of values recorded as they are increasing in magnitude are different from those when they are decreasing in magnitude; seen in some instruments.

incidence (of a condition) the number (percentage) of new cases of the disease that develop in a defined time period.

incomplete block designs each block in an experiment does not contain the entire set of treatments.

independent two events are independent if the probability of one occurring is not affected by the occurrence of the other event.

independent variable the variable in a regression analysis which is used to predict the value of the dependent or response variable. It is also called the regression, explanatory or predictor variable or the covariate.

inferential statistics that branch of statistics

concerned with drawing conclusions about a population using sample information.

instability or drift   a form of instrumental error in which the calibration varies.

instrumental error   inaccuracies introduced by the mechanical or electronic devices used to make the measurements.

intention to treat   the process of statistical analysis of data from an experiment in which animals which deviate from the protocol (withdrawals) are analysed as if they are still in the treatment groups to which they were originally assigned.

interaction   an interaction is present when two factors are not independent; then the difference in the response of interest between any two levels of one factor is not constant for different levels of the other factor.

interim analysis   a decision is made, before the fixed sample size investigation starts, to perform an analysis of the data at a predetermined time before the end of the investigation. Hence the term 'repeated significance test'.

interquartile range   the range of values which encloses the central 50% of the observations if the observations are arranged in rank order.

inverse sine   *see* arcsine transformation.

Kaplan-Meier survival curve   a survival curve based on known survival times and which incorporates censored data.

kappa coefficient   *see*   Cohen's kappa coefficient.

Kendall's tau   a non-parametric correlation coefficient.

Kolmogorov-Smirnov test   a test which can be used to test whether data come from a particular distribution (e.g. the Normal) or whether two groups of data come from the same distribution.

Kruskal–Wallis one-way ANOVA   a non-parametric equivalent to the one-way ANOVA, used to compare independent groups of observations.

kurtosis   a term used to describe the peakedness of a unimodal frequency curve.

laboratory experiment   a particular form of experimental study in the laboratory in which

the experimental intervention is highly regulated and controlled.

learning objectives   task-oriented terms indicating what you should be able to 'do' when you have mastered the concepts to test your growing understanding; if you are able to perform the tasks specified in the learning objectives, you have understood the concepts.

level   a particular category of a qualitative variable or factor, e.g. dose levels of a drug, different treatments.

level of significance   *see* significance level.

Levene's test   a parametric test used to investigate the equality of variance in two or more groups.

limits of agreement   the range of values between which most (usually 95%) of the differences between pairs of observations lie.

linear   straight line.

linear correlation coefficient   a measure of the linear association between two variables.

linear regression analysis   a formal process of estimating the coefficients of the linear regression equation and making inferences from it.

linear regression equation   describes the linear relationship between two variables when one variable is dependent on the other.

logistic regression   *see*   multiple logistic regression.

logistic (logit) transformation   the transformation, $\log_e\{p/(1-p)\}$, of the proportion, p, used to linearize a sigmoid curve.

Lognormal distribution   a continuous probability distribution. If data which are skewed to the right are log transformed, and the resulting distribution is Normal, the data are said to approximate a Lognormal distribution.

logrank test   a non-parametric test which compares survival curves.

longitudinal study   one in which we investigate changes over time.

lower quartile   the 25th percentile.

Mann-Whitney U test   a non-parametric test used to compare two groups of independent observations. It produces the same result as the Wilcoxon rank sum test.

Mantel–Haenszel method   the correct approach to combining the results contained in contingency tables which relate to different strata of the population.

McNemar's test a test, based on the Chi-squared test, which compares two proportions in paired data.

mean *see* arithmetic mean.

mean square the sum of squares divided by the degrees of freedom; an estimate of variance.

measure of agreement describes how well pairs of observations conform to one another; it may be calculated as the SD of the differences between pairs of measurements.

measure of dispersion a measure of how widely scattered the observations are in either direction from their average.

measure of location some form of average which measures the central tendency of the data set.

median a measure of location. It is the central value in the set of observations which have been arranged in rank order.

median survival time the time which corresponds to a survival probability of 0.5 in survival analysis.

meta-analysis (overview) a systematic approach to combining the information from several independent studies of a given condition in order to arrive at a statistical summary of the numerical results.

method agreement also called reproducibility – concerned with gauging the similarity of different methods of measurement, e.g. different observers using the same technique, or a single observer using different techniques.

method of least squares a mathematical technique for finding the best fitting line through a series of points. It relies on minimizing the sum of the squared deviations from the line.

modal group or **modal class** the group or class of a frequency distribution which contains more observations than any other class.

mode the most commonly occurring observation in a set of observations.

model definition of probability *see a priori* probability.

multicollinearity *see* collinearity.

multiple comparisons the process of performing many hypothesis tests in a data set; it re-sults in increasing the risk of a Type I error unless adjustments are made.

multiple correlation coefficient (*R*) the square root of the coefficient of determination. *R* measures the association between the observed values of the dependent variable and the values of it obtained from the equation.

multiple linear logistic regression often called *logistic regression* – a model in which interest is centred on the dependency of binary response variable on a number of explanatory variables. This binary variable indicates whether or not an individual possesses a characteristic; the logistic regression shows the linear relationship between the explanatory variables and the logit transformation of the proportion of individuals with the characteristic.

multiple linear regression equation often called *multiple regression* – a mathematical expression which describes the linear relationship between two or more explanatory variables and a dependent variable.

multiplication rule the probability of two independent events occurring is the product of the probability of each event.

multi-stage sampling a simple random sample of clusters is selected from a population of clusters. In two-stage sampling, a simple random sample of units is selected for observation from the selected clusters. This process can be extended to encompass more stages.

multivariate analysis a general term traditionally used to describe a number of techniques which examine several response or dependent variables simultaneously, when every individual takes a value for each of the variables.

natural pairing litter mates, or some other biological association, provide the experimental material.

negative control the animal receives no active treatment. A negative control group is a group of such animals.

negative predictive value (NPV) the proportion of animals with a negative test result (i.e. shown by the test not to have the disease) which are disease-free.

Newman–Keuls test a multiple comparisons test of the means in independent groups.

nominal scale   the distinct categories which define the variable are unordered and each can be assigned a name, e.g. coat colour.

non-parametric tests   often called *distribution-free tests* – methods which make no assumptions about the underlying data distributions.

Normal or **Gaussian distribution**   a continuous probability distribution. It is a bell-shaped distribution and is approximated by many biological variables.

Normal plot   a diagram scaled in such a way that Normally distributed data are exhibited as a straight line. Deviations from the straight line suggest that the data are not Normally distributed.

null hypothesis (H_0)   the term given to the proposition that is under test in a hypothesis testing procedure. In general, it is expressed in terms of no treatment effect, e.g. no difference in means.

numerical measure   a characteristic which takes a quantitative value.

observational study   we merely observe the animals in the study and record the relevant measurements on those animals; we make no attempt to intervene, for example, by administering treatments or withholding factors which we feel may affect the course of the condition.

odds of exposure   the ratio of the probability of being exposed to the probability of being unexposed.

odds ratio   the ratio of two odds, usually the odds of exposure in the diseased group divided by the odds of exposure in the control group; an estimate of the relative risk.

one-sample *t*-test   a parametric test based on the *t*-distribution used to test H_0 that the true mean takes a particular value.

one-sided test   a hypothesis test in which the *P*-value is determined by referring the test statistic to only a single tail of a theoretical distribution. The *a priori* decision to make a test one-sided relies on the specification of the alternative hypothesis which must indicate the direction of the treatment effect based on the impossibility of the effect occurring in the other direction.

one-tailed probability   the *P*-value resulting from a one-sided test such that all the probability of interest is contained in only a single tail area of the theoretical distribution.

one-tailed test   see one-sided test.

one-way ANOVA   an extension of the two-sample *t*-test when we wish to compare the means of more than two independent groups of observations.

one-way repeated measures ANOVA   may be regarded as an extension of the paired *t*-test when means are to be compared in three or more groups of related observations.

ordered variable   a categorical variable which has some basis of order or ranking in the various categories, e.g. body condition scores, age categories.

ordinal scale   the categories which constitute the variable have some intrinsic order but the intervals between the various categories cannot be interpreted in a consistent manner.

outcome variable   *see* dependent variable.

outlier   an observation whose value is highly inconsistent with the main body of the data.

overview   *see* meta-analysis.

paired observations   each observation in one group is paired or individually matched with an observation in the other group.

paired *t*-test   a parametric test based on Student's *t*-distribution used to investigate paired data in two groups.

parallel group design   each individual animal receives only one treatment, and treatment comparisons are made between groups of animals rather than within animals.

parameter   a characteristic in the population, such as the mean or SD, which describes a particular feature of a distribution.

parametric test   this investigates a hypothesis about the parameter(s) of a distribution and makes assumptions about the underlying form of the distribution of the observations, e.g. that it is Normal, or that there is equality of variance.

partial regression coefficient   the coefficient in the multiple regression equation which corresponds to a particular explanatory variable. It is generally different from the regression coefficient which would be obtained by regressing the dependent variable on that explanatory variable alone, omitting the other explanatory variables from the equation altogether. It is sometimes called the *regression coefficient*.

Pearson's product moment correlation coefficient *see* correlation coefficient.

percentage point the upper percentage point (percentile) is the value of the variable which has $p\%$ of the distribution of the variables to the right of it. The lower percentage point has $p\%$ to the left of it. For a two-tailed test, we consider the percentage of the distribution in both tails, i.e. to the right and left of the relevant percentage points.

percentiles the values of the variable which divide the total frequency into 100 equal parts.

pharmaceutical and agrichemical industries industrial and commercial companies whose products may raise issues concerned with risks to human health derived from farming, e.g. drug residues in carcasses at slaughter, pesticides and fertilizer residues in plants.

pictogram a diagram, often used to display the frequency distribution of a data set, in which the frequency in a category is indicated by some measure (e.g. the height, number of repeated images) of a pictorial representation of a relevant object.

pie chart a diagram used to display the frequency distribution of a data set. It is a circle divided into segments with each segment portraying a different category of the qualitative variable. The area of a segment is proportional to the percentage of individuals in that category.

pilot study a small-scale preliminary investigation.

placebo a pharmacologically inert substance identical in appearance to the test treatment, which dissociates the pharmacological effect of treatment from any suggestive element (the placebo effect) imposed by the receipt of treatment.

placebo effect the response induced by suggestion on the part of the animal attendants or investigators when the animal receives a placebo (dummy) treatment.

Poisson distribution a discrete probability distribution of the count of the number of events occurring randomly in time or space at a constant rate on average.

polynomial a non-linear or curvilinear relationship described by a regression equation in which the degree of the polynomial is determined by the power of the explanatory variable(s), e.g. for the explanatory variable, x, the quadratic equation includes the term x^2, the cubic equation includes the term x^3, etc.

population the complete finite (real) or infinite (hypothetical) collection of observational units.

population survey an observational study of the entire population, e.g. a census.

positive control in clinical trials, a standard therapy against which a novel therapy is compared. In laboratory studies, it is a treatment inducing the maximum response.

positive predictive value (PPV) the proportion of animals with a positive test result (i.e. shown by the test to have the disease) which have the disease.

power (of a test) the probability that a test will reject the null hypothesis when the null hypothesis is false; it is the chance of detecting as statistically significant a true treatment effect of a given size.

power-efficiency a way of comparing the power of a parametric test and that of its non-parametric equivalent. It is the extent to which the sample size of the non-parametric test needs to be increased to make it as powerful as its parametric equivalent.

precision refers to how well repeated observations agree with one another.

predictive value *see* positive predictive value and negative predictive value.

predictor variable *see* independent variable.

prevalence (of a condition) the number (percentage) of cases of the disease that exist at a specific instant in time (point prevalence) or in a defined interval of time (period prevalence).

probability the chance of a particular event occurring.

probability density function the curve, defined by a mathematical formula which describes the relative frequency distribution of the population. The total area under the curve is one, and the proportion of observations between any two limits is the area under the curve between these limits.

probability distribution   a theoretical distribution which we specify mathematically, and use to calculate the theoretical probability of an event occurring.

probability sampling   *see* random sample.

proportion   the ratio of the number of events of interest to the total number of events.

proportional or **scale error**   a technical error in which the magnitude of the inaccuracy in measurement increases (or decreases) with the magnitude of the value.

prospective longitudinal study   the study is conducted forwards in time from a defined starting point.

publication bias   the tendency for journals to accept only significant results for publication, thereby giving undue weight to positive treatment effects in meta-analyses.

published scientific literature   information available to the student and professional from the work of others and published in scientific journals, textbooks and magazines, and electronically (e.g. on the Internet).

P-**value**   the *P*-value in a hypothesis test is the probability of obtaining the observed results (or more extreme results) if the null hypothesis is true.

qualitative/categorical variable   an individual belongs to any one of two or more distinct categories of the variable.

quality control   ensuring that processes and procedures are carried out in a consistently satisfactory manner so that the results are trustworthy.

quantitative variable   consists of numerical values on a well-defined scale.

random allocation   assigning of animals to groups (e.g. treatments) in a randomized manner (i.e. the process is based on chance). Also referred to as randomization.

random error   the recorded values are evenly distributed above and below the true value; it is due to unexplained sources.

randomization   this is the same as random allocation. In addition, a set of objects is said to be randomized if they are arranged in random order.

randomized block   a particular ANOVA design in which each of the treatments in the investigation is randomly allocated to the units within a 'block', the complete design comprising a number of such blocks.

randomized controlled trial (RCT)   a clinical trial which incorporates at least one control group, and which uses randomization to allocate the animals to the different treatment and control groups.

random sample   a selection made from the population such that every individual in the sample has an equal chance of selection, and the selection of one individual has no influence on the selection of subsequent individuals.

random selection   the process whereby individuals are chosen to be included in a random sample.

random variable   a variable which can take various values with given probabilities. All the values that the random variable can take, with their associated probabilities, comprise the probability distribution of the random variable.

range   the difference between the largest and smallest observations in a data set.

rank order   a systematized arrangement of the data values in ascending or descending order.

ranks   the successive numbers, starting at 1, assigned to the values of the observations in a data set which have been arranged in ascending (or descending) order. Thus, the rank of the smallest observation is 1, of the next smallest is 2, etc.

raw data   *see* readings.

readings   primary measurements taken from individual animals or biological samples (*see also* values, raw data).

real (or finite) population   the individuals in the population actually exist (cf. hypothetical population).

receiver operating characteristic curve (ROC curve) a plot of the sensitivity of a test against (1 – specificity); it is used to choose the cut-off value of a continuous variable which will lead to the optimal diagnostic or screening test.

reference interval *see* reference range.

reference range or **reference interval** the range of values of a variable which defines the healthy population, usually calculated as the interval which encompasses the central 95% of the observations; if the data are Normally distributed, it is defined by the mean ± 1.96SD.

regression coefficient this usually refers to the coefficient which corresponds to the explanatory variable in a simple linear regression equation, i.e. it is the gradient or slope of the line (β estimated by b), and represents the average change in the dependent variable for a unit change in the explanatory variable. Sometimes, the constant term (the intercept) in simple linear regression is also referred to as a regression coefficient. Furthermore, the partial regression coefficient in a multiple regression equation is sometimes called the regression coefficient.

regression of *y* on *x* the equation (usually a linear model) which describes the relationship between a dependent variable, *y*, and an explanatory variable, *x*.

regression to the mean a phenomenon whereby animals which may have been selected for study because they had extreme measurements on the variable of interest, are likely to have measurements which are closer to the average if the measurement is repeated on a second occasion.

regressor variable *see* independent variable.

relative frequency distribution shows the proportion or percentage of observations in each class or category of the distribution.

relative risk the ratio of two risks, usually the ratio of the risk of disease in the 'exposed' group to the risk of disease in the 'unexposed' group. It provides a measure of the strength of the association between the disease and the exposure to the factor. If the relative risk is unity, then exposure to the factor does not affect the animal's chance of developing the disease; if it is greater than unity it indicates the increased risk associated with 'exposure'.

repeatability the extent to which replicate measurements in identical circumstances of a particular technique or instrument or observer are the same.

repeated measures design an experimental design where each animal is investigated at every level of a factor, so the effects of interest are examined on a within-animal basis; e.g. when each animal receives all treatments or is investigated at a number of time-points. *See also* one-way repeated measures ANOVA.

repeated significance tests hypothesis tests performed at intermediate stages of a trial. *See also* interim analysis.

replication we take more than one measurement on the variable of interest on each individual.

reproducibility *see* method agreement.

residual in general, the residual is the difference between two quantities; in regression, it is the difference between the observed value of the response variable and its value predicted by the model.

residual mean square *see* residual variance.

residual variance that part of the total variance of a variable which remains after the effect of certain factors has been removed; it measures the variability which cannot be explained by the model. The residual variance is the residual mean square in an ANOVA.

response variable *see* dependent variable.

restricted randomization *see* blocked randomization.

retrospective longitudinal study the study is conducted by looking backwards in time from a defined starting point.

risk of disease represents the probability that an animal will develop the disease in the stated time period.

robust a hypothesis test is robust if the probabilities of the Type I and Type II errors are hardly affected when the assumptions underlying the test are not fulfilled.

rounding error inaccuracy introduced due to rounding off the number string to a lesser number of decimal places.

runs test   a non-parametric test used to investigate randomness of a binary variable in a single group.

sample   a subgroup drawn from the population.

sample size   the number of individuals included in an investigation when a subgroup of the population is studied.

sample survey   an observational study which uses sample data to provide information, and subsequently draws conclusions, about the population from which the sample was taken.

sampling distribution of the mean   the distribution of the sample means; it is a hypothetical distribution obtained by taking all possible repeated samples of a given size from a population, and calculating the sample mean in each sample. These sample means can be plotted to show the distribution in diagrammatic form.

sampling distribution of the proportion   the distribution of the sample proportions; it is a hypothetical distribution obtained by taking all possible repeated samples of a given size from a population, and calculating the sample proportion in each sample.

sampling error   that part of the error in the estimate of a population parameter which is present because we have taken only a sample of observations from the population, and are not looking at it in its entirety.

sampling units   the population is divided into non-overlapping parts called units (e.g. individual animals, different herds); the sampling process involves selecting a subgroup of these units from the population. The units may then be called sampling units.

sampling variation   describes the fact that the values of a statistic (e.g. the sample mean which estimates the population mean) will not be identical in different samples. The variance and the SD of the sampling distribution of the statistic describe this sampling variation (the SD of the sampling distribution is called the standard error of the statistic).

scatter diagram   a two-dimensional plot in which each axis represents the scale of measurement of one of two variables; each point represents the coordinates for a value on both the scales.

Scheffe's test   a multiple comparisons test of means of three or more independent groups.

self-pairing   the animal acts as its own control in a clinical trial, and so receives both treatments in random order.

sensitivity   the effectiveness of a diagnostic test to identify animals with the disease.

sequential trial   the sample size is not fixed in advance but depends on the results as they become available. A formal approach to the analysis has to be devised; it takes into account considerations such as the significance level and precision, and depends on stopping rules which allow the trial to terminate in favour of a particular treatment if certain conditions are met.

serial correlation   a measurement of serial dependence in a sequence of observations, such as a time series. Its presence implies that the deviations about any long-term trends are associated.

Shapiro–Wilk W test   a test of Normality of a data set.

significance level   a cut-off for the P-value such that the null hypothesis will be rejected if the P-value from a hypothesis test falls below this cut-off value; this value is decided upon before the test is conducted and is often chosen as 0.05. Then if $P < 0.05$, we say that the test is significant at the 5% level. The significance level is the probability associated with the Type I error.

sign test   a non-parametric test used to investigate data in a single group, or from related pairs of subjects.

simple randomization   we randomly allocate animals to the different treatment groups without using any refinements or restrictions.

simple random sampling   a method of sampling in which every unit in the population has an equal chance of being selected.

single-blind   only one of these two parties – the carer or the assessor – is blind to the treatment that an animal receives in a clinical trial.

skewed to the left (negatively skewed)   the frequency distribution is not symmetrical but has an extended left-hand tail.

skewed to the right (positively skewed) the frequency distribution is not symmetrical but has an extended right-hand tail.

skewness a term used to describe the asymmetry of a frequency distribution.

Spearman's rank correlation coefficient a non-parametric equivalent to Pearson's product moment correlation coefficient; it measures the association (not necessarily linear) between two variables which may be ordinal.

specificity the effectiveness of a diagnostic test to identify non-diseased animals.

square of the correlation coefficient (r^2) the proportion of the variance of one variable explained by its linear relationship with another variable. It is sometimes called the coefficient of determination.

stability concerns the long-term repeatability of measurements.

standard deviation (SD) a measure of spread which may be regarded as an average of the deviations of the observations from the arithmetic mean. It is equal to the square root of the variance.

standard deviation of the proportion it is the standard deviation of the sampling distribution of a proportion, and is usually called the standard error of the proportion. It is a measure of the precision of p as an estimate of π.

standard error of measurement an estimate of the variability of the individual measurements in a repeatability study; it is equal to the square root of half the variance of the differences between pairs of measurements.

standard error of the estimate a measure of the precision of the sample statistic as an estimate of the population parameter. It is equal to the standard deviation of the sampling distribution of the statistic.

standard error of the mean the standard deviation of the sampling distribution of the mean; it is a measure of the dispersion of the sample means and of the precision of the sample mean as an estimate of the population mean.

standardized difference used in the calculations of sample size required for a hypothesis test; it is based on the meaningful treatment effect (one which we should not like to overlook) divided by the relevant standard deviation.

Standardized Normal Deviate (SND), z a variable which follows the Normal distribution with a mean of zero and a standard deviation of unity.

Standard Normal distribution a Normal distribution with a mean of zero and a standard deviation of one (unity).

statistic an estimate of the population parameter made from the sample. Sometimes called a sample statistic, although since a statistic always relates to the sample, strictly, the word 'sample' is redundant.

statistical inference the process of generalizing to the population from the sample; it enables us to draw conclusions about certain features of a population when only a subgroup of that population – the sample – is available for investigation.

statistical significance the result of a hypothesis test is statistically significant if the decision is made to reject the null hypothesis; statistical significance should be contrasted with biological importance.

statistics defined narrowly, this is the skills of data manipulation and analysis, but generally in biological science it is taken to mean a wider numerical approach to the science (*see* biometry).

stem-and-leaf diagram a diagram, generally computer generated, which shows the distribution of a data set; the stem is the core value of the observations (e.g. the unit value before the decimal place) and each leaf is a sequence of ordered single digits, one for each observation, which follow the core value (e.g. the first decimal place).

stepwise selection the process of determining an optimal regression equation; it is essentially a step-up procedure which starts with one variable and adds more variables successively, but it allows the variables in the equation to be dropped according to defined statistical criteria specified by the computer package.

stratified randomization   we divide the population into different strata according to the categorization of the key potentially confounding variables; then, within each stratum, we randomly allocate animals to each of the treatment groups.

stratified sampling   the population is divided into strata and a simple random sample of units is selected from each stratum.

Student's *t*-distribution   *see* *t*-distribution.

subjective probability   personal view of probability which is to regard it as a measure of the strength of belief an individual has that a particular event will occur.

summary measure   a quantity which reduces a set of measurements to a single value which is representative of that set. For example, it may be a biological or clinically relevant quantity which describes an important feature of a series of measurements over time for an individual (e.g. the maximum response); use of summary measures considerably simplifies the analysis of such data by reducing a series of values for each individual to a single quantity.

sum of squares   the sum of the squared deviations of each observation from the mean; it is used in the calculations of mean squares in the analysis of variance.

survey   we examine an aggregate of animals or other such units in an observational study in order to derive values for or estimates of various parameters in the population.

survival analysis   the analysis of the time to a critical event, e.g. death, in a group of animals in which there may be censored data.

symmetrical distribution   the shape of the distribution to the right of a central value is a mirror image of that to the left of the central value.

systematic error   one in which the recorded value is consistently above (or below) its true value.

systematic review   a qualitative clearly defined examination of published and unpublished results which collates the information to answer questions, often about the effectiveness of a treatment.

systematic sampling   a method of selecting a sample of elements from the population; a random start point in the frame is chosen (the *k*th element) and then a selection is made of every *k*th element thereafter; apart from the choice of the initial element, this is not random sampling.

***t*-distribution**   discovered by 'Student', a pseudonym for W.S. Gossett, it is a continuous probability distribution; the distribution is symmetrical about the mean, and is characterized by the degrees of freedom. As the degrees of freedom increase, it becomes more like the Normal distribution.

***t*-test**   *see* single group, paired and unpaired *t*-test; these are significance tests based on Student's *t*-distribution.

table   an orderly arrangement, usually of numbers or words in rows and columns, which exhibits a set of facts in a distinct and comprehensive way.

tails   of a frequency distribution represent the frequencies at the extremes of the distribution.

technical variations or errors   variability in the measurements due to a variety of instrumental causes and to human error.

test statistic   a quantity which follows a theoretical distribution and which forms the basis for performing a hypothesis test. By referring the computed value of the test statistic to the appropriate probability distribution, we can determine the *P*-value and decide whether we have enough evidence to reject the null hypothesis.

theoretical probability distribution   determined from a mathematical model.

time series   a long series of measurements made at many successive points in time. Usually, the successive observations are dependent so that the magnitude of one value influences the magnitude of the next, i.e. we have an autoregressive series.

transformation   a mathematical manipulation (e.g. taking the log) of each value in the entire data set in an attempt to produce a new data set which conforms to the particular requirements of the analysis, e.g. Normality, a linear relationship, or constant variance.

treatment effect   a parameter specification of

the treatment comparison of interest, e.g. the difference in means between the treatment and control groups.

two-sample *t*-test   *see* unpaired *t*-test.

two-sided test   a hypothesis test in which the *P*-value is determined by relating the test statistic to both tails of a theoretical distribution. The *a priori* decision to make a test two-sided relies on the specification of the alternative hypothesis which does not indicate the direction of the treatment effect.

two-tailed probability   the *P*-value resulting from a two-sided test in which all the probability of interest is contained in both tails (i.e. the sum of the right- and left-hand tail areas) of the probability distribution.

two-tailed test   *see* two-sided test.

two-way ANOVA   an analysis of data which examines the effect of two factors on a response variable, when each of these factors possesses two or more levels.

Type I error   we reject the null hypothesis when it should not be rejected, i.e. when it is true. The probability of making a Type I error is the significance level of the test.

Type II error   we fail to reject the null hypothesis when it should be rejected, i.e. when it is false.

unbiased   free from bias or systematic error.

unbiased estimate (of the population parameter)   the mean of the sampling distribution of the sample statistic coincides with the population parameter which the statistic is estimating.

unimodal   a distribution which has a single mode or modal group.

univariate analysis   the analysis of data which comprises a single dependent or response variable.

unpaired *t*-test   a parametric test based on Student's *t*-distribution used to compare the

means in two independent groups. It is also called the *two-sample t-test*.

upper quartile   the 75th percentile.

validity   concerned with determining whether the measurement is actually measuring what it purports to be measuring.

values   *see* readings.

variable   a characteristic which can take values which vary from individual to individual or group to group, e.g. height, weight, sex (M or F).

variance   a measure of dispersion. It is the square of the standard deviation.

variance ratio test (*F*-test)   a parametric test, based on the *F*-distribution, used to compare two variances.

Wilcoxon rank sum test   a non-parametric test used to compare the distributions of data in two independent groups. It produces the same result as the Mann-Whitney *U* test, and may be used as the non-parametric alternative to the two-sample *t*-test.

Wilcoxon signed rank test   a non-parametric test used to compare the distribution of data in related groups of paired observations. It may be used as the non-parametric alternative to the paired *t*-test.

withdrawal   an animal which, having been included in a trial, fails to adhere to the protocol, perhaps because of side-effects or intractability.

Yates' correction   an adjustment applied to the Chi-squared test statistic when it is used to test a hypothesis in a 2×2 contingency table. It makes the discrete distribution of the test statistic a better approximation to the continuous Chi-squared distribution.

zero error   a technical error whereby the instrument fails to register a true zero reading.

Index